An Illustrated Review of the

NERVOUS SYSTEM

An Illustrated Review of the

NERVOUS SYSTEM

Glenn F. Bastian

HarperCollinsCollegePublishers

Acquisitions Editor: Bonnie Roesch
Cover Designer: Kay Petronio
Production Manager: Bob Cooper
Printer and Binder: Malloy Lithographing, Inc.
Cover Printer: The Lehigh Press, Inc.

AN ILLUSTRATED REVIEW OF THE NERVOUS SYSTEM

by Glenn F. Bastian

Library of Congress Cataloging-in-Publication Data

Bastian, Glenn F.
    An illustrated review of the nervous system / Glenn F. Bastian.
      p.   cm.
    Includes bibliographical references.
    ISBN: 0-06-501705-6
    1. Neurophysiology—Outlines, syllabi, etc. 2. Neuroanatomy—
Outlines, syllabi, etc. I. Title.
QP361.B33 1993
612.8—dc20
                              93–3825
                                CIP

94 95 96 97 9 8 7 6 5 4 3 2

To Katherine

CONTENTS

LIST OF TOPICS & ILLUSTRATIONS

Text: One page of text is devoted to each of the following topics. *Illustrations are listed in italics.*

PREFACE

An Illustrated Review of Anatomy and Physiology is a series of ten books written to help students effectively review the structure and function of the human body. Each book in the series is devoted to a different body system. This book reviews the nervous system.

My objective in writing these books is to make very complex subjects accessible and unthreatening by presenting material in manageable size bits (one topic per page) with clear, simple illustrations to assist the many students who are primarily visual learners. Designed to supplement established texts, they may be used as a student aid to jog the memory, to quickly recall the essentials of each major topic, and to practice naming structures in preparation for exams.

INNOVATIVE FEATURES OF THE BOOK

(1) Each major topic is confined to one page of text.

A unique feature of this book is that each topic is confined to one page and the material is presented in outline form with the key terms in boldface or italic typeface. This makes it easy to quickly scan the major points of any given topic. The student can easily get an overview of the topic and then zero in on a particular point that needs clarification.

(2) Each page of text has an illustration on the facing page.

Because each page of text has its illustration on the facing page, there is no need to flip through the book looking for the illustration that is referred to in the text ("see Figure X on page xx"). The purpose of the illustration is to clarify a central idea discussed in the text. The images are simple and clear, the lines are bold, and the labels are in a large type. Each illustration deals with a well-defined concept, allowing for a more focused study.

PHYSIOLOGY TOPICS (1 text page : 1 illustration)
Each main topic in physiology is limited to one page of text with one supporting illustration on the facing page.

ANATOMY TOPICS (1 text page : several illustrations)

For complex anatomical structures a good illustration is more valuable than words. So, for topics dealing with anatomy, there are often several illustrations for one text topic. For example, the basic information concerning the cranial nerves can be stated on one page of text, but it is necessary to have a series of illustrations to show the origin and distribution of all 12 pairs of cranial nerves.

(3) Unlabeled illustrations have been included.

In Part II, all illustrations have been repeated without their labels. This allows a student to test his or her visual knowledge of the basic concepts.

(4) Pronunciation Guide has been included.

Phonetic spelling of unfamiliar terms is listed in a separate section, unlike other textbooks where it is usually found in the glossary or spread throughout the text. The student may use this guide for pronunciation drill or as a quick review of basic vocabulary.

(5) A glossary that pertains to only the nervous system has been included.

Most textbooks have glossaries that include terms for all of the systems of the body. It is convenient to have all of the key terms for the nervous system in a single glossary.

ACKNOWLEGEMENTS

I would like to thank the reviewers of the manuscript for this book who carefully critiqued the text and illustrations for their effectiveness: William Kleinelp, Middlesex County College and Robert Smith, University of Missouri, St. Louis. Their help and advice is greatly appreciated. I am greatly indebted to my editor Bonnie Roesch for her willingness to try a new idea, and her support throughout this project. I invite students and instructors to send any comments and suggestions for enhancements or changes to this book to me, in care of HarperCollins, so that future editions can continue to meet your needs.

Glenn Bastian

An
Illustrated
Review
of the
NERVOUS SYSTEM

Introduction

INTRODUCTION / Nervous System Organization

ANATOMICAL ORGANIZATION

Anatomically (structurally), the nervous system has 2 principal divisions: CNS & PNS.

Central Nervous System   (CNS)

The CNS consists of the brain and the spinal cord.

   (1) Brain : cerebrum, diencephalon, brain stem, & cerebellum.

   (2) Spinal Cord : continuation of the brain stem; extends from the base of the skull to the
                 1st lumbar vertebra.

Peripheral Nervous System   (PNS)

The PNS consists of the nerves—the cranial nerves and the spinal nerves.

   (1) Cranial Nerves : there are 12 pairs of cranial nerves emerging from the brain.

   (2) Spinal Nerves : there are 31 pairs of spinal nerves emerging from the spinal cord.

FUNCTIONAL ORGANIZATION

Principal Functions of the Nervous System

(1) Sensory : detecting changes in the internal and external environments.

(2) Integrative : analyzing sensory information and deciding how to respond.

(3) Motor : sending instructions (nerve impulses) to muscles and glands.

    The neurons (nerve cells) that carry out the above functions are of 3 basic types: Sensory neurons (also called afferent neurons) carry information about changes in the internal and external environments to the brain or spinal cord. Association neurons (also called interneurons or connecting neurons) analyze sensory information and decide how to respond; they are located in the CNS. Motor neurons (also called efferent neurons) carry instructions from the CNS to muscles and glands.

Subdivisions of the PNS

The peripheral nervous system may be subdivided into the somatic nervous system (SNS) and the autonomic nervous system (ANS). Actions carried out by the SNS are voluntary, while actions carried out by the ANS are usually involuntary and automatic. Sensations in the SNS are consciously perceived, while sensations in the ANS are usually not consciously perceived.

Somatic Nervous System   (SNS)

(1) Sensory Neurons Sensory neurons of the SNS carry impulses into the CNS from :
   receptors for general senses (touch, pressure, vibration, temperature, pain, & proprioception)
   and *receptors for special senses* (smell, taste, vision, hearing, & equilibrium).

(2) Motor Neurons Motor neurons of the SNS carry impulses away from the CNS to :
   skeletal muscles (only).

Autonomic Nervous System   (ANS)

(1) Sensory Neurons Sensory neurons of the ANS carry impulses to the CNS from :
   visceral receptors (receptors located in the internal organs of the ventral body cavity).

(2) Motor Neurons Motor neurons of the ANS carry impulses from the CNS to :
   smooth muscle, cardiac muscle, & glands.

    The motor (efferent) portion of the ANS has 2 principal divisions: sympathetic and parasympathetic. In general, impulses from one division stimulate a given organ, while impulses from the other division inhibit the organ. For example, stimulation by the sympathetic division <u>increases</u> heart rate; stimulation by the parasympathetic division <u>decreases</u> heart rate.

NERVOUS SYSTEM ORGANIZATION

CNS
Central N.S.

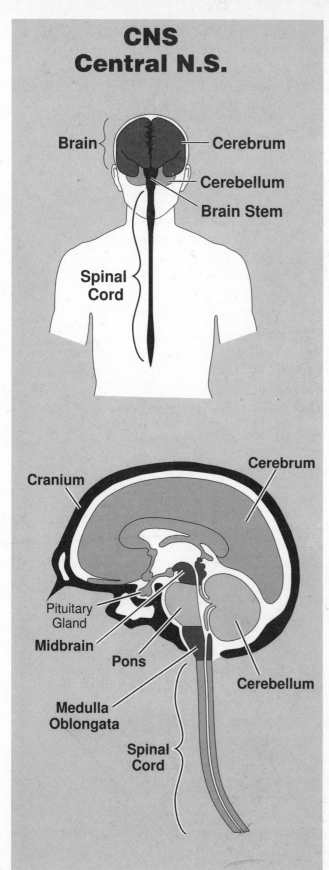

Brain
Cerebrum
Cerebellum
Brain Stem
Spinal Cord

Cranium
Cerebrum
Pituitary Gland
Midbrain
Pons
Cerebellum
Medulla Oblongata
Spinal Cord

PNS
Peripheral N.S.

Cranial Nerves

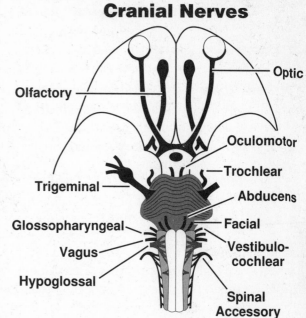

Olfactory
Optic
Oculomotor
Trochlear
Trigeminal
Abducens
Glossopharyngeal
Facial
Vagus
Vestibulo-cochlear
Hypoglossal
Spinal Accessory

Spinal Nerves

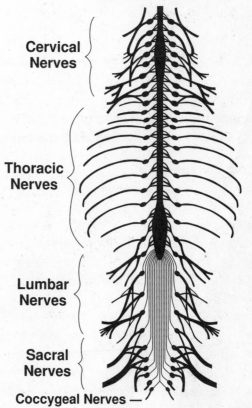

Cervical Nerves
Thoracic Nerves
Lumbar Nerves
Sacral Nerves
Coccygeal Nerves

3

INTRODUCTION / Neuron Parts

Nerve tissue consists of 2 cell-type classifications: neurons (nerve cells) and neuroglia (also called glia). Nerve cells transmit electrochemical signals (nerve impulses); neuroglia insulate, nourish, support, and protect the neurons.

The human nervous system contains at least 10 billion neurons and 100 - 500 billion neuroglial cells. Most neurons have 3 main parts : cell body, dendrites, and axon.

THE BASIC PARTS

(1) Cell Body (also called perikaryon or soma)

The cell body includes the nucleus and the cytoplasm immediately surrounding it. Its membrane is receptive to stimuli from other neurons. The cytoplasm in this region contains the normal cell organelles : mitochondria, ribosomes, Golgi complex, etc. It also contains other structures that are characteristic of neurons, including :

Chromatophilic Substance (Nissl bodies) : rough endoplasmic reticulum.
Neurofibrils : filaments providing support and shape for the cell body.
Lipofuscin Pigment : yellowish brown granules; end products of lysosomal activity.

(2) Dendrites (*dendron* = tree, branches)

Dendrites are highly branched processes that extend out from the cell body. They are specialized for receiving stimuli from the environment, specialized sensory organs, or from other neurons.

(3) Axon

The axon is a single process specialized for conducting nerve impulses to other cells (nerve, muscle, and gland cells). Special structures of the axon include :

Axon Hillock : the cone-shaped region where the axon joins the cell body.
Initial Segment : the first portion of the axon.
Trigger Zone : the junction of the axon hillock and the initial segment; where nerve impulses start.
Axon Collateral : a side branch along the length of an axon.
Axon Terminals : the branched end portions of an axon.
Synaptic End Bulb : enlarged region at the end of an axon terminal; contains synaptic vesicles.
Synaptic Vesicle : a membrane-enclosed sac filled with molecules of neurotransmitter.
(in the PNS the neurotransmitter is acetylcholine or norepinephrine)

Related Terms

Neurolemmocyte (Schwann cell)
A neurolemmocyte is a type of neuroglial cell found only in the PNS. Many neurolemmocytes are associated with a single axon. They insulate, nourish, and support axons.

Neurofibral node (node of Ranvier)
The space between two adjacent neurolemmocytes, where the axon is exposed to the surrounding tissue fluid, is called the neurofibral node.

Axonal Transport
There are two mechanisms for transporting materials in an axon.
Slow axonal transport conveys the cytoplasm (axoplasm) in only one direction, from the cell body toward the axon terminals. It supplies materials for growing and regenerating axons.
Fast axonal transport conveys material in both directions along the surfaces of microtubules. It supplies materials that form the plasma membrane (axolemma), synaptic end bulbs, and synaptic vesicles.

NEURON (nerve cell)

Neurons carry impulses to other neurons, muscle cells, & gland cells.

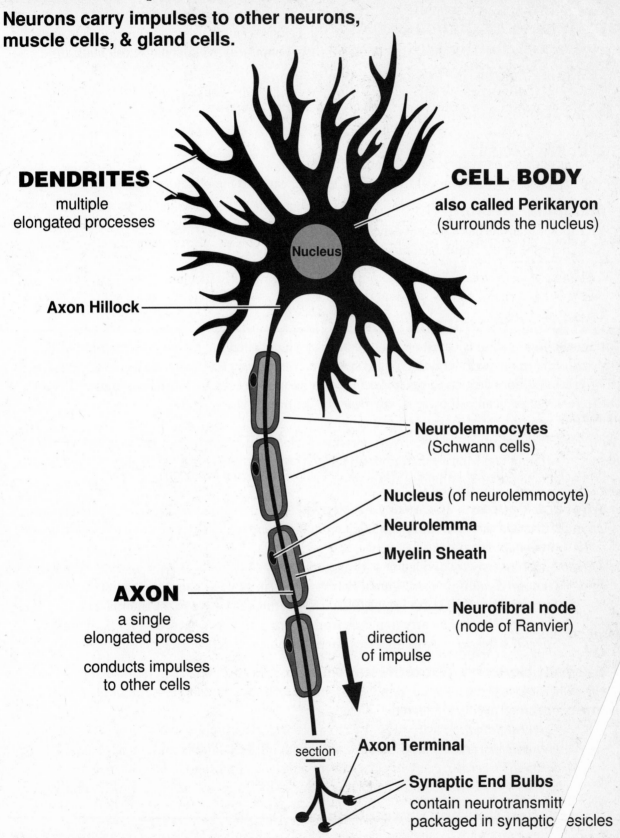

DENDRITES
multiple
elongated processes

CELL BODY
also called Perikaryon
(surrounds the nucleus)

Nucleus

Axon Hillock

Neurolemmocytes
(Schwann cells)

Nucleus (of neurolemmocyte)

Neurolemma

Myelin Sheath

AXON
a single
elongated process

conducts impulses
to other cells

Neurofibral node
(node of Ranvier)

direction
of impulse

section

Axon Terminal

Synaptic End Bulbs
contain neurotransmitt
packaged in synaptic esicles

5

INTRODUCTION / Neuron Classification

STRUCTURAL CLASSIFICATION
Structural classification is based on the number of processes extending from the cell body.

Unipolar Neurons (Pseudounipolar Neurons)
Unipolar neurons have a single process extending from the cell body.
Sensory neurons are of this type.

Bipolar Neurons
Bipolar neurons have one dendrite and one axon.
They are found in the retina of the eye, the internal ear, and the olfactory mucosa.

Multipolar Neurons
Multipolar neurons have several dendrites and one axon.
Most neurons in the brain and spinal cord are of this type.
Motor neurons and most *association neurons* are of this type.

FUNCTIONAL CLASSIFICATION
Functional classification is based on the direction in which a neuron transmits a nerve impulse.
Neurons found in the peripheral nervous system are of two basic functional types :
(1) Afferent neurons carry impulses *toward* the central nervous sytem (brain or spinal cord).
(2) Efferent neurons carry impulses *away from* the central nervous system.
All afferent neurons carry sensory information, so they are also called *sensory* neurons.
All efferent neurons affect the activity of muscles or glands; they are also called *motor* neurons.
Sensory = Afferent and Motor = Efferent. In this text *sensory* and *motor* are the terms most frequently used when referring to these types of neurons.

Afferent Neurons (Sensory Neurons)
Afferent neurons carry incoming impulses from the internal and external environments into the CNS (brain or spinal cord).
Afferent neurons may by divided into 4 categories:
> *General Somatic :* carry impulses from the skin, skeletal muscles, & joints.
> *Special Somatic :* carry impulses from the retina of the eye & the internal ear.
> *General Visceral :* carry impulses from internal organs & receptors for body fluids.
> *Special Visceral :* carry impulses from the tongue & olfactory mucosa.

Efferent Neurons (Motor Neurons)
Efferent neurons carry outgoing impulses from the CNS to effectors (muscles or glands).
Efferent neurons may be divided into 3 categories:
> *General Somatic :* carry impulses to most skeletal muscles.
> *General Visceral :* carry impulses to smooth muscle, cardiac muscle, & glands.
> *Special Visceral :* carry impulses to certain skeletal muscles.
> > (certain skeletal muscles in the face, jaw, neck, larynx, & pharynx)

Association Neurons (Interneurons)
Association neurons are located in the central nervous system. They carry nerve impulses from one neuron to another inside the brain or spinal cord. They establish interrelationships with other neurons, forming complex neuronal circuits.

NEURON CLASSIFICATION

Brain

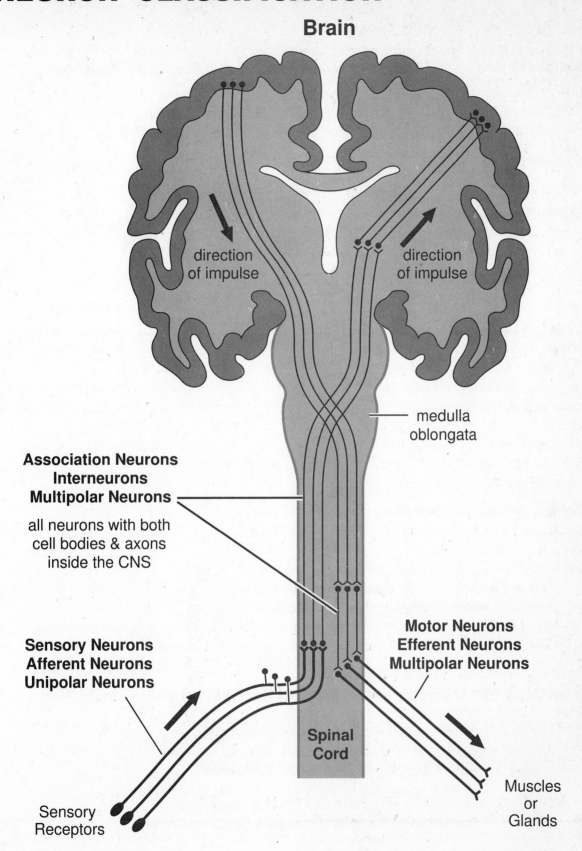

direction of impulse

direction of impulse

medulla oblongata

Association Neurons
Interneurons
Multipolar Neurons

all neurons with both cell bodies & axons inside the CNS

Sensory Neurons
Afferent Neurons
Unipolar Neurons

Motor Neurons
Efferent Neurons
Multipolar Neurons

Spinal Cord

Sensory Receptors

Muscles or Glands

TYPES OF NEURONS
based on structure

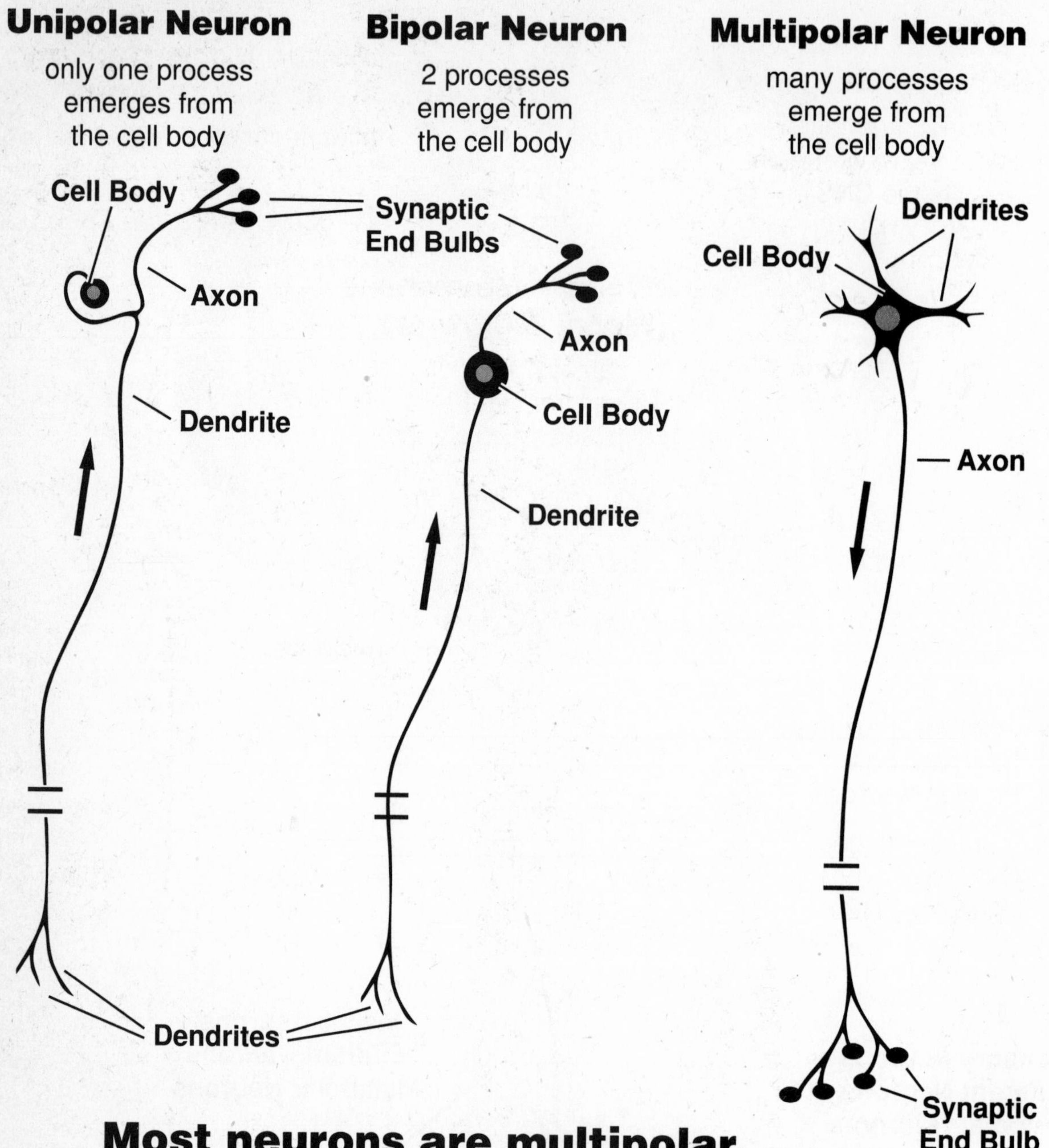

Unipolar Neuron

only one process
emerge from
the cell body

Cell Body

Synaptic
End Bulbs

Axon

Dendrite

Dendrites

Bipolar Neuron

2 processes
emerge from
the cell body

Axon

Cell Body

Dendrite

Multipolar Neuron

many processes
emerge from
the cell body

Dendrites

Cell Body

Axon

Synaptic
End Bulb

Most neurons are multipolar.

UNIPOLAR : afferent neurons (sensory neurons)

BIPOLAR : found in eye, ear, & olfactory mucosa

MULTIPOLAR : all efferent neurons (motor neurons)
              most association neurons (interneurons)

TYPES OF NEURONS
based on function

Afferent Neurons (Sensory Neurons)

carry information about the environment to the CNS

Efferent Neurons (Motor Neurons)

carry information away from the CNS to muscles and glands

Association Neurons (interneurons)

integrate incoming information and "decide" how to respond

(found only in the CNS)

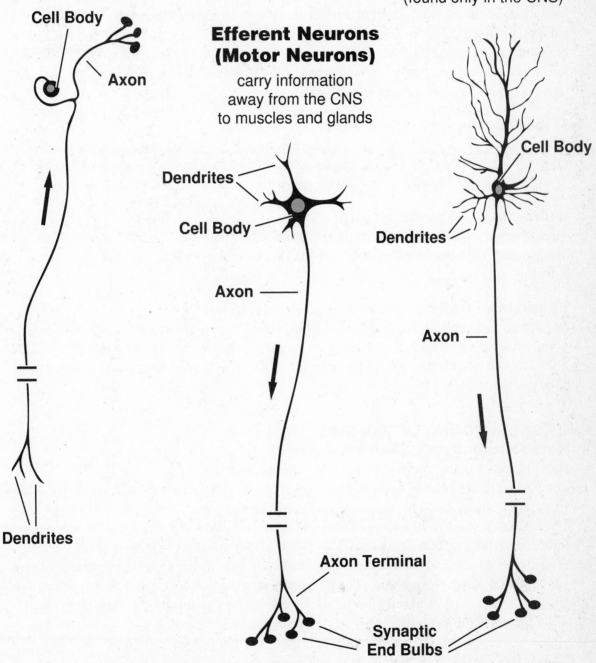

Cell Body

Axon

Dendrites

Cell Body

Axon

Cell Body

Dendrites

Axon

Dendrites

Axon Terminal

Synaptic End Bulbs

9

INTRODUCTION / Neuroglia

In addition to neurons, the nervous system contains neuroglia, also called glia. There are 10 to 50 times as many neuroglia as neurons. However, since neuroglia are much smaller than neurons, they occupy only half the total volume of the brain and spinal cord.

NEUROGLIA FOUND IN THE CNS

Astrocytes   *(neurotransmitter metabolism & potassium balance)*

Astrocytes are the largest of the neuroglia. Many of their numerous, long processes have expanded ends that attach to the walls of capillaries, forming a sheath around them. They participate in the metabolism of neurotransmitters and maintain the proper balance of potassium that is needed for the generation of nerve impulses. They also help to form the blood-brain barrier that regulates the passage of substances into the brain. Processes of astrocytes also form a layer that separates the neurons of the brain and spinal cord from the membrane (the pia mater) that surrounds them.

Oligodendrocytes   *(form myelin)*

Oligodendrocytes are analogous to the neurolemmocytes of peripheral nerves — both form myelin. The processes of a single oligodendrocyte can myelinate as many as 15 axons. The myelin sheath insulates the axons and increases the speed of impulse transmission.

Microglia   *(phagocytic; eat bacteria)*

Microglia have small, elongated cell bodies and short processes covered by numerous small expansions. They are found in both gray matter and white matter. They are phagocytic (eat bacteria).

Ependymal Cells   *(movement of cerebrospinal fluid)*

Ependymal cells line the ventricles of the brain and the central canal of the spinal cord. Most ependymal cells possess *cilia* that assist in the circulation of the cerebrospinal fluid (CSF). They have an abundant supply of mitochondria, which is needed to produce energy for ciliary action.

NEUROGLIA FOUND IN THE PNS

Neurolemmocytes (Schwann Cells)

(form myelin sheath; support, protect, & nourish neurons)

The plasma membranes of neurolemmocytes form myelin sheaths around axons in the PNS. The myelin sheath insulates the axons and increases the speed of impulse transmission.
Myelinated Nerve Fibers   A nerve fiber is said to be *myelinated* when it is wrapped in many layers of plasma membrane. As many as 500 neurolemmocytes may be involved in the myelination of one long axon, and each neurolemmocyte forms a sheath consisting of up to 100 layers of plasma membrane. The plasma membrane has an unusually high percentage of fat; thus, it serves as an excellent insulating material. It also allows the axon to transmit nerve impulses more rapidly.

Satellite Cells   *(support neuron cell bodies in ganglia of the PNS)*

Satellite cells are flattened cells that surround and support neuron cell bodies in ganglia.

NEUROGLIAL CELLS
neuroglia of the CNS

Astrocytes

functions :
regulate interstitial fluid composition
maintain blood-brain barrier
provide structural framework
repair damaged neural tissue

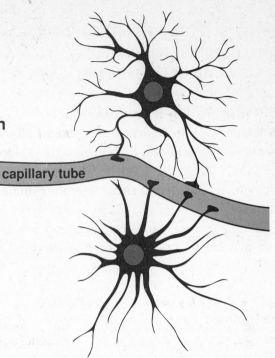

capillary tube

Oligodendrocytes

functions :
myelinate axons
provide structural framework

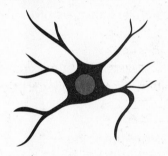

Microglia

function :
phagocytize pathogens
& cellular debris

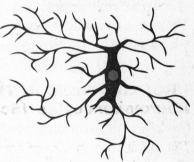

Ependymal Cells

epithelial cells that line brain ventricles
& central canal of spinal cord

function :
assist in secretion & circulation of CSF

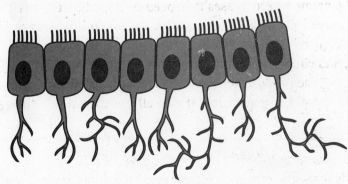

NEUROLEMMOCYTES

Many neurons have neurolemmocytes (Schwann cells) wrapped around their axons.
The neurolemmocytes help to insulate, nourish, and support the axons; they also increase the velocity of impulse transmission.

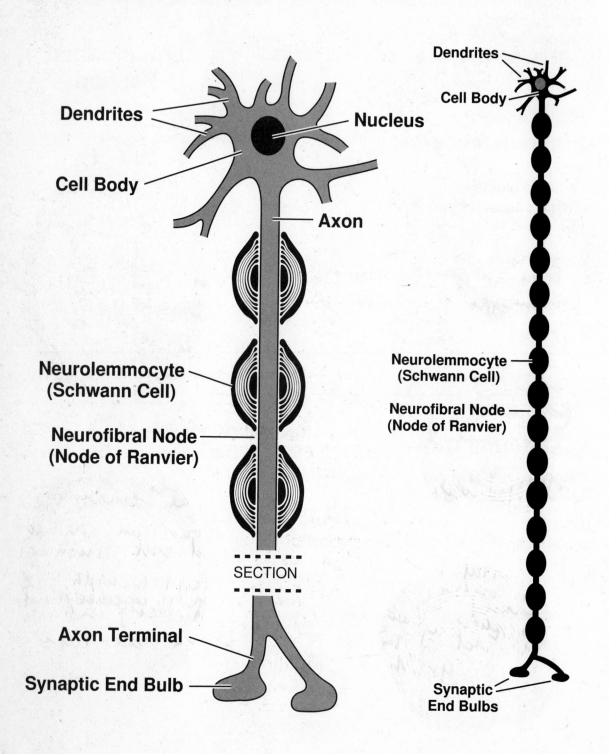

Dendrites

Nucleus

Cell Body

Axon

Neurolemmocyte
(Schwann Cell)

Neurofibral Node
(Node of Ranvier)

SECTION

Axon Terminal

Synaptic End Bulb

Dendrites

Cell Body

Neurolemmocyte
(Schwann Cell)

Neurofibral Node
(Node of Ranvier)

Synaptic
End Bulbs

MYELIN SHEATH : myelination

A neurolemmocyte (Schwann cell)
wrapping around an axon,
forming a myelin sheath

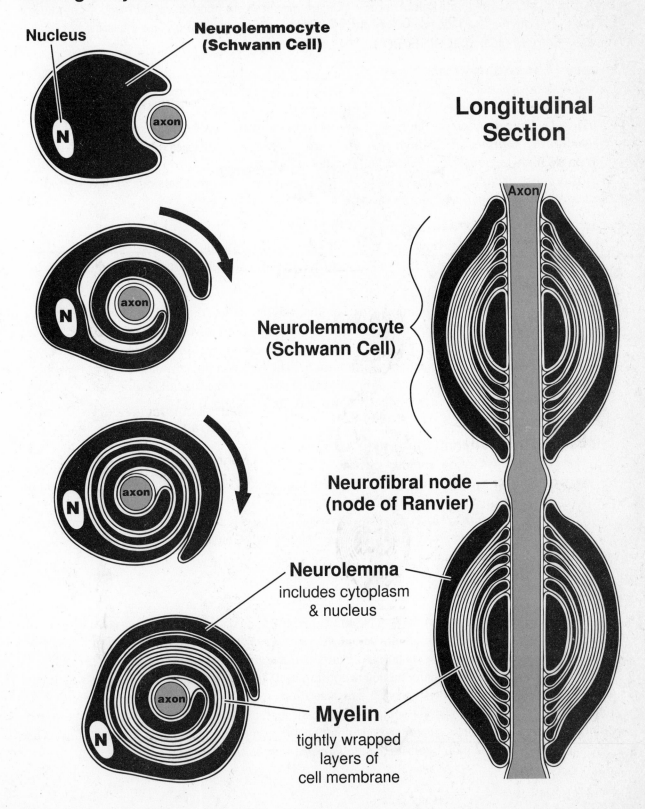

Nucleus

Neurolemmocyte
(Schwann Cell)

N

axon

Longitudinal
Section

Axon

Neurolemmocyte
(Schwann Cell)

N

axon

Neurofibral node —
(node of Ranvier)

N

axon

Neurolemma

includes cytoplasm
& nucleus

axon

N

Myelin

tightly wrapped
layers of
cell membrane

INTRODUCTION / Pathways & Tracts

PATHWAYS

The route followed by a nerve impulse as it travels through the nervous system is called a nerve pathway. A pathway includes the nerve fibers in nerves, which are organized in bundles called *fascicles*, and the nerve fibers inside the brain and spinal cord, which are organized in bundles called *tracts*. Bundles of nerve fibers linking the two halves of the brain are called *commissures*. There are 2 basic types of pathways : sensory (ascending) and motor (descending).

Sensory (Ascending) Pathways

Sensory pathways start at sensory receptors and end in the cerebral cortex of the brain.
A sensory pathway consists of a series of three neurons :
First-order neurons (sensory neurons) : extend from the sensory receptor into the CNS.
Second-order neurons (association neurons) : carry sensory impulses to the thalamus (an integrating center in the region of the brain called the diencephalon).
Third-order neurons (association neurons) : carry impulses from the thalamus to the cerebral cortex, where conscious sensation is produced.

Motor (Descending) Pathways

Motor pathways start in the brain and terminate at muscles or glands.
There are two general motor pathways : direct (pyramidal) and indirect (extrapyramidal).

Direct (Pyramidal) Pathways

Direct pathways carry nerve impulses from the cerebral cortex "directly" to lower motor neurons. In the spinal cord association neurons may connect upper and lower motor neurons.
Upper motor neurons : carry impulses from the cerebral cortex "directly" to lower motor neurons located in the spinal cord or brain stem. The fibers of upper motor neurons pass through two bulges called *pyramids* located on the ventral surface of the medulla oblongata.
Lower motor neurons : carry impulses from the CNS to skeletal muscles, resulting in precise, voluntary movements.

Indirect (Extrapyramidal) Pathways

Indirect pathways follow complex circuits. They carry nerve impulses to lower motor neurons by way of other parts of the brain (including the motor cortex, basal ganglia, thalamus, cerebellum, reticular formation, and nuclei in the brain stem).
Upper motor neurons : carry impulses from nuclei of the brain stem to lower motor neurons.
Lower motor neurons : carry impulses from the CNS to skeletal muscles; muscle responses are semivoluntary and automatic.

TRACTS

Bundles of nerve fibers (axons) in the CNS are called tracts. Tracts containing nerve fibers that carry impulses up the spinal cord to the brain are called *sensory (ascending) tracts*; tracts containing nerve fibers that carry impulses down the spinal cord from the brain are called *motor (descending) tracts*.

In the spinal cord a tract is usually named according to its location in the spinal cord, its origin, and its termination. For example, fibers carrying pain sensations from the skin are located in the lateral portions of the spinal cord (the lateral white columns); these tracts originate at some level of the spinal cord (where the sensory neuron enters) and terminate in a region of the brain called the thalamus. Thus, the tracts that contain these pain fibers are called *lateral spinothalamic tracts*.

PATHWAYS
Sensory & Direct Motor Pathways

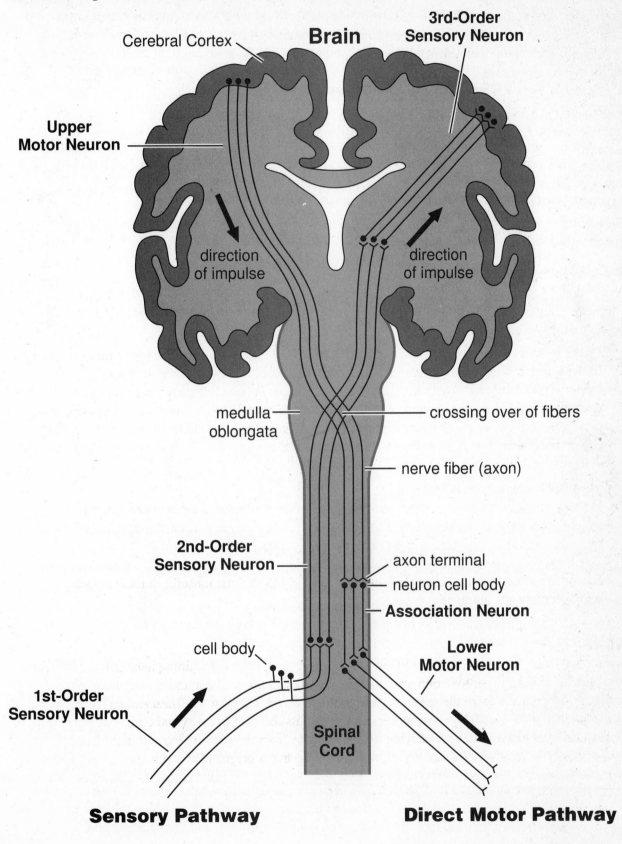

Cerebral Cortex

Brain

3rd-Order
Sensory Neuron

Upper
Motor Neuron

direction
of impulse

direction
of impulse

medulla
oblongata

crossing over of fibers

nerve fiber (axon)

2nd-Order
Sensory Neuron

axon terminal

neuron cell body

Association Neuron

cell body

Lower
Motor Neuron

1st-Order
Sensory Neuron

Spinal
Cord

Sensory Pathway

Direct Motor Pathway

INTRODUCTION / Ganglia & Nuclei

GANGLIA *(located in the PNS)*

A cluster of neuron cell bodies outside the brain or spinal cord (in the PNS) is called a ganglion (plural: ganglia). In a ganglion the axon terminal of one neuron (the preganglionic neuron) forms a synapse (point of contact) with the cell body of a second neuron (the postganglionic neuron). There are 4 basic types of ganglia.

Posterior Root Ganglia (Dorsal Root Ganglia)

Posterior root ganglia contain the cell bodies of sensory neurons. They are located very near the spinal cord in the posterior (dorsal) roots of the spinal nerves. When part of a cranial nerve, they are called *craniospinal ganglia*. Examples of craniospinal ganglia are the spiral and vestibular ganglia; they are part of the 8th cranial nerve (vestibulocochlear nerve), which carries impulses from the internal ear to the brain.

Sympathetic Trunk Ganglia (Sympathetic Division)

Sympathetic trunk ganglia form a chain of ganglia on each side of the vertebral column from the neck to the coccyx. They contain the cell bodies of postganglionic sympathetic neurons. They are also called *paravertebral ganglia* and *sympathetic chain ganglia*.

Prevertebral Ganglia (Sympathetic Division)

Prevertebral ganglia are located anterior to the vertebral column and close to the abdominal arteries. They contain the cell bodies of postganglionic sympathetic neurons. They are also called *collateral ganglia*.

Terminal Ganglia (Parasympathetic Division)

Terminal ganglia are located near or inside visceral effectors (internal organs). They consist of clusters of cell bodies of postganglionic parasympathetic neurons. They are also called *intramural ganglia*.

NUCLEI *(located in the CNS)*

A cluster of neuron cell bodies in the brain or spinal cord (in the CNS) is called a nucleus.
The CNS nuclei are isolated regions of gray matter that are located in the white matter of the brain and spinal cord. The neurons in a given nucleus perform a specific function.
Some examples of nuclei are:

   Basal Ganglia (Cerebral Nuclei or *Basal Nuclei)* The basal ganglia are several groups of nuclei located within the white matter of the cerebral hemispheres. They include the caudate nucleus, lenticular nucleus (putamen & globus pallidus), substantia nigra, subthalamic nuclei, and red nuclei. They are also called the *cerebral nuclei* and the *basal nuclei*. They integrate semi-voluntary, automatic movements such as walking, swimming, and laughing.

   Thalamus The thalamus consists of a pair of oval masses, one on each side of the 3rd ventricle in the diencephalon. It is mostly gray matter made up of many nuclei. These nuclei are concerned with a wide variety of functions, including language, memory, emotion, and the integration and relay of sensory impulses to the cerebral cortex.

   Hypothalamus The hypothalamus is the region of the diencephalon located below the two halves of the thalamus; it consists of a variety of nuclei and nuclear areas. Some of the functions controlled by these nuclei are: thirst, hunger, hormone production, and fear and rage reactions. These nuclei make up the single most important control area for the internal environment.

   Brain Stem The nuclei for most of the cranial nerves are in the brain stem. It also contains nuclei that control breathing, the force and rate of heart contractions, and blood vessel diameter.

   Cerebellum The cerebellar nuclei are regions of gray matter located deep within the cerebellum. They are concerned with balance, proprioception (self-awareness), and the planning and coordination of complex muscular activities.

GANGLIA & NUCLEI
(clusters of neuron cell bodies)

A cluster of neuron cell bodies in the PNS
(outside the brain or spinal cord)
is called a ganglion.

A cluster of neuron cell bodies in the CNS
(inside the brain or spinal cord)
is called a nucleus.

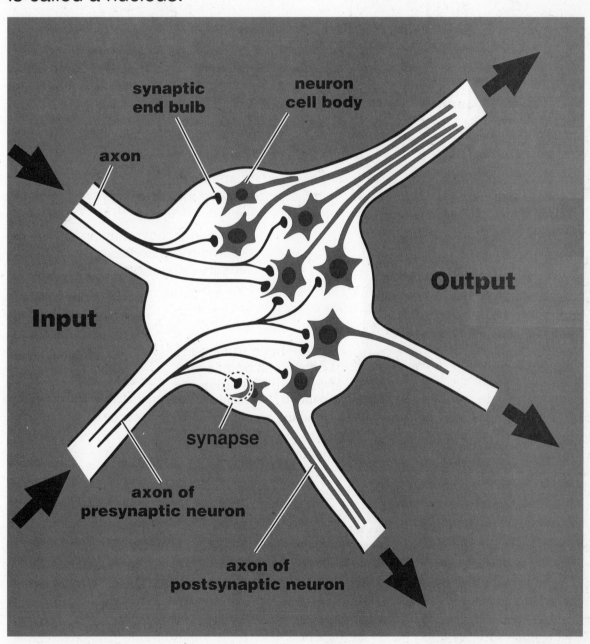

GANGLIA
Ganglia are clusters of neuron cell bodies in the PNS.

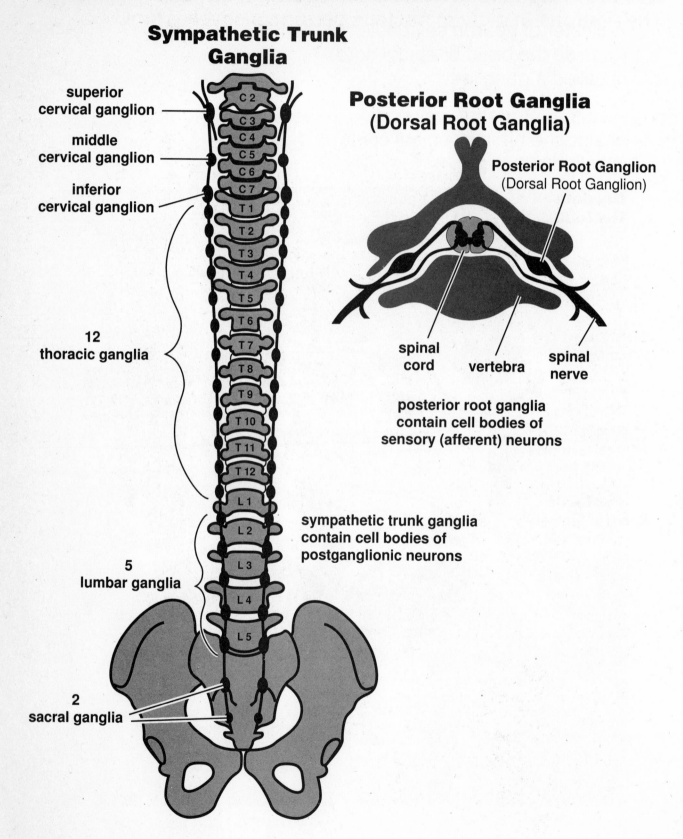

Sympathetic Trunk Ganglia

superior cervical ganglion

middle cervical ganglion

inferior cervical ganglion

12 thoracic ganglia

5 lumbar ganglia

2 sacral ganglia

C 2
C 3
C 4
C 5
C 6
C 7
T 1
T 2
T 3
T 4
T 5
T 6
T 7
T 8
T 9
T 10
T 11
T 12
L 1
L 2
L 3
L 4
L 5

Posterior Root Ganglia
(Dorsal Root Ganglia)

Posterior Root Ganglion
(Dorsal Root Ganglion)

spinal cord

vertebra

spinal nerve

posterior root ganglia contain cell bodies of sensory (afferent) neurons

sympathetic trunk ganglia contain cell bodies of postganglionic neurons

NUCLEI (in the brain)

Nuclei are clusters of neuron cell bodies in the CNS.
The neurons in a given nucleus perform a specific function.

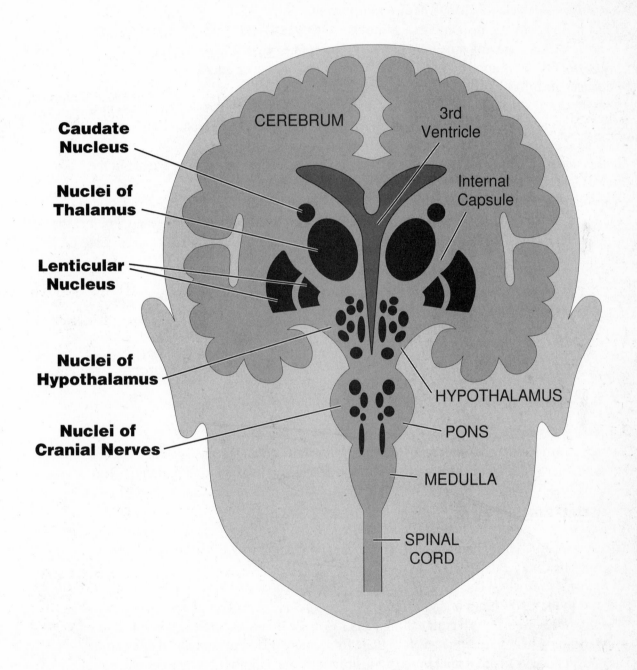

Caudate Nucleus

Nuclei of Thalamus

Lenticular Nucleus

Nuclei of Hypothalamus

Nuclei of Cranial Nerves

CEREBRUM

3rd Ventricle

Internal Capsule

HYPOTHALAMUS

PONS

MEDULLA

SPINAL CORD

INTRODUCTION / The Reflex Arc

Definitions

External Environment : conditions outside the body.
Internal Environment : conditions inside the body;
the chemical and physical characteristics of the body fluids.
Stimulus : a detectable change in the environment.
Reflex : an automatic response to a stimulus.
  Basic reflexes are unlearned, involuntary, "built in."
  Learned reflexes appear to be innate (hereditary), but occur only because a great deal of conscious effort has been spent to learn them.
Homeostasis : the stable, relatively constant, conditions of the internal environment.
Factors such as blood pressure, plasma glucose, pH, and body temperature must stay within a narrow range of values.
Homeostatic Mechanism : the sequence of events that keeps a specific variable in the internal environment relatively constant.
Negative Feedback : Homeostatic mechanisms are also called negative feedback control systems because the response counteracts (has a negative effect on) the original stimulus; the response tends to push the variable in the direction opposite to the original change (back to its original value).

Types of Reflexes

Somatic Reflexes Somatic reflexes result in the contraction of *skeletal muscles*. Examples are: blinking, ducking, sneezing, withdrawal from painful stimuli.
Autonomic Reflexes Autonomic reflexes result in the contraction of *smooth muscle* or *cardiac muscle* or the secretion of *glands*. Examples are: control of heart rate, pupil dilation and contraction, digestive tract contractions and secretions.

The Reflex Arc

The reflex arc is the basic structural and functional unit of the nervous system. The nervous system functions by responding to changes in the external and internal environments. The sequence of events by which the nervous system responds to a stimulus can be simplified and generalized. The pathway of the response has 5 basic components:

(1) Receptor The receptor is the specialized ending of a sensory neuron or a sense organ; it detects a specific kind of environmental change and responds by initiating a nerve impulse in a sensory neuron.
(2) Sensory Pathway The sensory (afferent) pathway carries a nerve impulse from a sensory receptor to the CNS (brain or spinal cord). It may include sensory and association neurons.
(3) Integrating Center The integrating center is made up of association neurons in the CNS. An association neuron often receives signals from many different sources; it adds up the various bits of information and sends out instructions via a motor neuron to effector cells.
(4) Motor Pathway The motor (efferent) pathway carries the instructions from the CNS to the effector (muscle or gland). It may include association neurons and motor neurons.
(5) Effector The effector is a muscle or a gland that contracts or secretes, thus causing the response that is called a reflex. The response usually counteracts the original stimulus—it has a negative feedback effect.

THE REFLEX ARC

The reflex arc is the basic structural and functional unit of the nervous system.

It summarizes the main steps involved in a nervous system response to a stimulus.

Thermostat

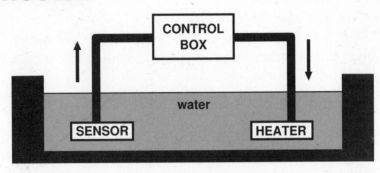

Reflex Arc

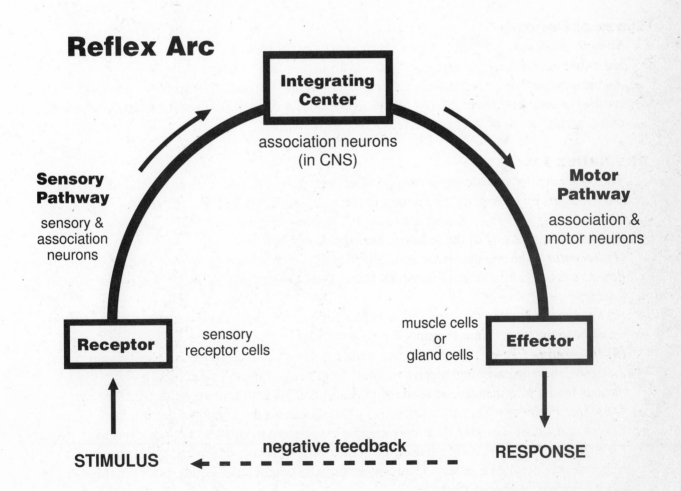

Nerve Impulse

Principles of Electricity *24*
 1. Charged Particles : electrons & ions
 2. Electrical Forces : voltage & electric potential
 3. Current (flow of charged particles) : current = voltage / resistance

Electrical Nature of Cells *26*
 1. Ion Channels : leakage channels & gated channels
 2. Membrane Potentials

Resting & Equilibrium Potentials *28*
 1. Generating a Resting Potential
  Concentration Gradients
  Membrane Permeability
 2. Equilibrium Potentials : sodium & potassium

Graded & Action Potentials *30*
 1. Graded Potentials
  Generator Potentials
  Postsynaptic Potentials : EPSPs & IPSPs
 2. Action Potential
  Voltage-Gated Ion Channels
  All-or-None Response
  Refractory Period
  Sequence of Events : Depolarization & Repolarization
  Restoring Concentration Gradients

Action Potential Propagation (Nerve Impulse) *32*
 1. Local Decremental Currents : extracellular & intracellular flow
 2. Positive-Feedback Cycle
 3. One-Way Propagation
 4. Types of Conduction : continuous & saltatory

Conduction Velocity & Frequency *34*
 1. Velocity of Impulses : fiber diameter, degree of myelination
 2. Frequency of Impulses (limited by the refractory period)
 3. Fiber Classification by Size : A fibers, B fibers, & C fibers
 4. Amount of Neurotransmitter Released (frequency of action potentials)

NERVE IMPULSE / Principles of Electricity

CHARGED PARTICLES
Electrons

Electrons are negatively charged particles that are present in all atoms. Atoms are electrically neutral because they have an equal number of positively charged and negatively charged particles : every atom has an equal number of positive protons and negative electrons.

Ions

Anions & Cations   An ion is an atom or group of atoms that has lost or gained one or more electrons. If it has lost electrons (negative charges), the atom becomes positively charged and is called a cation; if it has gained electrons, it becomes negatively charged and is called an anion.

Acids & Salts   Molecules are made up of atoms that are chemically combined, so, like atoms, they are electrically neutral. However, some molecules have a tendency to dissociate when placed in water. For example, acids dissociate to release positively charged hydrogen ions (protons); salts, such as sodium chloride, dissociate into positive metal ions (sodium) and negative nonmetal ions (chloride).

Phosphate, Carboxyl, & Amino Groups   Phosphate groups ($—H_2PO_4$) are attached to organic molecules, such as ATP; carboxyl groups ($—COOH$) and amino groups ($—NH_2$) are attached to proteins. Phosphate groups and carboxyl groups tend to lose protons and become negatively charged; amino groups tend to gain a proton and become positively charged.

ELECTRICAL FORCES
Interaction of Charged Particles

opposite charges attract; like charges repel :   An electrical force draws opposite charges together and causes like charges to move away from each other.

Magnitude of Electrical Force

Voltage and Electric Potential   Two terms are used interchangeably for the magnitude of an electrical force : *voltage* and *electric potential*. An electrical force is measured in volts, thus the term "voltage." An electrical force is a potential source of energy, so the term "electric potential" refers to how much stored energy is available due to the electrical force.

Quantity of Charge and Closeness of Charge   Two factors determine the magnitude of an electrical force : *quantity of charge* and *closeness of charge*. The magnitude of the force acting between electrical charges increases when the quantity of charge is increased and when the charged particles are moved closer together.

CURRENT

Amount of Flow   Current is defined as the movement or flow of electrical charges. An electrical current conducted through a metal wire is due to the flow of electrons; an electrical current conducted through water is due to the flow of ions. The amount of flow depends on the voltage (electric potential) and the nature of the material through which the charges move.

Insulators   Insulators are materials that have high resistance to flow.

Conductors   Conductors are materials that have low resistance to flow.

Ohm's Law :   Ohm's Law expresses the relationship between current, voltage, and resistance.
current (I) = voltage (V) / resistance (R)

CHARGED PARTICLES

Electrons

hydrogen $_1H^1$

carbon $_6C^{12}$

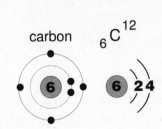

nitrogen $_7N^{14}$

oxygen $_8O^{16}$

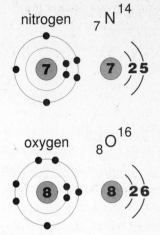

Major Ions in Body Fluids :

Na^+	sodium	K^+	potassium
Ca^{++}	calcium	Mg^{++}	magnesium
Cl^-	chloride	SO_4^{-2}	sulfate
HCO_3^-	bicarbonate	PO_4^{-3}	phosphate

Molecules with Ionized Groups

Phosphate Group

$$R-O-\overset{\overset{OH}{|}}{\underset{\underset{O}{\|}}{P}}-OH \longrightarrow R-O-\overset{\overset{O^-}{|}}{\underset{\underset{O}{\|}}{P}}-O^- + 2H^+$$

charge
charge

Carboxyl Group

$$R-\overset{}{\underset{\underset{O}{\|}}{C}}-OH \longrightarrow R-\overset{}{\underset{\underset{O}{\|}}{C}}-O^- + H^+$$

charge

Amino Group

$$R-N\overset{H}{\underset{H}{<}} + H^+ \longrightarrow R-\overset{\overset{H}{|}}{\underset{\underset{H}{|}}{N}}-H^+$$

charge

NERVE IMPULSE / Electrical Nature of Cells

Batteries Cells are like miniature batteries: they contain oppositely charged particles separated by an insulating material. The charged particles are ions and charged organic molecules; the insulating material is the phospholipid layer of the plasma membrane.

Membrane Potential The voltage across a plasma membrane is called the *membrane potential*; the value for resting cells varies from + 5 to − 100 millivolts, depending on the type of cell.

Polarized Cells A cell that exhibits a membrane potential is said to be polarized.

ION CHANNELS

The plasma membranes of all cells contain proteins that function as ion channels. Although all plasma membranes have ion channels, only the plasma membranes of *excitable cells* (nerve and muscle cells) have ion channels that have the ability to respond to certain stimuli by producing impulses (action potentials).

When the ion channels of excitable cells are open, they provide conduction pathways for the flow of ions, just as an electrical wire connected to the two terminals of a battery allows the flow of electrons if the switch is "on."

There are 2 basic types of ion channels in nerve cells : leakage channels and gated channels.

Leakage Channels Leakage channels are always open.

Gated Channels Gated channels open or close when activated by specific types of stimuli.

Chemically Gated activated by : chemicals, such as neurotransmitters, hormones, & foods.
   locations : neuron cell bodies & dendrites; receptors for taste & smell in the mouth.

Mechanically Gated activated by : mechanical vibration & pressure.
   locations : receptors that detect mechanical distortions; touch & pressure receptors in skin.

Light-Gated activated by : light.
   locations : rods & cones in the retina of the eye.

Voltage-Gated activated by : changes in the voltage (membrane potential).
   locations : highly concentrated at the axon trigger zone & the neurofibral nodes.

Excitability : the presence of voltage-gated ion channels in nerve and muscle plasma membranes gives these cells the property of excitability — the ability to respond to certain stimuli by producing impulses (nerve and muscle action potentials).

MEMBRANE POTENTIALS

Resting Membrane Potential When a neuron is at rest (not being stimulated or "excited") the voltage across the membrane ranges between − 40 and − 90 mV; a typical value is − 70 mV.

Equilibrium Potentials An equilibrium potential is a hypothetical value for a particular type of ion. It is the membrane potential that would result in a net diffusion of zero for that ion. The equilibrium potential for potassium ions is − 90 mV; for sodium ions it is + 60 mV.

Graded Potentials Graded potentials vary in magnitude and duration. They occur when chemically, mechanically, or light-gated ion channels open or close. The greater the stimulus the more gated ion channels open or close, and the greater the change in the membrane potential; the ion channels remain activated as long as the stimulus persists.

Action Potentials If a graded potential reaches a certain critical level (called threshold), it will activate voltage-gated ion channels and trigger an action potential. During an action potential a segment of membrane depolarizes (− 70 mV to 0 mV), reverses polarization (0 to + 30 mV), and then repolarizes (+ 30 to − 70 mV).

VOLTAGE electric potential energy

BATTERY

Batteries contain opposite charges
separated by an insulating material.

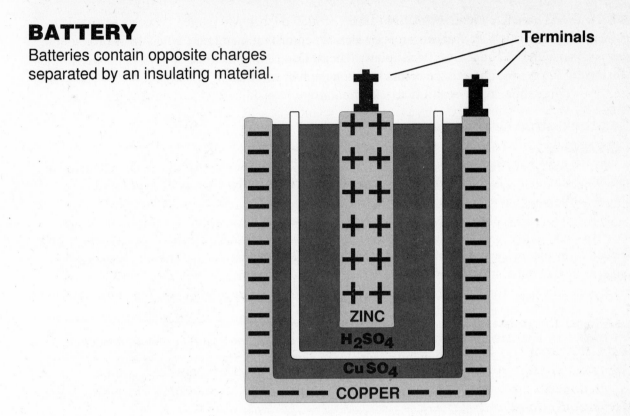

HUMAN CELL

All cells are positive on the outside relative to
the inside. The opposite charges are insulated by
the high fat content of the plasma membrane.

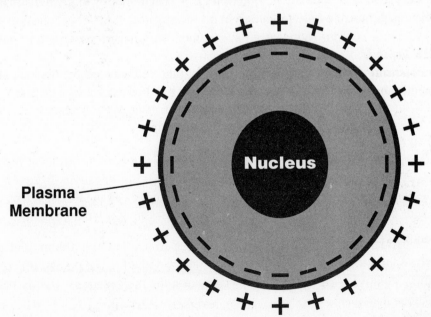

NERVE IMPULSE / Resting & Equilibrium Potentials

GENERATING A RESTING POTENTIAL

The resting potential is the electrical difference across a neuron cell membrane when the neuron is "resting" or inactive; it is equal to -70 millivolts. The neuron resting membrane potential is determined by 2 factors: (1) ion concentration gradients between the ICF and ECF.
(2) membrane permeability to specific ions.

Concentration Gradients   *Sodium (10 : 1)   Potassium (30 : 1)*

The resting membrane potential exists because of the distribution of charged particles in the fluids inside and outside the cell (the ICF & ECF). Both fluid compartments have many charged particles: sodium, potassium, chloride, magnesium, and calcium ions; bicarbonates, phosphates, sulfates, amino acids, and proteins.

Sodium ions (Na^+) and potassium ions (K^+) are present in the highest concentrations, so they have the greatest effect on the membrane potential. There are 10 times as many sodium ions outside the cell as inside, so the concentration force tends to move sodium ions <u>into</u> the cell; there are 30 times as many potassium ions inside the cell as outside, so the concentration force tends to move potassium ions <u>out</u>. The concentration gradients for sodium and potassium ions is maintained by the active transport of these ions by the *sodium-potassium pump*.

Membrane Permeability   *sodium ion channels closed; potassium ion channels open*

When a neuron is at rest the sodium ion channels are closed, so the membrane is relatively impermeable to sodium; the potassium ion channels are open, so the membrane is highly permeable to potassium. The cell membrane of a resting neuron is 50 to 75 times more permeable to potassium than it is to sodium, so potassium ions diffuse relatively easily out of the cell, while the flow of sodium ions is blocked by the impermeable membrane.

EQUILIBRIUM POTENTIALS

To understand why the resting potential is equal to -70 mV, it is helpful to understand equilibrium potentials. The equilibrium potential is the membrane potential at which the concentration force for a particular ion is in equilibrium with the electrical force; in other words, the concentration force is equal in magnitude to the electrical force but opposite in direction. It is based on a *hypothetical* situation : it assumes that the membrane is permeable only to the ion in question and that the concentration gradient for that ion is the same as it is for neurons (concentration gradients vary in different types of cells).

Sodium Equilibrium Potential

In this hypothetical situation the Na^+ ions would diffuse <u>into</u> the cell until the membrane potential reached $+60$ mV (the increase of positive charges inside the cell would decrease its negativity from -70 to $+60$ mV). At this point the electrical force repelling the positive charges would equal the concentration force driving Na^+ ions into the cell; the net movement of sodium ions would be zero.

Potassium Equilibrium Potential

In this hypothetical situation the K^+ ions would diffuse <u>out</u> of the cell until the inside of the cell reached -90 mV (loss of positive charges inside the cell would increase its negativity from -70 to -90 mV). At this point the electrical force attracting positive K^+ ions into the cell would equal the concentration force driving K^+ ions out of the cell; the net movement of potassium ions would be zero.

Neuron Resting Potential   Because resting neurons are permeable to potassium ions and relatively impermeable to sodium ions, the resting potential is almost equal to the potassium equilibrium potential. It is slightly more positive (-90 up to -70 mV), because the membrane is slightly permeable to sodium ions and some ions leak in.

EQUILIBRIUM POTENTIALS

RESTING POTENTIAL

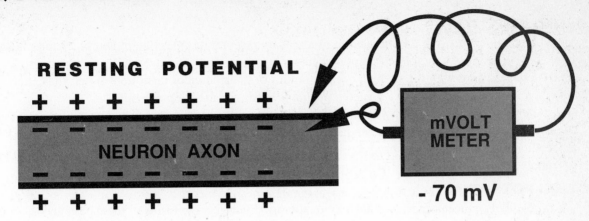

+ + + + + + +

NEURON AXON

$-$ $-$ $-$ $-$ $-$ $-$

$-$ $-$ $-$ $-$ $-$ $-$

+ + + + + + +

mVOLT METER

$-$ 70 mV

SODIUM EQUILIBRIUM POTENTIAL

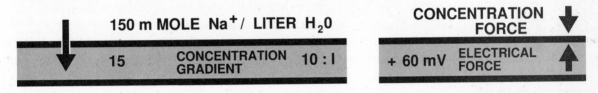

150 m MOLE Na$^+$ / LITER H$_2$0

15   CONCENTRATION GRADIENT   10 : 1

CONCENTRATION FORCE

+ 60 mV   ELECTRICAL FORCE

POTASSIUM EQUILIBRIUM POTENTIAL

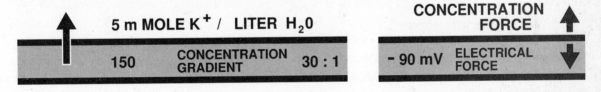

5 m MOLE K$^+$ / LITER H$_2$0

150   CONCENTRATION GRADIENT   30 : 1

CONCENTRATION FORCE

$-$ 90 mV   ELECTRICAL FORCE

RESTING POTENTIAL

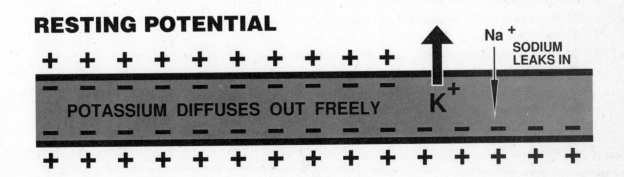

+ + + + + + + + + + +

POTASSIUM DIFFUSES OUT FREELY   K$^+$

Na$^+$ SODIUM LEAKS IN

+ + + + + + + + + + + + + +

NERVE IMPULSE / Graded & Action Potentials

GRADED POTENTIALS

A graded potential results from the stimulation of a sensory receptor or the action of neurotransmitters on the cell body and dendrites of a motor neuron or association neuron. The magnitude of the change in membrane potential (voltage) varies with the strength of the stimulus or the amount of neurotransmitter; thus, it is called a *graded* potential. The function of a graded potential is to trigger an action potential.

Generator Potentials Graded potentials that occur at sensory receptors are called generator potentials.

Postsynaptic Potentials Graded potentials that occur on the cell bodies and dendrites of motor and association neurons are called postsynaptic potentials; they may be excitatory (excitatory postsynaptic potentials / EPSPs) or inhibitory (inhibitory postsynaptic potentials / IPSPs).

ACTION POTENTIAL

An action potential is a membrane potential that temporarily reverses: the inside of the membrane becomes positive relative to the outside, then returns to the resting potential.

Voltage-Gated Ion Channels During an action potential voltage-gated ion channels open and close, controlling the movement of sodium and potassium ions through the membrane ion channels.

A single gate controls the flow of K^+ through each voltage-gated K^+ channel.

Each voltage-gated Na^+ channel has two separate gates:

(1) *Activation Gate :* opens when the ion channel is activated (membrane potential reaches threshold).

(2) *Inactivation Gate :* is open when the neuron is at rest (inactivated ion channel).

All-or-None Response Action potentials occur maximally or not at all. Under normal conditions the duration and magnitude is always the same: the entire action potential lasts only 1 millisecond (1/1000 second) and during this fraction of a second the membrane potential changes from -70 to $+30$ and back to -70 mV (a magnitude of 100 mV).

Refractory Period During an action potential, while the sodium or potassium ion channels are open, the membrane is *refractory* (unresponsive to stimuli).

Sequence of Events

Resting Membrane   *-70 mV   (Resting Stage)*

Na^+ activation gate : closed.

Na^+ inactivation gate : open.

K^+ gate : closed.

Depolarization   *-70 mV to $+30$ mV*

Graded Potential A graded potential depolarizes the membrane from -70 mV to -55 mV.

Threshold Potential $= -55$ mV.

Na^+ activation gate : opens quickly (Na^+ diffuses into the neuron).

Na^+ inactivation gate : slowly begins to close.

K^+ gate : slowly begins to open.

Repolarization   *$+30$ mV to -70 mV*

Reversal Potential $= +30$ mV.

Na^+ activation gate : slowly begins to close.

Na^+ inactivation gate : closes (blocks the diffusion of Na^+ into the neuron).

K^+ gate : opens (K^+ diffuses out of the neuron).

Resting Potential $= -70$ mV.

Na^+ activation gate : closes.

Na^+ inactivation gate : opens.

K^+ gate : slowly begins to close (K^+ continues to leak out, resulting in hyperpolarization; -90 mV).
    As voltage-gated K^+ channels close, the membrane returns to the resting level (-70 mV).

Restoring Concentration Gradients The loss of sodium and potassium concentration gradients is prevented by the continuous action of the sodium-potassium pump, an active transport system in the membrane that pumps sodium ions out of the cell and potassium ions in.

VOLTAGE – GATED ION CHANNELS
Changes in voltage-gated channels during an action potential

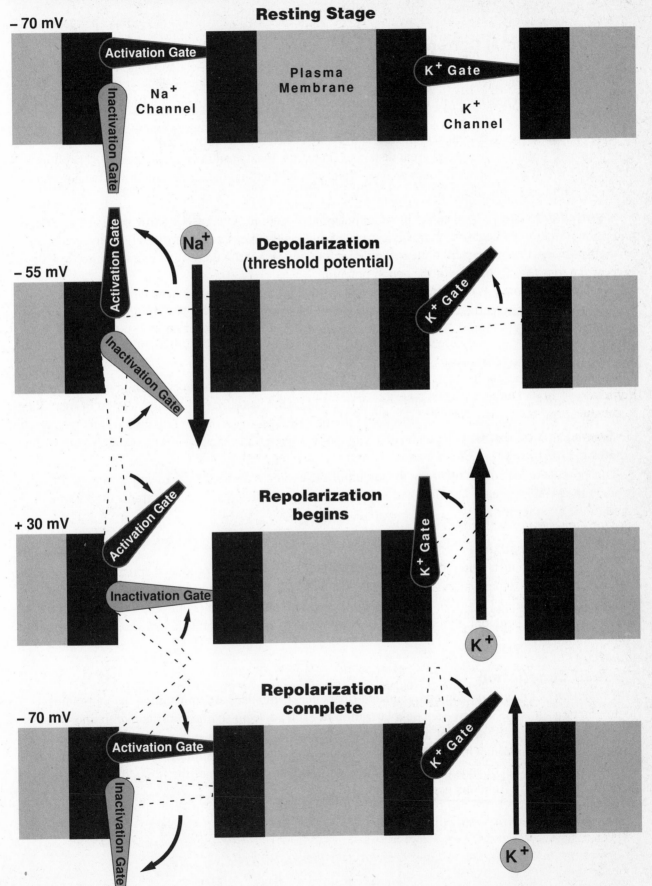

NERVE IMPULSE / Action Potential Propagation

Nerve Impulse : self-propagating action potentials traveling along an axon.

Local Decremental Currents

When an action potential occurs on a segment of axon, it produces local currents which depolarize the adjacent membrane. The local currents produced by an action potential are always strong enough to bring the adjacent membrane to its *threshold potential*, so a new action potential will fire on the adjacent membrane.

The currents are called local decremental currents. The term "local" differentiates these currents from the nerve impulses that travel great distances on axons; local currents are confined to very short distances (1 to 2 mm). The term "decremental" refers to the fact that the amplitude of the local currents decreases with increasing distance.

Extracellular Flow   When an action potential occurs, sodium ions rush into the cell. As a result, a region of relatively negative charge is generated outside the membrane. Positively charged ions in the nearby ECF are attracted to the negative region; consequently, there is an extracellular flow of positive ions <u>toward</u> the site of the action potential.

Intracellular Flow   At the same time there is an intracellular flow of positive ions <u>away from</u> the site of the action potential due to the increased concentration of positive sodium ions on the inside of the membrane.

Positive-Feedback Cycle

The local decremental currents generate a threshold potential on the adjacent membrane and this triggers a *positive-feedback cycle* : voltage-sensitive Na^+ channels open, making the section of membrane highly permeable to sodium ions; the ions rush into the cell, and a new action potential occurs. Once threshold is achieved and the positive feedback cycle is triggered the sequence is the same for all action potentials.

This process repeats itself all along the length of the axon membrane, until an action potential finally occurs at the axon terminal. The final action potential triggers the release of neurotransmitter, which is stored in the axon terminal.

One-Way Propagation

As action potentials are propagated along an axon, the local currents produced spread out in all directions, but a nerve impulse travels in only one direction. The portion of plasma membrane that has recently been depolarized is still in a *refractory* state, which means that it is temporarily incapable of producing an action potential. For this reason nerve impulses never travel back toward a region that has just been depolarized.

Types of Conduction

Continuous Conduction   On unmyelinated fibers nerve impulses are transmitted by continuous conduction. It is the step-by-step depolarization of each adjacent segment of the membrane. An action potential in one segment triggers an action potential in the adjacent membrane.

Saltatory Conduction   On myelinated fibers nerve impulses are transmitted by saltatory conduction. It is the propagation of an action potential along the exposed portions of the fiber. The action potentials seem to jump from one neurofibral node to the next.

A NERVE IMPULSE

PROPAGATED ACTION POTENTIALS

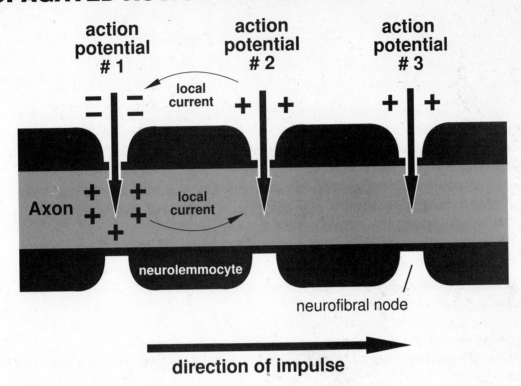

action potential # 1

action potential # 2

action potential # 3

local current

Axon

local current

neurolemmocyte

neurofibral node

direction of impulse

ACTION POTENTIALS
oscilloscope trace

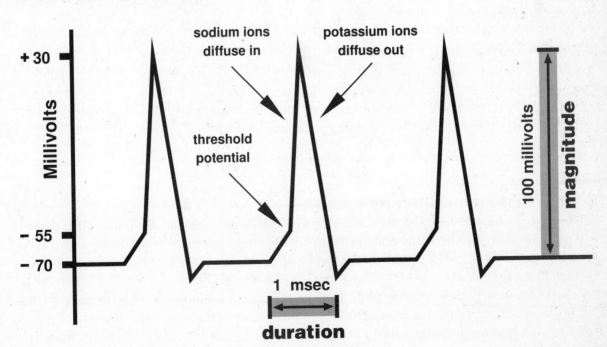

sodium ions diffuse in

potassium ions diffuse out

+ 30

threshold potential

Millivolts

- 55

- 70

1 msec

duration

100 millivolts

magnitude

NERVE IMPULSE / Conduction Velocity & Frequency

Velocity of Impulses

The velocity of a nerve impulse along a nerve fiber depends on 2 factors: fiber diameter and degree of myelination.

Fiber Diameter   The larger the fiber diameter the faster the propagation, because a large fiber offers less resistance to local intracellular current flow.

Degree of Myelination   The greater the degree of myelination the faster the propagation, because the fatty material in myelin makes it more difficult for local currents to leak in and out of the axon plasma membrane.

Frequency of Impulses

Refractory Periods   The refractory period is the time during which a neuron membrane is unresponsive to stimuli.

Absolute Refractory Period   The absolute refractory period coincides with an action potential and lasts for 1 millisecond.

Relative Refractory Period   The relative refractory period lasts for 10 to 15 milliseconds after the action potential has occurred; during this period the membrane will respond only to stimuli that are <u>above</u> threshold.

Even if the stimuli are above threshold (suprathreshold), the absolute refractory period limits the frequency of impulses to 1000 per second :

> 1 action potential / millisecond = 1000 action potentials / second.

And since a set amount of neurotransmitter is released every time an action potential occurs at an axon terminal, the absolute refractory period limits the amount of neurotransmitter that can be released over time.

Fiber Classification by Size

A Fibers   The largest diameter fibers are called A fibers. They are 5 to 20 micrometers in diameter and have brief absolute refractory periods. All are myelinated and conduct impulses from 12 to 130 meters per second. Examples are fibers of large sensory nerves that relay impulses associated with touch, pressure, joint position, and temperature.

B Fibers   Intermediate size fibers are called B fibers. They are less than 3 micrometers in diameter and all are myelinated. They conduct impulses up to 15 meters per second. Examples are sensory fibers that transmit impulses from the viscera (internal organs) and motor fibers that carry impulses to autonomic ganglia (general visceral neurons).

C Fibers   The smallest fibers are called C fibers. They are 0.5 to 1.5 micrometers in diameter and have the longest absolute refractory periods. All are unmyelinated fibers and they conduct impulses from 0.5 to 2 meters per second. Examples are motor fibers that carry impulses from autonomic ganglia to effectors and some sensory fibers that carry impulses for pain, touch, pressure, and temperature from the skin to the CNS.

Amount of Neurotransmitter Released

Frequency of Action Potentials   Since all action potentials are the same, the information transmitted by a nerve impulse depends mainly on the *frequency* of action potentials— how many arrive at the axon terminal per unit time. The greater the frequency of action potentials the greater the amount of neurotransmitter released.

Action potentials generally occur in bursts, because the graded potentials that initiate them are not used up after one action potential is completed. After the absolute refractory period is completed there is generally enough residual graded potential to constitute a suprathreshold stimulus, so another action potential occurs; the stronger the graded potential the longer the burst of action potentials.

NERVE IMPULSE : Velocity & Frequency

Velocity of Impulses
Impulses travel faster in large, myelinated axons.

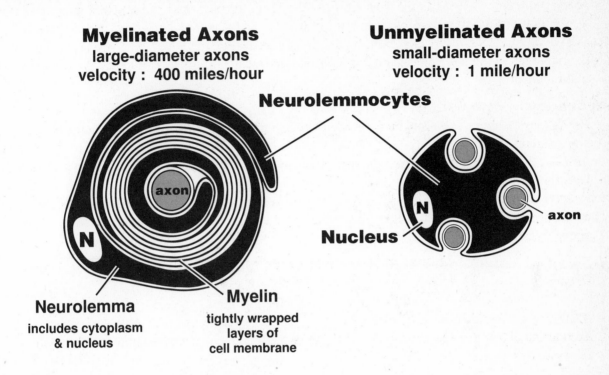

Myelinated Axons
large-diameter axons
velocity : 400 miles/hour

Unmyelinated Axons
small-diameter axons
velocity : 1 mile/hour

Neurolemmocytes

axon

Nucleus

axon

Neurolemma
includes cytoplasm
& nucleus

Myelin
tightly wrapped
layers of
cell membrane

Frequency of Impulses
The frequency of nerve impulses is limited by the refractory period.
During refractory periods new action potentials cannot be generated.

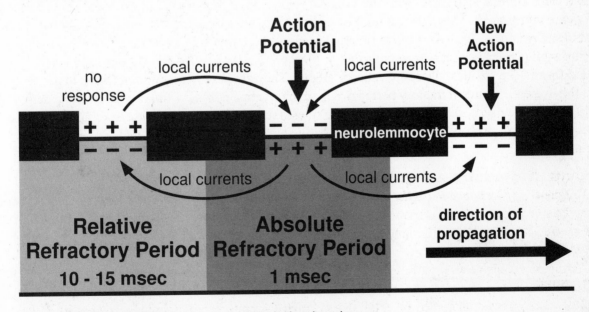

**Action
Potential**

**New
Action
Potential**

no
response

local currents

local currents

+ + +

− − −

neurolemmocyte

+ + +

− − −

+ + +

− − −

local currents

local currents

**Relative
Refractory Period**
10 - 15 msec

**Absolute
Refractory Period**
1 msec

**direction of
propagation**

repolarized region
(recent action potential)

depolarized region
(action potential in process)

Synapse

Synaptic Junctions *38*
    1. Types of Synaptic Junctions :
        chemical synapses
        electrical synapses (gap junctions)
    2. Presynaptic & Postsynaptic Neurons
    3. Excitatory & Inhibitory Synapses
    4. Structures
        synaptic end bulb
        synaptic cleft
        postsynaptic membrane

Synaptic Transmission *40*
    1. Sequence of Events
    2. One-Way Transmission
    3. Presynaptic Facilitation & Inhibition
    3. Removal of Neurotransmitter

Summation *42*
    1. Excitatory Synapse
    2. Inhibitory Synapse
    3. Temporal & Spatial Summation

Neurotransmitters *44*
    1. Chemical Classification :
        amino acids, biogenic amines, neuropeptides, & acetylcholine
    2. PNS Neurotransmitters : acetylcholine & norepinephrine
    3. CNS Neurotransmitters : GABA & catecholamines

Altered Synaptic Mechanisms *46*
    1. Drugs : agonists & antagonists
    2. Morphine Addiction
    3. Other Examples of Altered Synaptic Activity

Neuromuscular Junction *48*
    1. Structures
    2. End-Plate Potentials
    3. Altered Neuromuscular Transmission

Neuronal Circuits *50*
    1. Simple Series   4. Reverberating
    2. Diverging   5. Parallel After-Discharge
    3. Converging

SYNAPSE / Synaptic Junctions

Types of Synaptic Junctions

For an electrical signal to pass from one excitable cell to another it must cross a **synapse** (*synapsis* = point of contact).

Chemical Synapses If the two excitable cells are neurons, the junction between them is a chemical synapse; the term "chemical" refers to the fact that the stimulation of the second (or postsynaptic) neuron is caused by a chemical released by the first (or presynaptic) neuron.
Junctions between neurons and muscle cells are called *neuromuscular junctions*; they also are chemical synapses and function in a way similar to synapses between neurons.

Electrical Synapses In electrical synapses ionic current spreads directly from one cell to another through tubular structures called *connexons*. A cluster of 100 or so connexons forms a pathway (connection) called a *gap junction* between adjacent cells. Gap junctions are common between cardiac muscle cells and between single-unit smooth muscle visceral cells.

Presynaptic & Postsynaptic Neurons

Presynaptic Neuron A neuron that conducts electrical signals <u>toward</u> a synapse is called a presynaptic neuron.

Postsynaptic Neuron A neuron that conducts electrical signals <u>away from</u> a synapse is called a postsynaptic neuron. The same neuron in a chain of interconnected neurons can be a postsynaptic neuron to one group of neurons and a presynaptic neuron to another group of neurons.

A single neuron may have thousands of synaptic junctions on its dendrites and cell body. A motor neuron cell body in the spinal cord may have as many as 15,000 synaptic junctions, while some association neurons in the brain have as many as 100,000 synaptic junctions. This allows signals from many different cells to converge on one neuron.

Excitatory & Inhibitory Synapses

Excitatory Synapse If the neurotransmitter released at a synapse tends to *depolarize* the postsynaptic membrane and bring it closer to threshold, the synapse is an *excitatory synapse*. Depolarization means that the electric potential across the membrane decreases; the outside becomes less positive relative to the inside of the cell.

Inhibitory Synapse If the neurotransmitter tends to *hyperpolarize* the postsynaptic membrane, it is an *inhibitory synapse*. Hyperpolarize means that the electric potential across the membrane increases; the outside becomes even more positive relative to the inside of the cell.

Structures A synaptic junction between neurons has 3 main parts: the synaptic end bulb, the synaptic cleft, and the postsynaptic membrane.

Synaptic End Bulb : At the end of each axon terminal is an enlarged knob or swelling called the synaptic end bulb; it contains membrane-enclosed bubbles called synaptic vesicles, which contain molecules of neurotransmitter. Each synaptic vesicle is about 25 nm (nanometers) in diameter.

Synaptic Cleft : The narrow gap between the axon terminal of the presynaptic neuron and the cell body or dendrite of the postsynaptic neuron is filled with extracellular fluid and is called the synaptic cleft.

Postsynaptic Membrane : The membrane across the synaptic cleft (belonging to the dendrite or cell body of the postsynaptic neuron) is called the postsynaptic or subsynaptic membrane. Embedded in the outer surface of this membrane are molecules of receptor proteins that combine with neurotransmitter molecules and trigger depolarization or hyperpolarization of the postsynaptic membrane.

SYNAPSE : contact point between neurons

Presynaptic & Postsynaptic Neurons

Presynaptic Neurons : conduct impulses toward a synapse
Postsynaptic Neurons : conduct impulses away from a synapse

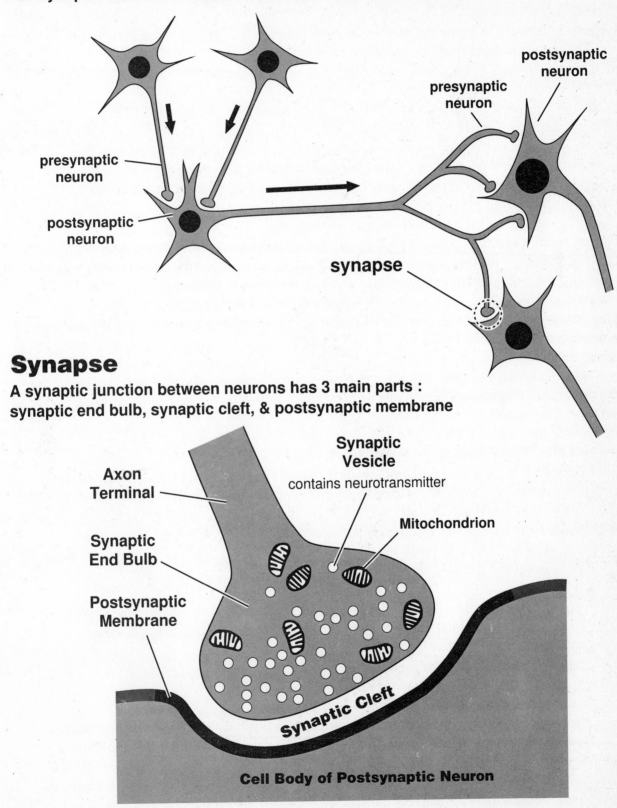

Synapse

A synaptic junction between neurons has 3 main parts :
synaptic end bulb, synaptic cleft, & postsynaptic membrane

SYNAPSE / Synaptic Transmission

Sequence of Events

At chemical synapses the electrical activity of one neuron influences the electrical activity of a second neuron by means of a chemical messenger (neurotransmitter). The sequence of events is the following :

(1) *Action Potential :* A nerve impulse reaches the axon terminal of a presynaptic neuron; the membrane is depolarized by an action potential.

(2) *Calcium Channels :* Depolarization of the axon terminal during the action potential causes voltage-sensitive calcium ion channels to open.

(3) *Calcium Diffusion :* Calcium ions diffuse into the axon terminal from the ECF.

(4) *Exocytosis :* The increase in calcium ions causes some synaptic vesicles to fuse with the plasma membrane; they release neurotransmitter into the synaptic cleft by exocytosis.

(5) *Neurotransmitter Diffusion :* Neurotransmitter molecules diffuse across the synaptic cleft and bind to the receptors embedded in the outer surface of the postsynaptic membrane.

(6) *Receptor Activation :* The neurotransmitter-receptor complexes cause specific ion channels to open; they are called *chemically-gated ion channels.*

(7) *Postsynaptic Potential :* Graded postsynaptic potentials are generated by the diffusion of ions in and out of the postsynaptic cell. At excitatory synapses there is a net flow of positive ions <u>into</u> the cell; at inhibitory synapses there is a net flow of positive ions <u>out of</u> the cell.

(8) *Local Currents :* If the local currents produced by the graded potentials are strong enough, the postsynaptic neuron will reach its threshold potential and an action potential will result — the second neuron will "fire."

One-Way Transmission
Because neurotransmitter is stored only on the presynaptic side of the synaptic cleft, the transmission of a nerve impulse between neurons can occur in only one direction.

Presynaptic Facilitation & Inhibition

Facilitation : the amount of neurotransmitter released from the end bulb of a presynaptic neuron is increased. The increased release of neurotransmitter is the result of an excitatory input from a third neuron that synapses near the end bulb of the presynaptic neuron.

Inhibition : the amount of neurotransmitter released from the end bulb of a presynaptic neuron is decreased. This is the result of an inhibitory input from a third neuron that synapses near the end bulb of the presynaptic neuron.

Removal of Neurotransmitter
As long as neurotransmitter remains in the synaptic cleft, it will continue to combine with receptors and activate the postsynaptic membrane. Removal of neurotransmitter may be accomplished in several ways :

(1) Diffusion into the extracellular fluid (ECF).

(2) Enzymatic degradation in the synaptic cleft.

(3) Reuptake by the presynaptic neuron.

Acetylcholine : The enzyme acetylcholinesterase, which is located on the outer surface of the postsynaptic membrane, splits acetylcholine into acetate and choline. The choline is actively transported back into the axon terminal and reused; the acetate diffuses into the ECF.

Norepinephrine (& Dopamine) : The activity of norepinephrine and dopamine diminishes as the neurotransmitters are actively transported back into the axon terminals.

SYNAPTIC TRANSMISSION
Sequence of Events

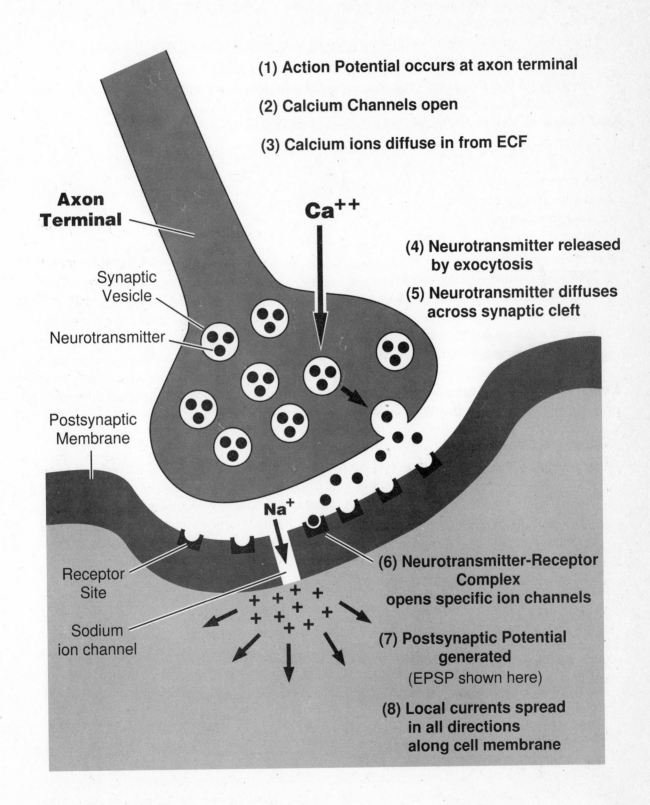

(1) Action Potential occurs at axon terminal

(2) Calcium Channels open

(3) Calcium ions diffuse in from ECF

Ca^{++}

Axon Terminal

(4) Neurotransmitter released by exocytosis

(5) Neurotransmitter diffuses across synaptic cleft

Synaptic Vesicle

Neurotransmitter

Postsynaptic Membrane

Na^+

Receptor Site

Sodium ion channel

(6) Neurotransmitter-Receptor Complex opens specific ion channels

(7) Postsynaptic Potential generated
(EPSP shown here)

(8) Local currents spread in all directions along cell membrane

SYNAPSE / Summation

Summation (an example) Touching a hot object usually triggers a withdrawal reflex; the hand automatically withdraws from the painful stimulus. However, through a conscious effort, the cerebral cortex can send inhibitory signals to block this response. Whether or not the motor neurons fire depends on which input is stronger, the inhibitory from the brain or the excitatory from the sensory input. The motor neuron involved adds up the opposing inputs and responds accordingly. This process of adding up different inputs is called summation or integration.

Receptors & Ion Channels Motor neurons and association neurons have 2 kinds of chemical synapses : excitatory and inhibitory. The type of synapse is determined by the type of receptor on the postsynaptic membrane and the type of ion channel that the receptor controls.

Trigger Zone The junction of an axon hillock and the initial segment of an axon is called the trigger zone, because it is at this location where nerve impulses are "triggered." It is the region where the local currents generated by excitatory and inhibitory events are added together. If the summation reaches threshold, the first action potential occurs at the trigger zone. Voltage-gated ion channels are clustered most densely in this region.

Excitatory Synapse

At excitatory synapses the binding of neurotransmitter and receptor causes Na^+ channels to open.
Depolarization There is a net movement of positive Na^+ into the postsynaptic cell, which causes slight depolarization. This occurs each time an action potential reaches the axon terminal of the presynaptic neuron. The activity is called an *excitatory postsynaptic event* and the result is an *excitatory postsynaptic potential (EPSP)*. Its effect is to increase the likelihood that the postsynaptic membrane will reach threshold. An EPSP generates local currents that cause positively charged ions to flow toward the trigger zone of the axon. If the local currents are strong enough, threshold potential will be reached at the trigger zone and the axon will "fire."

Inhibitory Synapse

At inhibitory synapses the combination of neurotransmitter and receptor causes K^+ channels to open.
Hyperpolarization There is a net movement of positive potassium ions *out of* the postsynaptic cell, which causes a slight hyperpolarization. It is called an *inhibitory postsynaptic event* and the result is called an *inhibitory postsynaptic potential (IPSP)*. Its effect is to lessen the likelihood that the postsynaptic membrane will reach threshold. An IPSP generates local currents that cause positively charged ions to flow away from the trigger zone of the axon, causing hyperpolarization.

Summation

One EPSP is not enough to trigger an action potential on a postsynaptic neuron. A single EPSP on a motor neuron is estimated to be only 0.5 mV, whereas the threshold potential varies from 15 to 25 mV. A single neuron may receive hundreds of excitatory and inhibitory signals at the same time; whether or not it fires depends on the summation of the two types of signals.

Temporal Summation If two or more synaptic events occur at the same location in rapid succession, the effects are added together. Input signals arrive at different times.
Spatial Summation When two or more synapses fire simultaneously (at different locations) the effects are added together. The closer the synapses are to the trigger zone the greater their effects on the membrane potential of that region.

SUMMATION

**One synaptic event will not cause a postsynaptic neuron to fire.
A postsynaptic neuron fires when many excitatory & inhibitory inputs
are added together (summated).**

**A motor neuron cell body may have
15,000 synaptic junctions.**

(only 10 are shown)

Motor Neuron

Trigger Zone
action potentials
start here

**Initial
Segment**

Excitatory Synapse

At excitatory synapses, the binding
of neurotransmitter with receptor
causes sodium ion channels to open.

Sodium ions diffuse into the cell body,
generating an EPSP.

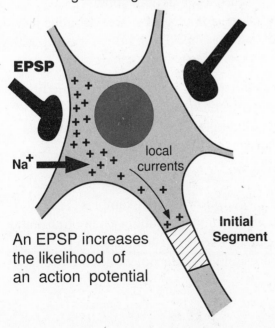

EPSP

Na^+

local
currents

Initial
Segment

An EPSP increases
the likelihood of
an action potential

Inhibitory Synapse

At inhibitory synapses, the binding
of neurotransmitter with receptor
causes potassium ion channels to open.

Potassium ions diffuse out of the cell body,
generating an IPSP.

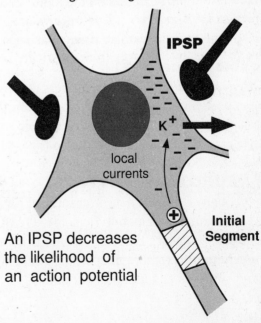

IPSP

K^+

local
currents

Initial
Segment

An IPSP decreases
the likelihood of
an action potential

43

SYNAPSE / Neurotransmitters

CHEMICAL CLASSIFICATION
(1) Amino Acids
inhibitory : GABA, Glycine

excitatory : Aspartate, Glutamate
(2) Biogenic Amines (produced in axon terminals)
Serotonin

Histamine

Catecholamines : Norepinephrine, Epinephrine, Dopamine
(3) Neuropeptides (produced in neuron cell bodies)
Endorphins

Enkephalins

Substance P
(4) Acetylcholine (produced in axon terminals)

PNS NEUROTRANSMITTERS
There are many different neurotransmitters present in the CNS, but in the PNS there are only two principal neurotransmitters : acetylcholine and norepinephrine.

Acetylcholine (ACh)
Cholinergic Fibers   All nerve fibers that release acetylcholine are called cholinergic fibers. All somatic motor neurons (leading to skeletal muscles) release acetylcholine; all preganglionic and postganglionic parasympathetic neurons and all preganglionic sympathetic neurons also release acetylcholine.

Although most postganglionic sympathetic neurons release norepinephrine, there are exceptions : acetylcholine is released by sympathetic neurons which innervate sweat glands and those which innervate some blood vessels in skeletal muscles (causing vasodilation).

Receptors : There are 2 types of receptors for acetylcholine.

Nicotinic receptors : The drug nicotine stimulates the receptors of all autonomic postganglionic neurons and the receptors on the motor end plates of neuromuscular junctions.

Muscarinic Receptors : The mushroom poison muscarine stimulates the acetylcholine receptors on smooth muscle, cardiac muscle, and gland cells.

Norepinephrine (NE)
Adrenergic Fibers   All nerve fibers that release norepinephrine are called adrenergic fibers. Most postganglionic sympathetic neurons release norepinephrine.

Receptors : There are 2 types of receptors for norepinephrine : alpha-adrenergic and beta-adrenergic receptors; classification is based on the drugs that stimulate them.

CNS NEUROTRANSMITTERS
There are many different neurotransmitters in the CNS. The following are examples :

GABA (gamma aminobutyric acid)   GABA is the most common inhibitory neurotransmitter in the brain. It causes IPSPs by opening chemically gated chloride ion channels.

Catecholamines (norepinephrine, epinephrine, & dopamine)   Catecholamines are excitatory at some synapses and inhibitory at others.

NEUROTRANSMITTERS
Neurotransmitters released by Motor Neurons

Motor Neurons   Effectors

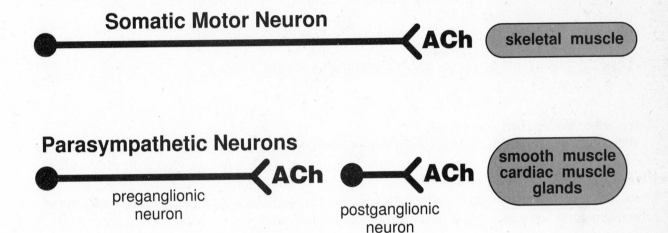

Somatic Motor Neuron
ACh — skeletal muscle

Parasympathetic Neurons
ACh — ACh
preganglionic neuron — postganglionic neuron

smooth muscle
cardiac muscle
glands

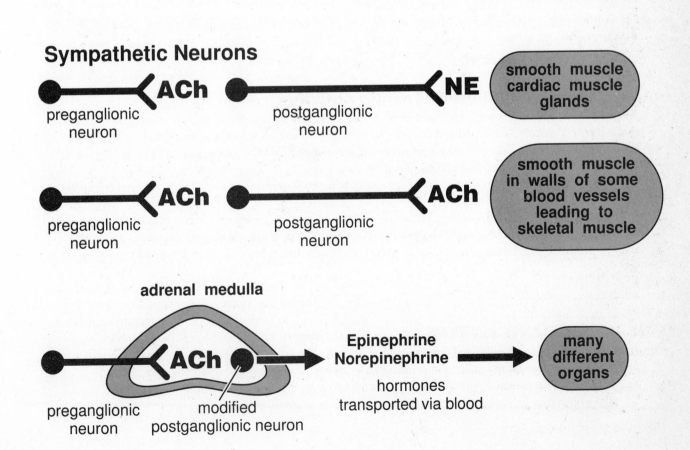

Sympathetic Neurons
ACh — NE
preganglionic neuron — postganglionic neuron

smooth muscle
cardiac muscle
glands

ACh — ACh
preganglionic neuron — postganglionic neuron

smooth muscle in walls of some blood vessels leading to skeletal muscle

adrenal medulla

ACh
preganglionic neuron — modified postganglionic neuron

Epinephrine
Norepinephrine

hormones transported via blood

many different organs

SYNAPSE / Altered Synaptic Mechanisms

Most drugs, poisons, and chemical messengers such as neuromodulators affect the nervous system by altering some aspect of synaptic transmission : the synthesis, release, action, re-uptake, or degradation of neurotransmitter.

Drugs

Drugs may be divided into 2 broad categories, those that mimic neurotransmitters and those that block the action of neurotransmitters.

Agonists : Agonists mimic neurotransmitters; they bind to receptor sites and produce a response similar to that of the neurotransmitter.

Antagonists : Antagonists block neurotransmitters; they bind to receptor sites but do not activate the postsynaptic membrane.

Morphine Addiction (an hypothesis)

Neurotransmitters called *endorphins* and *enkephalins* are released as a part of the normal functioning of the brain. They block the transmission of pain impulses in certain pathways. Normally only half of the receptors in the postsynaptic membranes are occupied by endorphin and enkephalin molecules. Morphine molecules bind to the same receptor sites, increasing the pain-inhibiting effects of the natural neurotransmitters and producing a "high." In response to this condition, the neurons decrease their synthesis of neurotransmitter, so it requires increased doses of morphine to achieve the same "high." This is called tolerance (for the drug). When no morphine is taken, the absence of any molecules in the postsynaptic receptors blocks all synaptic activity and causes withdrawal symptoms.

Opiate Drugs Opiate drugs (morphine, codeine, heroin) combine with the receptors normally used by endorphins and enkephalins and mimic the effects of these neurotransmitters. They have analgesic properties that diminish awareness of pain; they are also involved in neuronal pathways that are concerned with moods and emotions.

Other Examples of Altered Synaptic Activity :

Amphetamine Amphetamine causes an increase in the amount of dopamine released at synapses (especially in the limbic system). Amphetamine is a *dopamine agonist*. It causes the symptoms of schizophrenia.

Antipsychotic Drugs The anti-psychotic drugs used in the treatment of schizophrenia are *dopamine antagonists*; they combine with and block dopamine receptors.

Cocaine Cocaine enhances the effects of *norepinephrine* by preventing its normal inactivation (re-uptake by axon terminals) after it is released.

Lithium Carbonate Lithium causes a decrease in the amount of *norepinephrine* released from axon terminals. Lithium is an effective drug in the treatment of manias: it slows down thought processes and motor activity and normalizes mood. In bipolar disorders it reduces the severity of mood swings between depression and mania.

LSD LSD is a *serotonin antagonist*. Serotonin is a neurotransmitter important in pathways concerned with mood and states of consciousness; LSD is an hallucinogen that induces states resembling schizophrenia.

Mescaline Mescaline is a methylated derivative of *dopamine*. Enzymes in the brain convert mescaline into dopamine, increasing the activity at dopamine-mediated synapses; mescaline is an hallucinogenic drug.

Psilocin Psilocin is a methylated derivative of *serotonin*. Enzymes in the brain convert psilocin into serotonin, increasing the activity at serotonin-mediated synapses. Psilocin is an hallucinogenic drug.

Tricyclic Antidepressants Tricyclic antidepressants cause an increase in the amount of *norepinephrine* released from axon terminals. These drugs are used to treat depression.

MORPHINE ADDICTION (hypothesis)

Normal Release

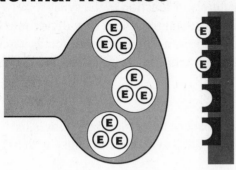

(E) = endorphin or enkephalin molecule
(M) = morphine molecule

Only 1/2 of the receptors are activated;

the normal release of endorphins creates
an analgesic and euphorigenic effect
in the pain-inhibitory pathways of the brain.

Drug Use

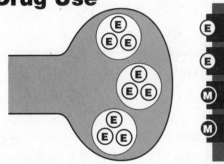

All of the receptors are activated;

there is an increased analgesic and
euphorigenic effect — a "high."

Tolerance

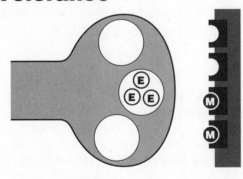

Once again, only 1/2 of the receptors are
activated; there has been a reduction
in the synthesis and release of endorphins
due to a negative-feedback mechanism;
the drug must be increased
to produce the same effects.

Withdrawal

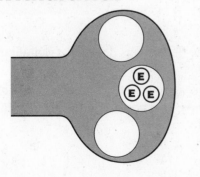

No receptors are activated;

the resulting absence of synaptic activity causes
withdrawal symptoms: anxiety, disturbed sleep,
abdominal cramps, muscle tremors, nausea.

SYNAPSE / Neuromuscular Junction

Structures

The contact point between a somatic motor neuron and a skeletal muscle fiber is called a *neuromuscular junction* or *myoneural junction*. It is very similar in structure and function to the synapse between two neurons. As the axon of a single motor neuron approaches a skeletal muscle, it may divide into several branches or up to several thousand branches; each branch forms a single neuromuscular junction with one muscle fiber. A single axon may innervate many muscle fibers, but each muscle fiber has only one neuromuscular junction.

A neuromuscular junction has three main parts :

Synaptic End Bulb   As an individual branch of an axon approaches a muscle fiber, it loses its myelin sheath and divides into several bulb-shaped structures called synaptic end bulbs, which contain vesicles filled with acetylcholine.

Synaptic Cleft   The synaptic cleft is the space between the synaptic end bulb and the membrane of the muscle fiber. It is the same as the synaptic cleft in a synapse between neurons.

Motor End Plate   The portion of muscle fiber membrane that corresponds to the postsynaptic membrane is called the motor end plate.

End-Plate Potentials

The events that occur during the transmission of an impulse from a motor neuron to a muscle fiber are similar to those which occur at other synapses. The main difference is the nature of the membrane potential produced, which is called the end-plate potential. Each nerve impulse that reaches the neuromuscular junction triggers the release of enough acetylcholine to generate an end-plate potential (EPP).

The mechanism that produces the EPP is similar to the one that produces an EPSP at a synapse, except the magnitude of the EPP is much greater: one EPP generates strong enough local currents to bring the adjacent muscle fiber membrane to threshold. The local currents spread in both directions along the muscle fiber and trigger action potentials that are propagated along the length of the muscle fiber in both directions (the neuromuscular junction is located toward the middle of most muscle fibers). The propagated muscle action potentials initiate a wave of contraction that moves along the muscle fiber.

Altered Neuromuscular Transmission

Just as drugs and toxins alter synaptic transmission between neurons, they also affect the transmission of impulses at neuromuscular junctions. The following are some examples:

Botulinum Toxin

Botulinum toxin, which is produced by the bacterium *Clostridium botulinum*, blocks the release of acetylcholine.

Curare

The South American Indian arrowhead poison called curare binds to acetylcholine receptor sites, blocking access.

Nerve Gases (Organophosphates)

Nerve gases inhibit the action of acetylcholinesterase, the enzyme that breaks down acetylcholine.

Myasthenia Gravis

Myasthenia gravis is an autoimmune disorder caused by antibodies directed against ACh receptors. The antibodies bind to the receptors and block the attachment of ACh. The skeletal muscles become weak and may eventually cease to function.

NEUROMUSCULAR JUNCTION

The contact point between a somatic motor neuron and a skeletal muscle is called a neuromuscular junction or a myoneural junction.

A single motor neuron axon may divide into hundreds or thousands of branches. Each axon branch innervates one skeletal muscle fiber.

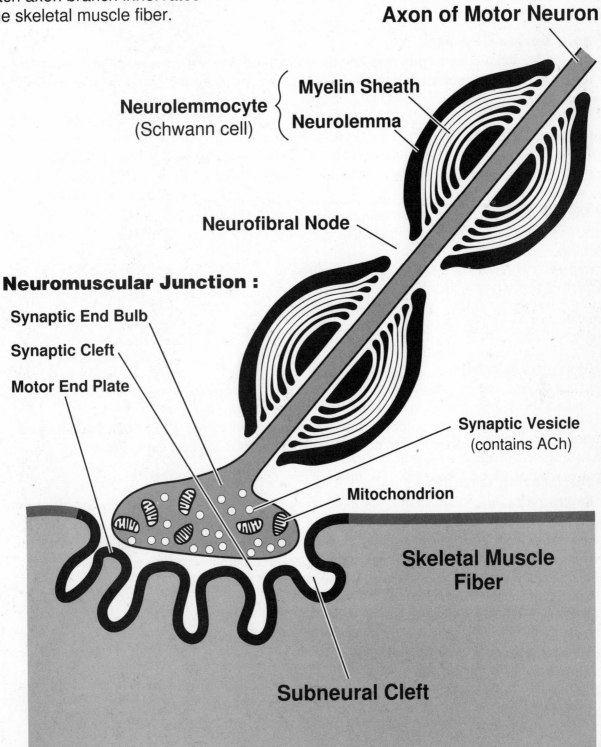

Axon of Motor Neuron

Neurolemmocyte
(Schwann cell)

Myelin Sheath

Neurolemma

Neurofibral Node

Neuromuscular Junction :

Synaptic End Bulb

Synaptic Cleft

Motor End Plate

Synaptic Vesicle
(contains ACh)

Mitochondrion

Skeletal Muscle Fiber

Subneural Cleft

SYNAPSE / Neuronal Circuits

Neuronal Pools   There are billions of neurons in the brain organized into complicated patterns called neuronal pools. Each neuronal pool is distinct from the others. Each neuronal pool contains thousands or millions of neurons and has a specific homeostatic role.

The neurons in neuronal pools are arranged in circuits. A circuit describes the basic pattern by which the neurons in a specific pool interact. There are 5 basic types of circuits:

Simple Series Circuits

In a simple series circuit a presynaptic neuron stimulates one neuron in a neuronal pool. That neuron then stimulates another neuron. It is a one-to-one chain reaction. Most neuronal circuits are more complex.

Diverging Circuits

In diverging circuits, a single presynaptic neuron synapses with several postsynaptic neurons or several effector cells (muscle or gland cells). In this type of circuit one neuron can influence the activities of several postsynaptic cells at the same time.

Motor Pathways : Upper motor neurons have their cell bodies in the cerebral cortex. The axons of these neurons can extend down the spinal cord and form branches that activate a pool of lower motor neuron cell bodies.

Sensory Pathways : First-order sensory neurons carry sensory impulses into the CNS. Inside the CNS their axons may branch and activate several second-order sensory neurons. The second-order sensory neurons transmit impulses to the thalamus where they may branch, activating several third-order neurons that carry impulses to several regions of the brain.

Converging Circuits

In converging circuits, several presynaptic neurons synapse with a single postsynaptic neuron. This causes increased stimulation or inhibition of the postsynaptic neuron.

Motor Pathways : Upper motor neurons originating in different regions of the brain may converge on a single lower motor neuron that transmits impulses to skeletal muscle fibers.

Reverberating Circuits

Reverberating circuits are similar to simple series circuits because the incoming impulse stimulates the first neuron, which stimulates the second, which stimulates the third, and so on. It is a chain reaction. But it differs from the simple series circuits because each neuron has branches that carry the impulse back to earlier neurons in the series. The output signal may last from several seconds to many hours, depending upon the complexity of the circuits.

Breathing, coordinated muscular activities, waking up, sleeping, and short-term memory are thought to be the result of reverberating circuits.

Parallel After-Discharge Circuits

In this type of circuit the axon of a single presynaptic neuron branches, stimulating a group of neurons. Each neuron in the group synapses with a common postsynaptic neuron, causing multiple EPSPs and IPSPs.

This type of circuit may be used for mathematical calculations.

NEURONAL CIRCUITS

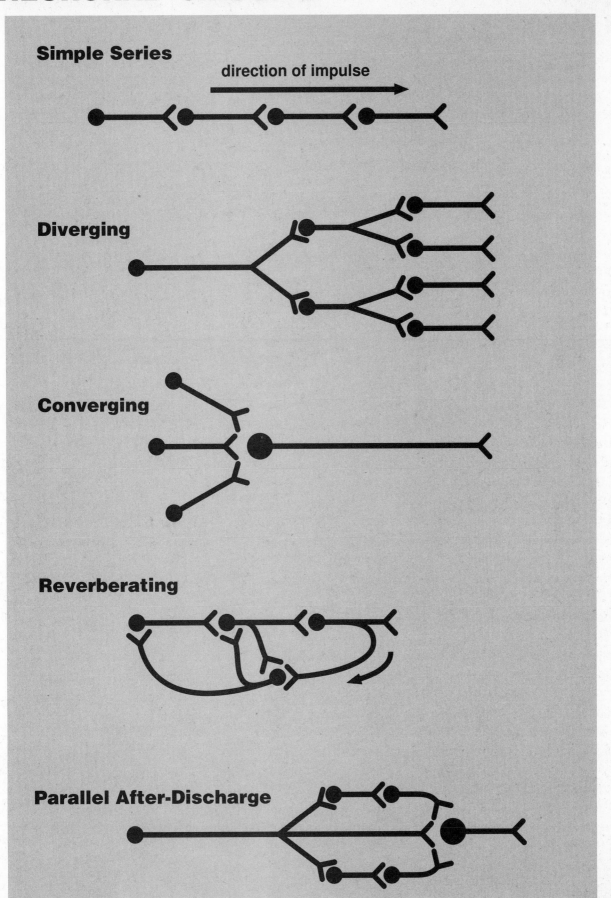

Simple Series

direction of impulse

Diverging

Converging

Reverberating

Parallel After-Discharge

The Brain

BRAIN / Embryonic & Fetal Development

NEURAL TUBE

Ectoderm   Nerve tissue develops from embryonic ectoderm.

Neural Plate   First a neural plate forms along the dorsal surface of the embryo.

Neural Groove   Then the edges of the plate thicken, forming the neural groove.

Neural Tube   The edges of the groove grow toward each other and fuse, forming the neural tube. This structure gives rise to the entire CNS, including neurons, neuroglia, ependymal cells, and the epithelial cells of the choroid plexus.

Neural Crest   Some cells lateral to the neural groove, making up the neural crest, undergo extensive migrations and give rise to most of the PNS.

PRIMARY VESICLES (the 4th week)

During the 3rd week the walls of the neural tube thicken and the section located in the head region of the embryo forms 3 distinct bulges :

(1) Prosencephalon (Forebrain)   The anterior bulge is called the forebrain; it develops into the cerebral hemispheres and the diencephalon.

(2) Mesencephalon (Midbrain)   The middle bulge is called the midbrain; it changes very little during the development of the brain.

(3) Rhombencephalon (Hindbrain) The posterior bulge is called the hindbrain; it develops into the pons, medulla, and cerebellum.

Cerebrospinal Fluid   The 3 bulges in the neural tube are called vesicles and are filled with a fluid that becomes the cerebrospinal fluid (*vesicle* = a small bladder or sac containing fluid).

SECONDARY VESICLES (the 5th week)

As development progresses, the neural tube undergoes several flexures (bends). By the 5th week of development, the 3 primary vesicles have subdivided into 5 secondary vesicles.

(1) Telencephalon   The forebrain divides into 2 lateral bulges that develop into the two cerebral hemispheres and the basal ganglia.

(2) Diencephalon   The posterior portion of the forebrain (between the forebrain and the midbrain) develops into a region called the diencephalon. Cells that make up the walls of the diencephalon ultimately form the thalamus, hypothalamus, pineal gland, and pituitary gland.

(3) Mesencephalon (Midbrain) The midbrain develops 4 prominent structures called the corpora quadrigemina (*corpus* = body; *quad* = four). The two nearest the diencephalon are called the superior colliculi; the two nearest the hindbrain are called the inferior colliculi.

(4) Metencephalon   The region of the hindbrain nearest to the midbrain is called the metencephalon; it develops into the pons (floor of the hindbrain) and the cerebellum (roof of the hindbrain).

(5) Myelencephalon   The region of the hindbrain nearest to the spinal cord is called the myelencephalon; it develops into the medulla.

Ventricles   The cavities within the vesicles develop into the 4 ventricles of the brain, where cerebrospinal fluid is produced by specialized capillary networks called choroid plexuses.

BRAIN : Neural Tube Development

Lateral Views

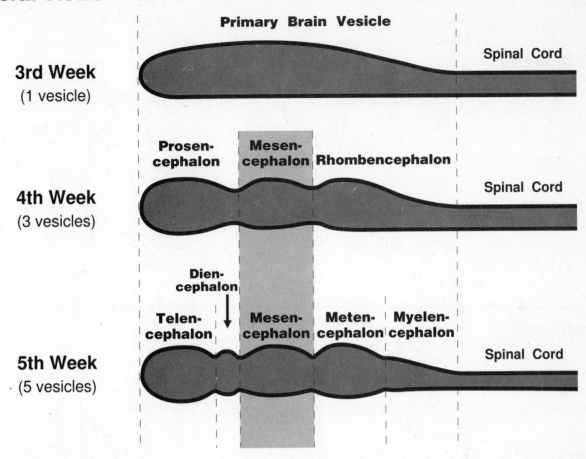

Primary Brain Vesicle

Spinal Cord

3rd Week
(1 vesicle)

Prosen-cephalon | **Mesen-cephalon** | **Rhombencephalon**

Spinal Cord

4th Week
(3 vesicles)

Dien-cephalon

Telen-cephalon | **Mesen-cephalon** | **Meten-cephalon** | **Myelen-cephalon**

Spinal Cord

5th Week
(5 vesicles)

Structures That Develop From Each Vesicle

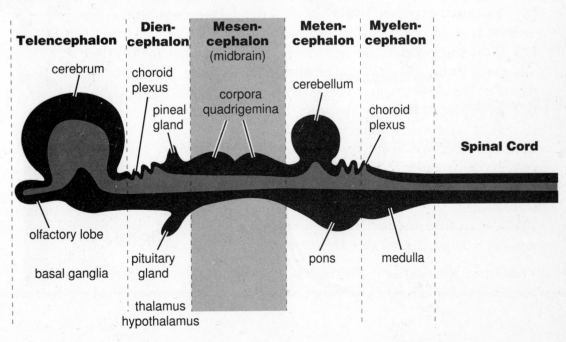

Telencephalon | **Dien-cephalon** | **Mesen-cephalon** (midbrain) | **Meten-cephalon** | **Myelen-cephalon**

cerebrum

choroid plexus

pineal gland

corpora quadrigemina

cerebellum

choroid plexus

Spinal Cord

olfactory lobe

pituitary gland

pons

medulla

basal ganglia

thalamus
hypothalamus

BRAIN : Embryonic Development

The neural tube is filled with cerebrospinal fluid (shaded areas).

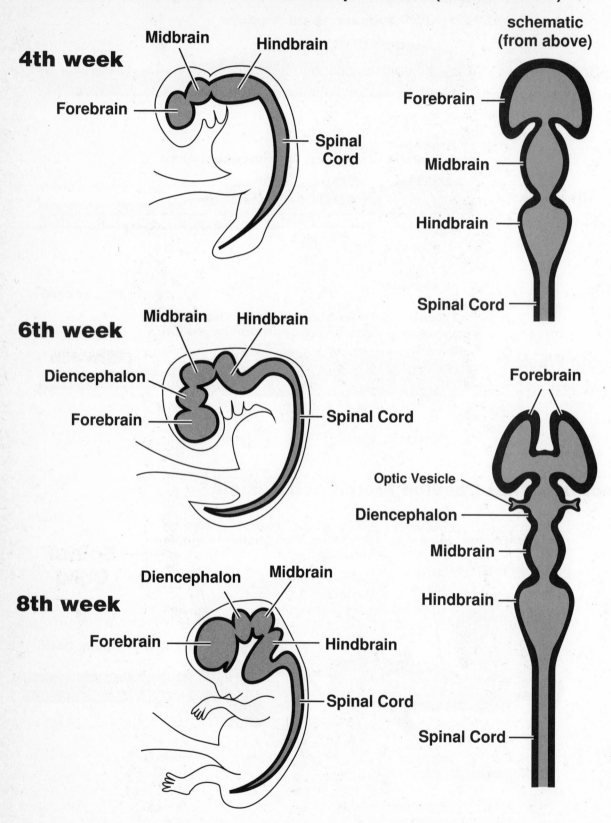

schematic (from above)

4th week

Midbrain
Hindbrain
Forebrain
Spinal Cord

Forebrain
Midbrain
Hindbrain
Spinal Cord

6th week

Midbrain
Hindbrain
Diencephalon
Forebrain
Spinal Cord

Forebrain
Optic Vesicle
Diencephalon
Midbrain
Hindbrain
Spinal Cord

8th week

Diencephalon
Midbrain
Forebrain
Hindbrain
Spinal Cord

BRAIN : 8th Week

By the end of the 8th week of embryonic development the CNS has 5 distinct regions :

Forebrain : develops into the cerebrum

Diencephalon : thalamus, hypothalamus, pituitary, & pineal glands

Midbrain : corpora quadrigemina (superior & inferior colliculi)

Hindbrain : pons, medulla, & cerebellum

Spinal Cord

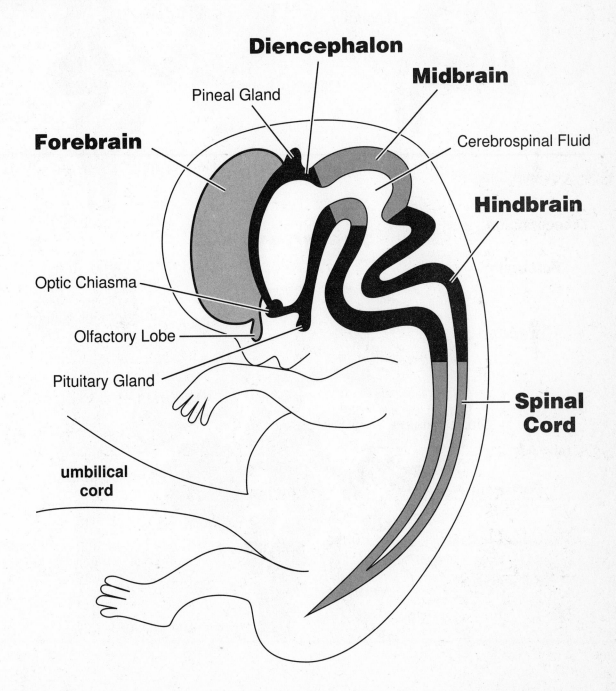

BRAIN : Fetal Development

2nd MONTH

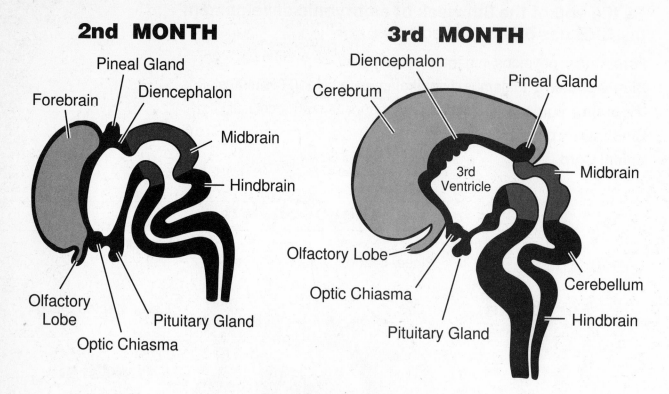

Forebrain
Pineal Gland
Diencephalon
Midbrain
Hindbrain
Olfactory Lobe
Optic Chiasma
Pituitary Gland

3rd MONTH

Diencephalon
Cerebrum
Pineal Gland
3rd Ventricle
Midbrain
Olfactory Lobe
Optic Chiasma
Cerebellum
Hindbrain
Pituitary Gland

7th MONTH

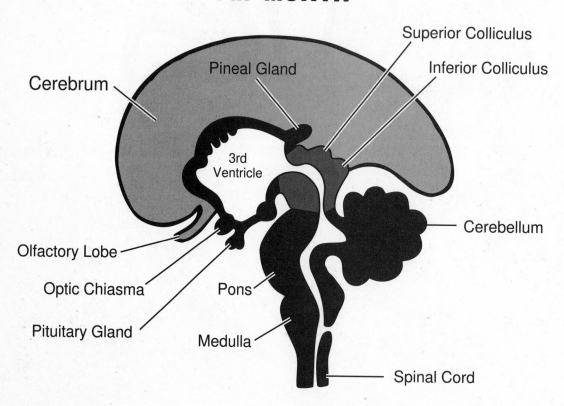

Cerebrum
Pineal Gland
Superior Colliculus
Inferior Colliculus
3rd Ventricle
Cerebellum
Olfactory Lobe
Optic Chiasma
Pons
Pituitary Gland
Medulla
Spinal Cord

58

MATURE BRAIN : the basic parts

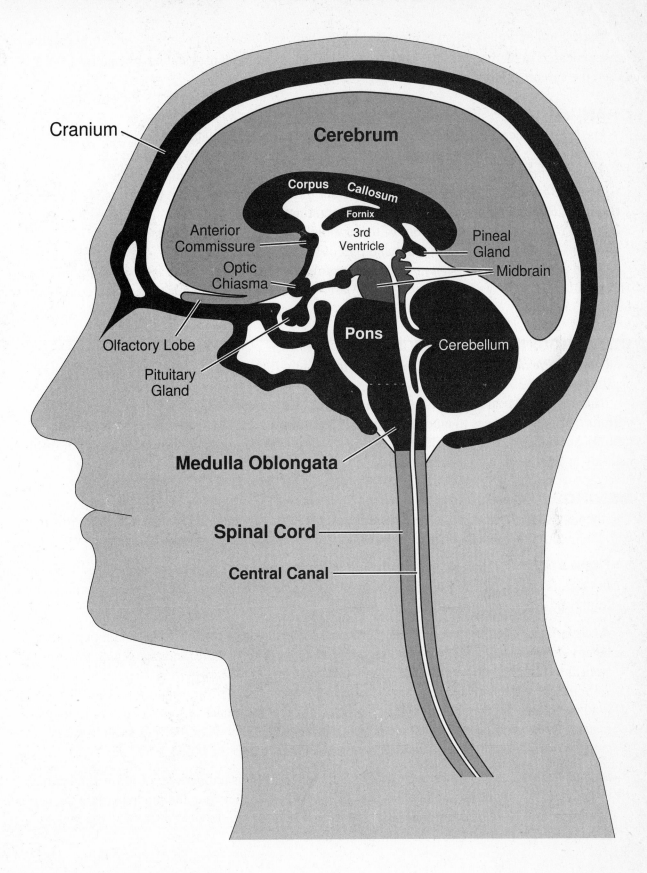

Cranium

Cerebrum

Corpus **Callosum**

Fornix

Anterior
Commissure

3rd
Ventricle

**Pineal
Gland**

Optic
Chiasma

Midbrain

Olfactory Lobe

Pons

Cerebellum

Pituitary
Gland

Medulla Oblongata

Spinal Cord

Central Canal

BRAIN / Protective Coverings

The central nervous system is protected by the bones of the cranium and the vertebral column. It is also encased in membranes of connective tissue called the meninges and cushioned by a fluid called the cerebrospinal fluid.

CRANIUM
The brain is encased in the cranium, which consists of 8 flat bones:

1 Frontal Bone : the anterior portion of the cranium in the region of the forehead.
1 Sphenoid Bone : the base of the cranium between the occipital and temporal bones.
1 Ethmoid Bone : the anterior portion of the floor of the cranium between the orbits.
1 Occipital Bone : the posterior portion of the cranium.
2 Parietal Bones : the sides and roof of the cranium.
2 Temporal Bones : the inferior sides and part of the floor of the cranium.

There are holes called *foramina* where the cranial nerves emerge, and a large opening in the base of the cranium called the *foramen magnum* ("large opening") through which the spinal cord emerges from the cranium.

CEREBROSPINAL FLUID (CSF)
Choroid Plexuses Cerebrospinal fluid is formed by filtration and secretion from networks of capillaries called choroid plexuses, which are located in the ventricles of the brain.

Blood-Brain Barrier The tissues of the choroid plexuses form the blood-brain barrier that permits certain substances to enter the fluid but prohibits others, thus protecting the brain from harmful substances. The fluid also serves as a shock-absorbing medium to protect the brain from banging against the inner walls of the cranium.

MENINGES (membranes)
The meninges are delicate, protective membranes that envelop the brain and spinal cord. Starting with the outermost layer, the meninges are named dura mater, arachnoid, and pia mater.

Dura Mater The dura mater is the tough, outer membrane next to the bony inner surface of the cranium. It is composed of dense connective tissue and is separated from the arachnoid by a thin, fluid-filled space called the *subdural space*.

Arachnoid The arachnoid is the membrane under the dura mater. It has 2 components: a layer next to the subdural space and a system of supporting fibers called *trabeculae* that form a web-like structure between the arachnoid and the pia mater. The cavities between the trabeculae form the *subarachnoid space*, which is filled with cerebrospinal fluid. In some areas the arachnoid perforates the dura mater, forming protrusions that terminate in venous sinuses in the dura mater. These protrusions, which are covered by endothelial cells of the venous sinuses, are called *arachnoid villi*. Their function is to reabsorb CSF into the blood.

Pia Mater The pia mater is the innermost membrane; it is a thin layer of loose connective tissue that is transparent and contains many blood vessels. Between the pia mater and the nerve tissue is a thin layer of neuroglial processes firmly attached to the pia mater. The pia mater follows all the irregularities of the surface of the CNS.

CRANIUM : bone plates covering the brain

Left Lateral View

S = SPHENOID BONE

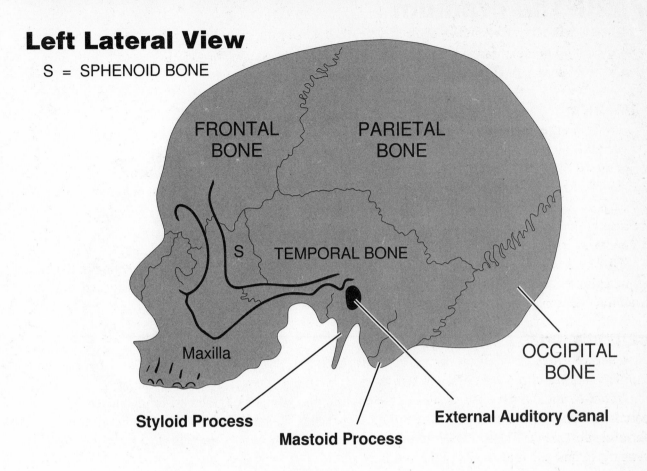

FRONTAL BONE

PARIETAL BONE

S   TEMPORAL BONE

Maxilla

OCCIPITAL BONE

Styloid Process

Mastoid Process

External Auditory Canal

Midsagittal section

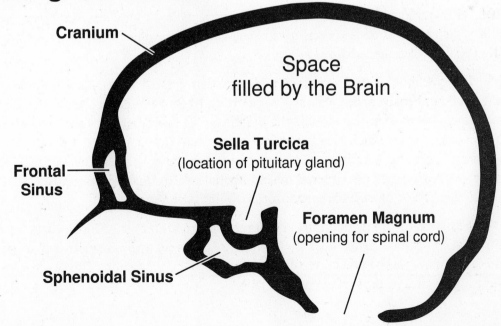

Cranium

Space
filled by the Brain

Sella Turcica
(location of pituitary gland)

**Frontal
Sinus**

Foramen Magnum
(opening for spinal cord)

Sphenoidal Sinus

BRAIN LOCATION
inside the cranium

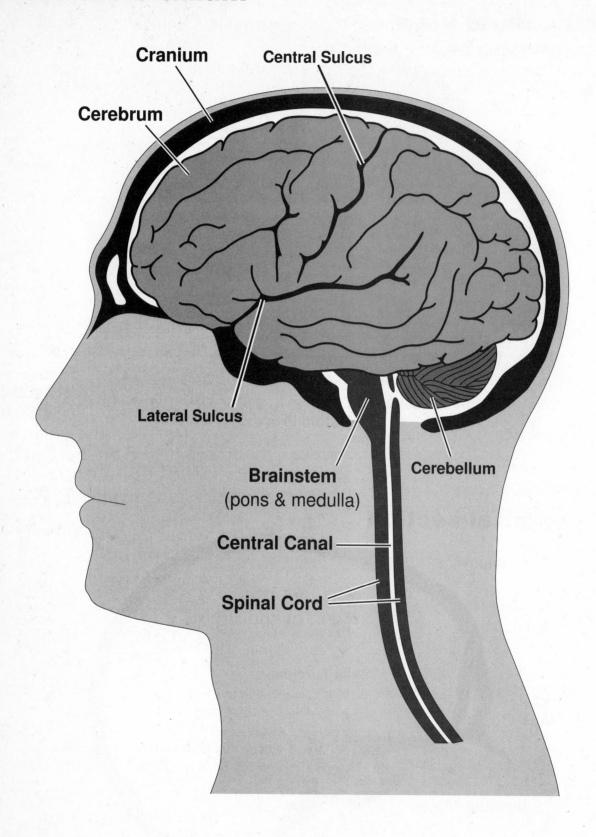

Cranium

Central Sulcus

Cerebrum

Lateral Sulcus

Brainstem
(pons & medulla)

Cerebellum

Central Canal

Spinal Cord

VENTRICLES IN THE BRAIN

There are 4 ventricles in the brain:
a lateral ventricle in each cerebral hemisphere (left & right lateral ventricles),
the 3rd ventricle in the diencephalon,
and the 4th ventricle between the pons & cerebellum.

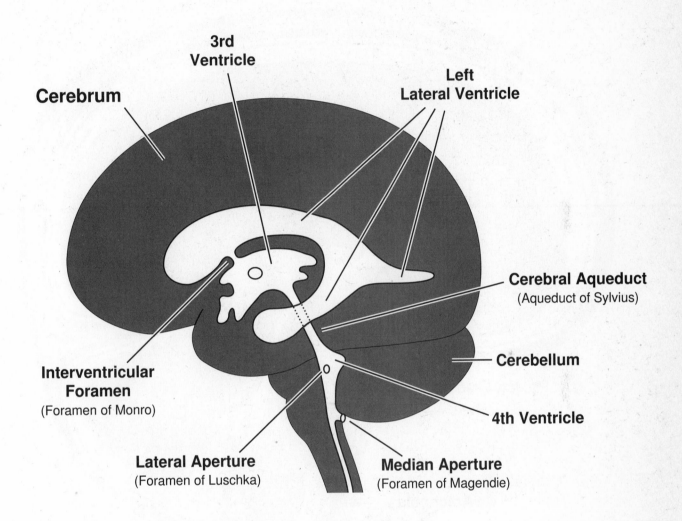

Choroid Plexuses

Networks of specialized capillaries are located
on the roof of each ventricle.
They produce cerebrospinal fluid (CSF)
and filter harmful materials (blood-brain barrier).

CEREBROSPINAL FLUID (CSF)

Cerebrospinal fluid is secreted by choroid plexuses.
It circulates through the brain and enters the superior sagittal sinus.

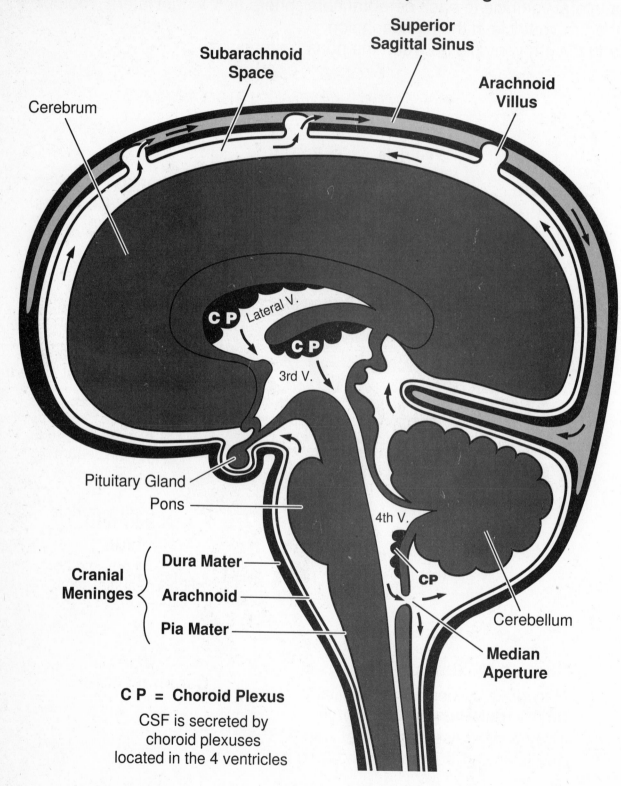

Superior
Sagittal Sinus

Subarachnoid
Space

Arachnoid
Villus

Cerebrum

C P   Lateral V.

C P

3rd V.

Pituitary Gland

Pons

Cranial
Meninges

Dura Mater

Arachnoid

Pia Mater

4th V.

CP

Cerebellum

Median
Aperture

C P = Choroid Plexus

CSF is secreted by
choroid plexuses
located in the 4 ventricles

MENINGES :
Dura Mater, Arachnoid, & Pia Mater

Frontal Section
through the brain

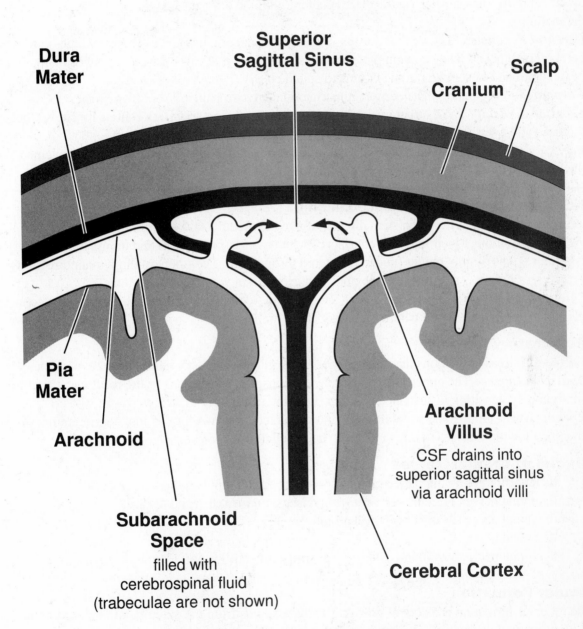

**Dura
Mater**

**Superior
Sagittal Sinus**

Scalp

Cranium

**Pia
Mater**

Arachnoid

**Arachnoid
Villus**

CSF drains into
superior sagittal sinus
via arachnoid villi

**Subarachnoid
Space**

filled with
cerebrospinal fluid
(trabeculae are not shown)

Cerebral Cortex

BRAIN / Midbrain & Pons

Brain Stem   The brain stem includes the midbrain, pons, & medulla oblongata.

MIDBRAIN (Mesencephalon)

The midbrain, or **mesencephalon** (*meso* = middle; *enkephalos* = brain), extends from the pons to the diencephalon; it is about the same length as the pons, 1 inch.

Structures found in the midbrain include :

Cerebral Aqueduct   (Aqueduct of Sylvius) The cerebral aqueduct passes through the midbrain, connecting the 3rd ventricle (in the diencephalon) with the 4th ventricle (between the pons and the cerebellum).

Cerebral Peduncles   The ventral portion of the midbrain contains a pair of fiber bundles called the cerebral peduncles. They contain motor and sensory fibers that carry impulses between upper parts of the brain and lower parts of the brain and spinal cord.

Corpora Quadrigemina   The corpora quadrigemina are two pairs of swellings on the roof.

Superior Colliculi   The 2 structures closest to the diencephalon are reflex centers for movements of the head and eyeballs in response to <u>visual</u> stimuli.

Inferior Colliculi   The 2 structures below the superior colliculi are reflex centers for movements of the head and trunk in response to <u>auditory</u> stimuli.

PONS (develops from the Metencephalon)

The pons is the section of the brain stem directly above the medulla and anterior to the cerebellum; like the medulla, it is about 1 inch long and consists of white matter (myelinated and unmyelinated nerve fibers) with regions of gray matter (nuclei) scattered throughout. The fibers run in 2 main directions:

Transverse Fibers : run between the pons and cerebellum via cerebellar peduncles.

Longitudinal Fibers : run up and down. They belong to the motor and sensory tracts that connect the spinal cord and medulla with upper parts of the brain.

Respiratory Centers

There are 2 areas in the pons that modify the discharge of respiratory neurons in the medulla.

Apneustic Center   The apneustic center causes the inspiratory neurons of the medulla to discharge continuously, resulting in sustained contraction of the inspiratory muscles.

Pneumotaxic Center   The pneumotaxic center produces intermittency of inspiratory neuron discharge, allowing muscles to relax and air to be expelled from the lungs by elastic recoil.

Nuclei of Cranial Nerves

The nuclei of the following paired cranial nerves are located in the pons :

    5th cranial nerve (Trigeminal) : chewing & sensations of the head & face.

    6th cranial nerve (Abducens) : eyeball movements.

    7th cranial nerve (Facial) : taste, salivation, & facial expression.

    8th cranial nerve (Vestibulocochlear) : hearing and equilibrium.

Reticular Formation

The reticular formation is a core of gray matter that extends from the medulla into the midbrain. It is made up of many thousands of small neurons arranged in complex, intertwining nets (*reticulum* = net). Located within it are nuclei and centers that regulate heart rate, blood pressure, respiration, and endocrine secretions.

RAS   The RAS (reticular activating system) is a complex polysynaptic pathway located in the reticular formation; activity in the RAS produces the conscious, alert state that makes perception possible.

BRAIN STEM : Midbrain, Pons, & Medulla

Midsagittal Section

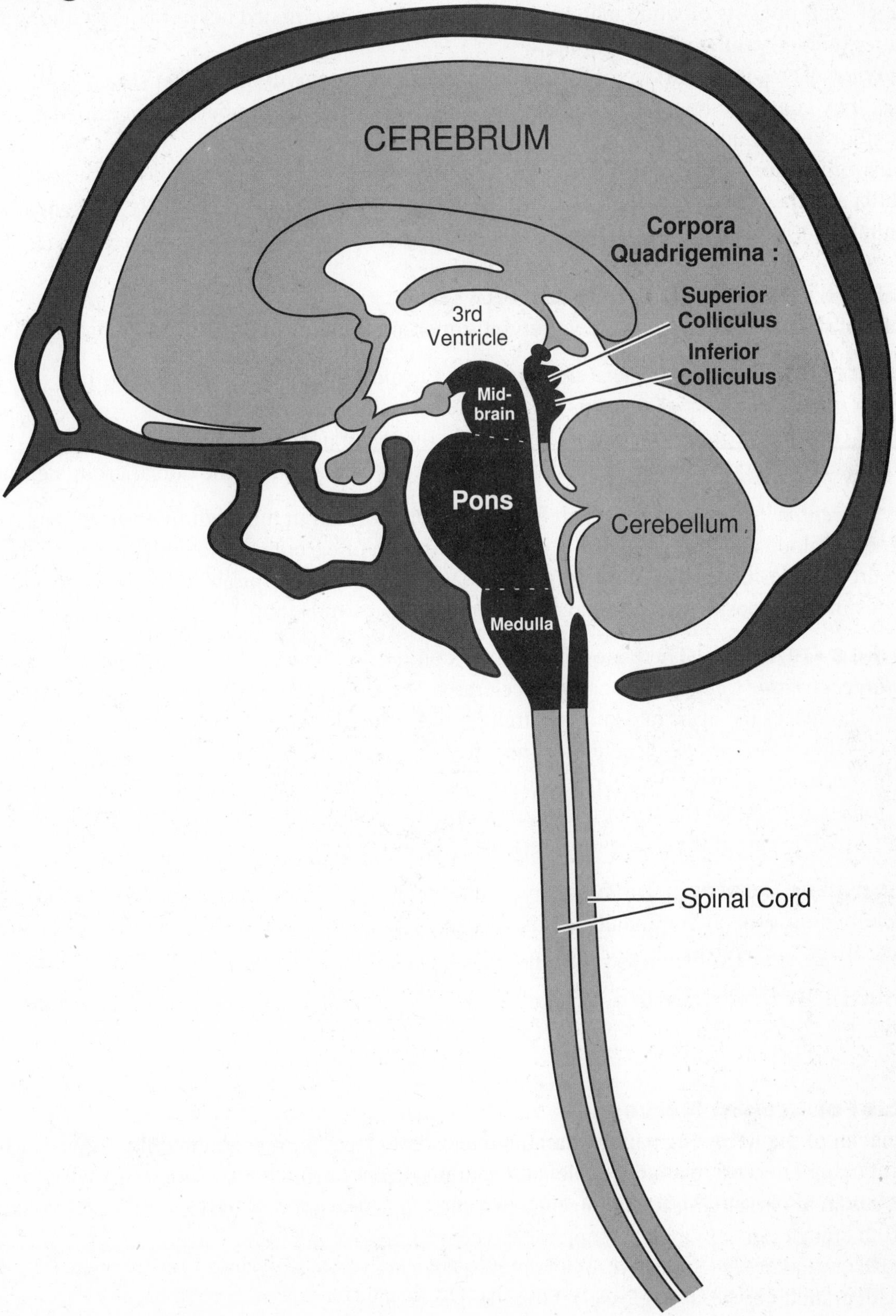

CEREBRUM

Corpora Quadrigemina :

Superior Colliculus

Inferior Colliculus

3rd Ventricle

Mid-brain

Pons

Cerebellum

Medulla

Spinal Cord

BRAIN / Medulla Oblongata

The medulla oblongata is a continuation of the spinal cord. It is located just above the large opening in the base of the cranium (the foramen magnum), and extends upward about an inch to meet the pons; it consists of white matter (myelinated and unmyelinated nerve fibers) with regions of gray matter (nuclei) scattered throughout.

Pyramids   The ventral surface of the medulla has 2 large, roughly triangular structures called the pyramids; they consist of bundles of descending nerve fibers carrying impulses that ultimately stimulate the skeletal muscles.

Decussation (crossing over of fibers)   Most of these fibers cross over just above the junction of the medulla and the spinal cord; thus, skeletal muscles on the right side of the body are controlled by nerve impulses originating in the left brain, and vice versa.

NUCLEI IN THE MEDULLA OBLONGATA

The nuclei of the medulla have a wide variety of important functions :

Respiratory Centers There are 2 groups of respiratory neurons in the medulla.
Dorsal Group :   a group of neurons responsible for automatic breathing.
Ventral Group :   a group of neurons that supply the respiratory muscles (intercostal and ipsilateral accessory); the discharge of these neurons is controlled by the dorsal group neurons.

Chemoreceptors   Chemoreceptors are groups of cells located in the medulla that are sensitive to changes in blood chemistry. A rise in the concentration of carbon dioxide or hydrogen ions or a large drop in the concentration of oxygen increases the level of respiratory center activity; changes in the opposite direction have a slight inhibitory effect.

Cardiac Centers   There are 2 centers for controlling the heart.
Cardioaccelerator Center   The cardioaccelerator center is a group of neurons that, when activated, increases the heart rate and the strength of contraction (the stroke volume); it sends impulses down the cardiac (accelerator) nerve; part of the sympathetic nervous system.
Cardioinhibitory Center   The cardioinhibitory center, when activated, slows down the heart rate (it has no effect on the stroke volume); it sends impulses to the pacemaker via the vagus nerve, which is part of the parasympathetic nervous system.

Vasomotor Center   The function of this center is to control the diameter of blood vessels, especially arterioles. It continually sends impulses via sympathetic nerves to the smooth circular muscle fibers in the walls of arterioles; it plays a major role in the regulation of blood pressure.

Nonvital Reflex Centers   There are also groups of neurons in the medulla that are responsible for coordinating nonvital reflexes such as swallowing, vomiting, coughing, sneezing, and hiccuping.

Nuclei of Cranial Nerves

The nuclei of the following paired cranial nerves are located in the medulla oblongata :
    8th cranial nerve (Vestibulocochlear) : hearing & equilibrium.
    9th cranial nerve (Glossopharyngeal) : swallowing, salivation, & taste.
    10th cranial nerve (Vagus) : supplies the heart, lungs, & digestive tract.
    11th cranial nerve (Spinal Accessory) : head & shoulder movements.
    12th cranial nerve (Hypoglossal) : tongue movements.

BRAIN STEM : Midbrain, Pons, & Medulla
(cranial nerves are numbered)

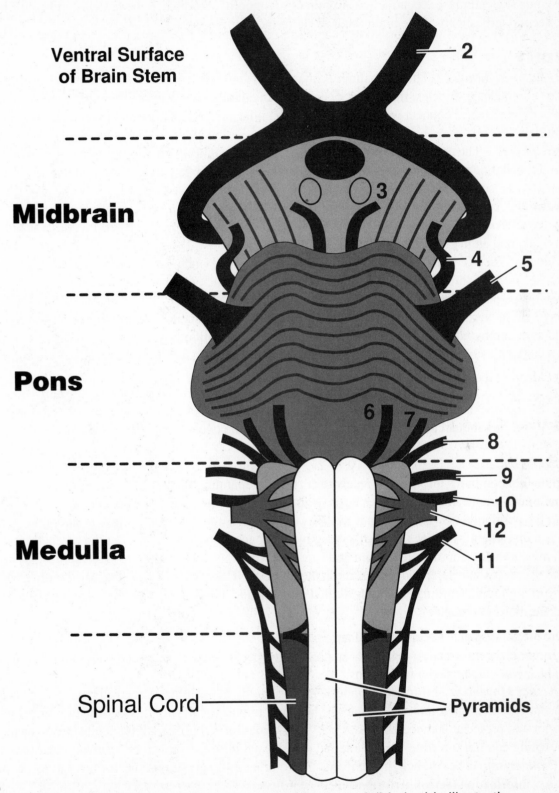

Ventral Surface of Brain Stem

2

Midbrain

3

4

5

Pons

6   7

8

9

10

12

11

Medulla

Spinal Cord

Pyramids

note : the 1st cranial nerves (olfactory nerves) are not visible in this illustration;
they emerge from olfactory bulbs that are located under the frontal lobes of the cerebrum.

BRAIN / Cerebellum

The cerebellum is located behind the pons and below the occipital lobes of the cerebrum. It controls subconscious skeletal muscle contractions required for smooth, coordinated movements and equilibrium. It is the second largest part of the brain (almost 1/8 of the brain's mass).

ANATOMY

Cerebellar Peduncles   The cerebellum is attached to the brainstem by 3 paired bundles of fibers called cerebellar peduncles: the superior cerebellar peduncles connect with the midbrain; the middle cerebellar peduncles connect with the pons; and the inferior cerebellar peduncles connect with the medulla.

Hemispheres   The cerebellum consists of 2 hemispheres connected by a region called the vermis. The cerebellar hemispheres and the vermis are more extensively folded and fissured than the cerebral hemispheres; so, for its size, the cerebellum has a very large surface area.

Cerebellar Cortex   The outer surface of the cerebellum is covered by a layer of gray matter called the cerebellar cortex; it has 3 layers: an external molecular layer, a Purkinje cell layer that is only one cell thick, and an internal granular layer.

Cerebellar Nuclei   Beneath the cerebellar cortex is the white matter with regions of gray matter (nuclei) scattered throughout. There are 4 deep cerebellar nuclei: the dentate, the globose, the emboliform, and the fastigial.

Vermis   The vermis is the region of the cerebellum that connects the 2 hemispheres. It has lobules, which are numbered from superior to inferior and each is identified by a name:
Lingula (L), Central (CL), Culmen (C), Declive (D), Folium (F), Tuber (T), Pyramis (P), Uvula (U), Nodulus (N).

Dura Mater   A section of the cranial dura mater called the *tentorium cerebelli* (tentorium = tent) extends over the cerebellum, separating it from the occipital lobes of the cerebrum. Another extension of the dura mater called the *falx cerebelli* separates the two cerebellar hemispheres.

FUNCTIONS

The cerebellum compares information received from two separate sources:
(1) From higher brain centers it receives information about what muscles *should* be doing.
(2) From the peripheral nervous system it receives information about what muscles *are* doing.
If there is a discrepancy between the two, corrective feedback signals are sent from the cerebellum via the thalamus to the cerebrum. New commands are sent from the cerebrum to the skeletal muscles involved to decrease the discrepancy and smooth the motion. The cerebellum is concerned with learning and performing rapid, coordinated, highly skilled movements; it also functions to maintain proper posture and equilibrium (balance).

There are four aspects to cerebellar function :

(1) Intentions   Information regarding planned movements is received from the motor cortex and basal ganglia via the nuclei in the pons.

(2) Actual Movement   Information about what is actually happening is received from proprioceptors (sensory receptors) in joints and muscles. The nerve impulses carrying this information travel in the anterior and posterior spinocerebellar tracts. The vestibulocerebellar tract transmits information concerning equilibrium from the the internal ear. Visual information is received from the eyes.

(3) Comparison   The cerebellum compares the command signals (intentions for movement) with the sensory information (actual performance).

(4) Corrective Feedback   The cerebellum sends out corrective signals to the nuclei in the brain stem and to the motor cortex via the thalamus.

CEREBELLUM

left lateral view

Corpus Callosum

Cerebellum

Optic Chiasma

Pituitary Gland

Pons

Medulla Oblongata

midsagittal section

Lobules of Vermis

L : lingula
CL : central
C : culmen
D : declive
F : folium

CL C D
L   F T
N U   P

T : tuber
P : pyramis
U : uvula
N : nodulus

dorsal view (section)

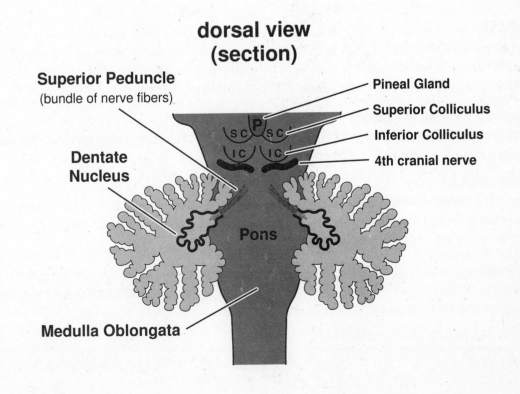

Superior Peduncle
(bundle of nerve fibers)

Pineal Gland

Superior Colliculus

Inferior Colliculus

4th cranial nerve

Dentate Nucleus

SC | P | SC
IC | IC

Pons

Medulla Oblongata

BRAIN / Thalamus

Diencephalon   The diencephalon is the region of the brain that develops between the forebrain (cerebral hemispheres) and the midbrain during the 5th week of embryonic development. The fluid-filled space inside the diencephalon becomes the 3rd ventricle.

The 2 main structures of the diencephalon are the *thalamus* and the *hypothalamus*. Nerve cells in the side walls of the diencephalon organize into nuclei that are collectively referred to as the thalamus; groups of nuclei that form below the thalamus are collectively referred to as the hypo-thalamus.

Thalamus   The thalamus consists of two oval masses of gray matter located above the mid-brain. Each mass is about 1 inch long and is organized into nuclei. The two masses form the side walls of the 3rd ventricle and are attached by a bridge of gray matter, the *intermediate mass*, that extends through the 3rd ventricle.

The thalamus can be divided into 3 regions : epithalamus, ventral thalamus, and dorsal thalamus. Each region is made up of nuclei with specific functions.
(1) Epithalamus   The epithalamus connects with the olfactory system (sense of smell).
(2) Ventral Thalamus   The functions of the ventral thalamus are unknown.
(3) Dorsal Thalamus   The functions of the dorsal thalamus include sensory relay, voluntary motor actions, arousal, language, recent memory, and emotion.

DORSAL THALAMUS
Nuclei of the dorsal thalamus are concerned with the following functions:

Sensory Relay
The thalamus is the principal relay station for sensory impulses on their way to the cerebral cortex. The dorsal thalamus contains nuclei for all sensations except smell.
Lateral Geniculate Nuclei : relay *visual* impulses to the visual cortex of the occipital lobes.
Medial Geniculate Nuclei : relay *auditory* impulses to the auditory cortex of the temporal lobe:
Ventral Posterior Nuclei : relay *general sensory* information from the skin and the muscles to the postcentral gyrus of the parietal lobes. These nuclei also relay taste sensations.

Voluntary Motor Actions
Ventral Lateral & Ventral Anterior Nuclei : receive input from the basal ganglia and the cerebellum and relay impulses to the motor cortex.

Arousal (RAS)
Midline & Intralaminar Nuclei : receive input from the RAS (reticular activating system). Impulses are relayed from this region of the thalamus to the cerebral cortex where they are responsible for the alerting and arousal effect of the RAS.

Language
Dorsolateral Nuclei : send impulses to the association areas of the cerebral cortex that are concerned with language.

Recent Memory & Emotion
Anterior Nuclei :   receive input from the mammillary bodies and relay impulses to parts of the limbic system that are concerned with recent memory and emotion.

DIENCEPHALON

Thalamus : develops from the side walls of the 3rd ventricle
Hypothalamus : develops from the floor of the 3rd ventricle

Location in the Mature Brain

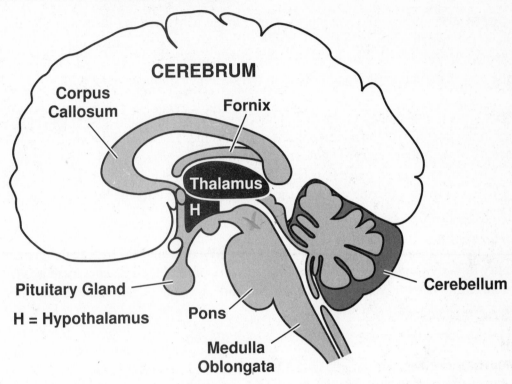

Location in the Embryonic Brain

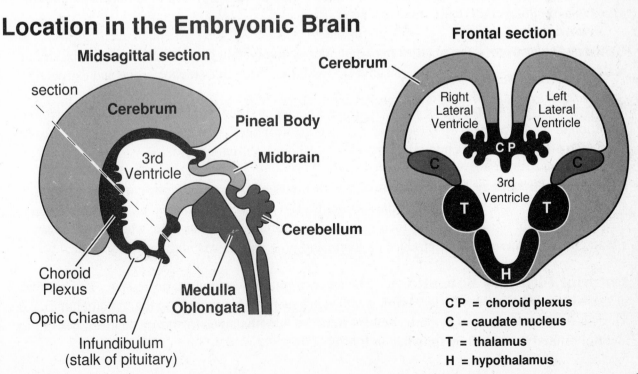

Midsagittal section

Frontal section

C P = choroid plexus

C = caudate nucleus

T = thalamus

H = hypothalamus

BRAIN / Hypothalamus

The hypothalamus is located in the diencephalon. It is the single most important region of the brain for regulating the internal environment—for maintaining homeostasis. It is also important for regulating basic drives such as eating, drinking, and sexual behavior.

Temperature   When cold receptors in the skin are activated, impulses travel to the posterior hypothalamus, which sends impulses to skeletal muscles that cause shivering; when heat receptors are activated, impulses travel to the anterior hypothalamus, which sends out impulses that cause sweating and vasodilation of blood vessels in the skin (heat radiates out).

Hunger   Food intake depends on the interaction of 2 hypothalamic areas: the hunger center (located in the lateral hypothalamus) and the satiety center (located in the ventromedial nucleus). The activity of the satiety center is governed by the level of glucose utilization of cells within that center. The cells are called *glucostats* because they monitor the level of glucose in the blood. When these cells are actively utilizing glucose, the satiety center inhibits the hunger center, and the individual has no appetite.

Thirst   *Osmoreceptors* are specialized cells located in the anterior hypothalamus that sense the osmolality of body fluids. When the osmotic pressure of the blood plasma increases (decreased water concentration), the osmoreceptors respond and stimulate nuclei in the lateral superior hypothalamus, which increases thirst.

Smell   The *mammillary bodies* are two rounded structures in the posterior portion of the hypothalamus that serve as relay stations in reflexes related to the sense of smell.

Fear & Rage Response   Emotions, especially fear and rage, stimulate lateral areas of the hypothalamus; the result is a general stress response that includes a rise in blood pressure, pupillary dilation, and piloerection (hairs stand on end).

Sexual Behavior   The anterior hypothalamus is involved in the control of sexual activity in males and females. These centers are activated by the sex hormones (testosterone and estrogen).

Endocrine Rhythms   The *suprachiasmatic nuclei* are involved in the control of the cyclic secretion of the hormone ACTH (adrenocorticotropic hormone). These nuclei receive input from the eyes and coordinate various body rhythms to the 24-hour light-dark cycle.

Posterior Pituitary Secretions   The hormones of the posterior pituitary gland are synthesized in neuron cell bodies located in the *supraoptic* and *paraventricular nuclei*, and transported down the axons of these neurons to their axon terminals in the posterior lobe, where they are secreted. Some of these neurons produce oxytocin and others produce antidiuretic hormone.

Anterior Pituitary Secretions   The anterior pituitary secretes 6 hormones. The secretion of these hormones is controlled by hormones that are secreted by neurons in the hypothalamus. These hormones are carried by portal vessels from the hypothalamus to endocrine gland cells in the anterior pituitary, which they stimulate or inhibit.

74

HYPOTHALAMUS : Principal Nuclei

Lateral View

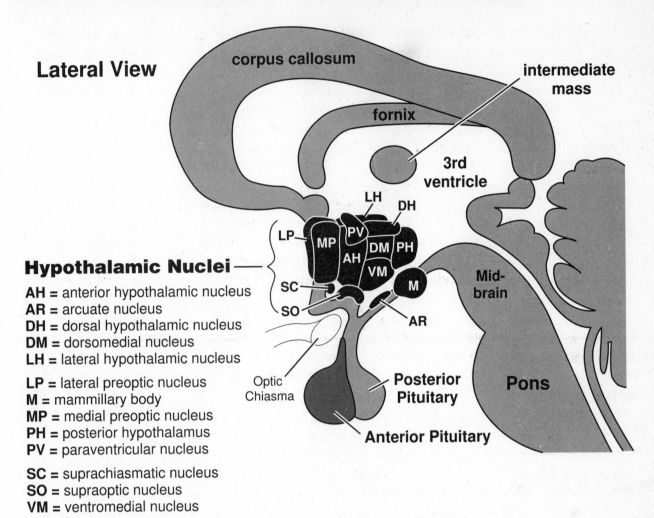

corpus callosum

intermediate mass

fornix

3rd ventricle

LH

DH

LP

MP

PV

DM

PH

AH

VM

SC

SO

M

AR

Mid-brain

Optic Chiasma

Posterior Pituitary

Pons

Anterior Pituitary

Hypothalamic Nuclei

AH = anterior hypothalamic nucleus
AR = arcuate nucleus
DH = dorsal hypothalamic nucleus
DM = dorsomedial nucleus
LH = lateral hypothalamic nucleus

LP = lateral preoptic nucleus
M = mammillary body
MP = medial preoptic nucleus
PH = posterior hypothalamus
PV = paraventricular nucleus

SC = suprachiasmatic nucleus
SO = supraoptic nucleus
VM = ventromedial nucleus

Frontal View

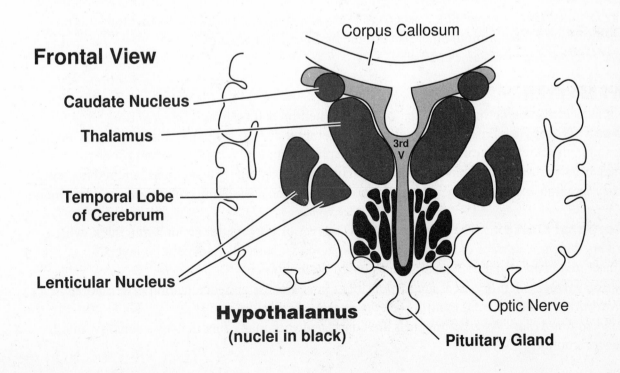

Corpus Callosum

Caudate Nucleus

Thalamus

Temporal Lobe of Cerebrum

3rd V

Lenticular Nucleus

Hypothalamus
(nuclei in black)

Optic Nerve

Pituitary Gland

BRAIN / Cerebral Hemispheres

Lateralization The cerebrum, the largest part of the brain, is made up of 2 deeply grooved hemispheres. Although the hemispheres appear to be bilaterally symmetrical, they have both structural and functional differences.

Left Hemisphere The left hemisphere is more important for right-hand control, spoken and written language, numerical and scientific skills, and reasoning.

Right Hemisphere The right hemisphere is more important for left-hand control, musical and artistic awareness, space and pattern perception, insight, and imagination.

Gyri & Sulci The surface of the cerebral hemispheres is covered by grooves (also called fissures or sulci) and ridges (also called gyri or convolutions). They serve as landmarks for locating specific regions of the cerebral cortex.

Lobes Each hemisphere is subdivided into 4 lobes, which are named for the cranial bones that cover them: *frontal, parietal, temporal,* and *occipital.* The lobes are more precisely defined by surface landmarks: the central sulcus separates the frontal lobe from the parietal lobe; the lateral sulcus separates the frontal lobe from the temporal lobe; and an imaginary line drawn from the parieto-occipital fissure to the pre-occipital notch separates the occipital lobes from the parietal and temporal lobes.

WHITE MATTER

White matter has a whitish appearance due to the fatty component of myelin. The myelinated nerve fibers (axons) that make up the white matter run in 3 principal directions:

Association Fibers Association fibers connect and transmit impulses between gyri in the same hemisphere.

Commissural Fibers Commissural fibers transmit impulses from the gyri in one cerebral hemisphere to the corresponding gyri in the opposite hemisphere. Three important commissural fibers are the *corpus callosum*, the *anterior commissure*, and the *posterior commissure*.

Projection Fibers Projection fibers form ascending and descending tracts that transmit impulses from the cerebrum to other parts of the brain and spinal cord.

The *internal capsule* is an example.

GRAY MATTER

Gray matter is made up primarily of densely packed neuron cell bodies.

Basal Ganglia Basal ganglia (also called cerebral nuclei) are paired masses of gray matter found in the cerebral hemispheres. Each hemisphere contains a caudate nucleus, lenticular nucleus (putamen and globus pallidus), substantia nigra, subthalamic nucleus, and red nucleus. They integrate semivoluntary, automatic movements such as walking, swimming, and laughing.

Cerebral Cortex The cerebral cortex is a layer of gray matter about 3 mm thick, which covers the entire surface of the cerebral hemispheres. It has 6 distinct cellular layers.

The cortex is divided into 3 general areas based on function:

Sensory Areas Sensory areas are responsible for awareness and localization of sensations.

Motor Areas Motor areas control skeletal muscle contractions.

Association Areas Association areas are concerned with many functions (personality, intelligence, emotions, etc.).

CEREBRUM
midsagittal section

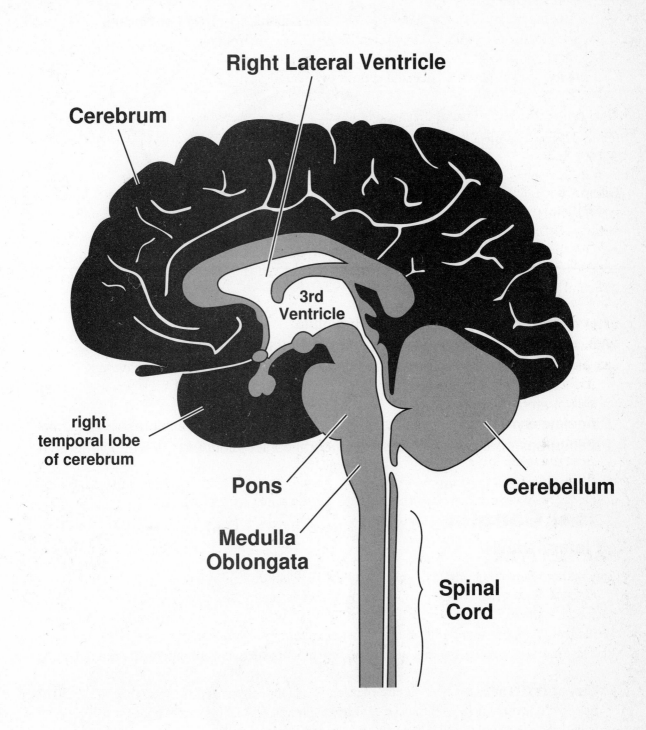

Right Lateral Ventricle

Cerebrum

3rd
Ventricle

right
temporal lobe
of cerebrum

Pons

Medulla
Oblongata

Cerebellum

Spinal
Cord

LIMBIC SYSTEM & BASAL GANGLIA

Limbic System
left lateral view

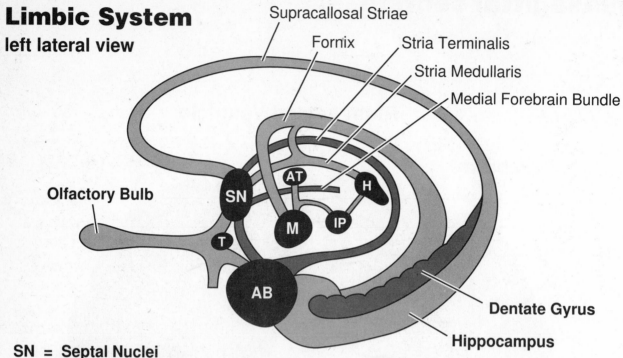

Supracallosal Striae

Fornix

Stria Terminalis

Stria Medullaris

Medial Forebrain Bundle

Olfactory Bulb

Dentate Gyrus

Hippocampus

SN = Septal Nuclei
T = Olfactory Tubercle
AB = Amygdaloid Body
M = Mammillary Body

H = Habenula
IP = Interpeduncular Nucleus
AT = Anterior Nucleus of Thalamus

not illustrated :
Cingulate Gyrus : region of the cerebral cortex superior to the supracallosal striae
Parahippocampal Gyrus : region of cerebral cortex inferior to the hippocampus

Basal Ganglia
left lateral view

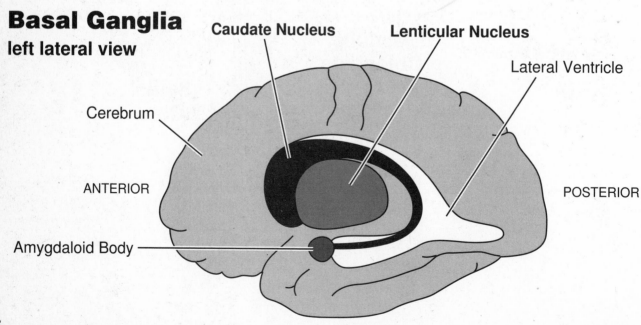

Caudate Nucleus

Lenticular Nucleus

Lateral Ventricle

Cerebrum

ANTERIOR

POSTERIOR

Amygdaloid Body

BRAIN : Horizontal Section

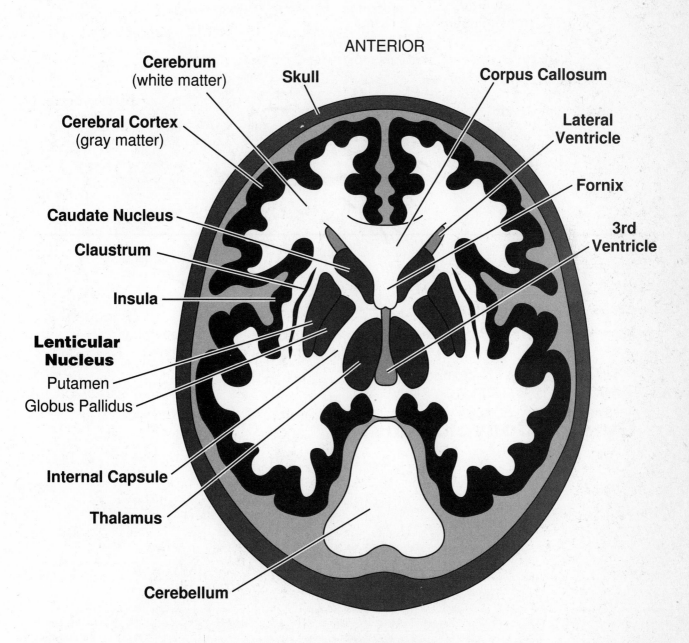

ANTERIOR

Cerebrum
(white matter)

Skull

Corpus Callosum

Cerebral Cortex
(gray matter)

Lateral
Ventricle

Caudate Nucleus

Fornix

Claustrum

3rd
Ventricle

Insula

**Lenticular
Nucleus**

Putamen

Globus Pallidus

Internal Capsule

Thalamus

Cerebellum

POSTERIOR

FISSURES AND GYRI (grooves & ridges)

Fissures (or Sulci)

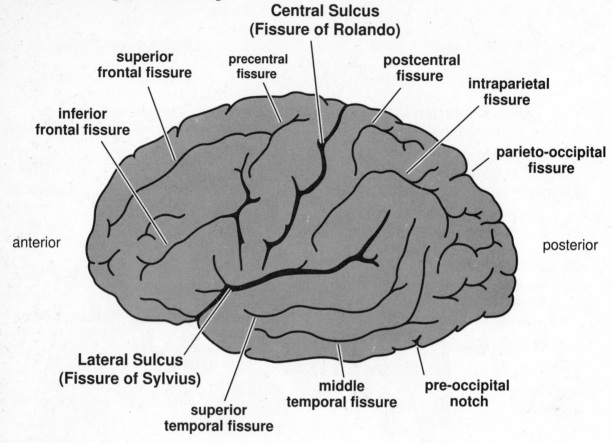

Central Sulcus
(Fissure of Rolando)

superior
frontal fissure

precentral
fissure

postcentral
fissure

intraparietal
fissure

inferior
frontal fissure

parieto-occipital
fissure

anterior

posterior

Lateral Sulcus
(Fissure of Sylvius)

middle
temporal fissure

pre-occipital
notch

superior
temporal fissure

Gyri (or Convolutions)

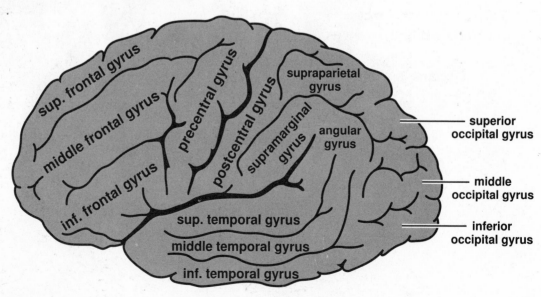

sup. frontal gyrus

middle frontal gyrus

precentral gyrus

postcentral gyrus

supraparietal
gyrus

supramarginal
gyrus

angular
gyrus

superior
occipital gyrus

inf. frontal gyrus

middle
occipital gyrus

sup. temporal gyrus

inferior
occipital gyrus

middle temporal gyrus

inf. temporal gyrus

CEREBRUM : 4 Lobes

Left Cerebral Hemisphere

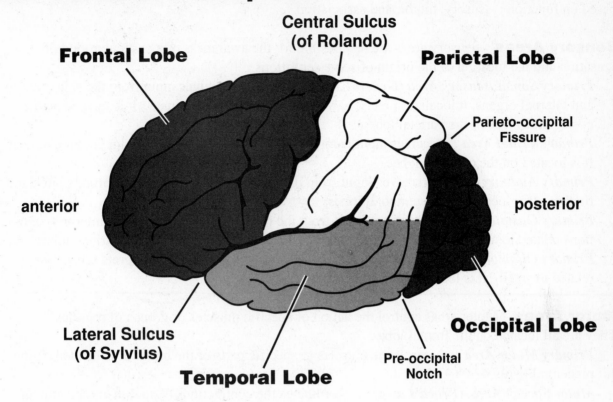

Central Sulcus (of Rolando)

Frontal Lobe

Parietal Lobe

Parieto-occipital Fissure

anterior

posterior

Lateral Sulcus (of Sylvius)

Occipital Lobe

Temporal Lobe

Pre-occipital Notch

View From Above

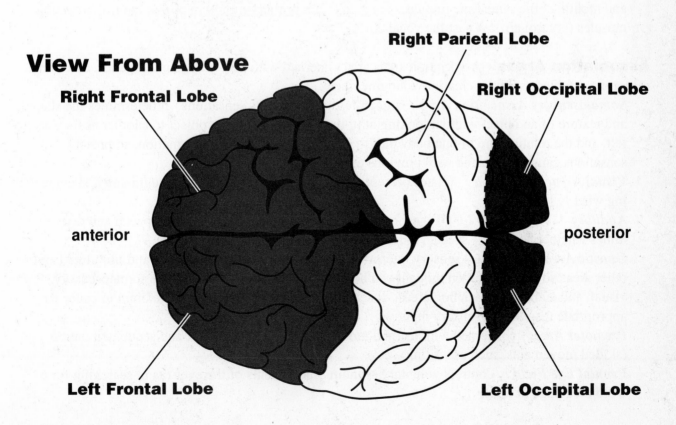

Right Parietal Lobe

Right Frontal Lobe

Right Occipital Lobe

anterior

posterior

Left Frontal Lobe

Left Occipital Lobe

BRAIN / Cerebral Cortex

The functions of the cerebral cortex are numerous and complex. It is divided into 3 main areas, based on function : sensory, motor, and association.

Sensory Areas   Sensory areas are responsible for the awareness of a particular kind of sensation and the location of the origin of some sensations.
   Primary Somatosensory Area (General Sensory Area) :   receives input from the skin, muscles, and internal organs; it localizes precisely where the sensations originate. It is located on the postcentral gyrus of the parietal lobes.
   Primary Visual Area :   receives input from the eyes; it interprets shape, color, and movement. It is located on the occipital lobes.
   Primary Auditory Area :   receives input from the internal ear (cochlea); it interprets pitch and rhythm. It is located on the temporal lobes.
   Primary Gustatory Area :   receives input from the taste buds of the tongue; it interprets sensations related to taste. It is located at the base of the postcentral gyrus on the parietal lobes.
   Primary Olfactory Area :   receives input from the olfactory bulbs; it interprets sensations related to smell. It is located on the temporal lobes.

Motor Areas   Motor areas control the action of specific muscles or groups of muscles. They are all located on the frontal lobes.
   Primary Motor Area :   controls the muscles in specific parts of the body. It is located on the precentral gyrus.
   Motor Speech Area (Broca's area) :   coordinates the contractions of speech and breathing muscles. Impulses are sent to the <u>premotor</u> areas that control muscles of the pharynx, larynx, and mouth; at the same time impulses are sent to the <u>primary motor</u> areas that control breathing muscles (control airflow past the vocal cords).

Association Areas   Association areas are concerned with personality, intelligence, emotions, reasoning, problem-solving, creativity, judgment, etc.
   Somatosensory Association Area :   integrates and interprets sensations. It determines the shape and texture of an object without looking at it, the orientation of one object to another as they are felt, and the relationship of one body part to another. It also stores information, so present sensations can be compared with previous experiences.
   Visual Association Area :   relates present to past visual experiences by recognizing and evaluating what is seen.
   Auditory Association Area (Wernicke's area) :   interprets the meaning of speech and determines whether a sound is speech, music, or noise.
   Gnostic Area :   integrates sensory interpretations from the association areas and impulses from other areas so that a common thought can be formed. It is located among the somatosensory, visual, and auditory association areas. It sends impulses to other parts of the brain to cause the appropriate response to sensory input.
   Premotor Area: concerned with learned motor activities of a complex and sequential nature (skilled movements, such as writing).
   Frontal Eye Field :   controls voluntary scanning movements of the eyes (as in searching for a word on a page of text).

CEREBRAL CORTEX
Sensory, Motor, & Association Areas

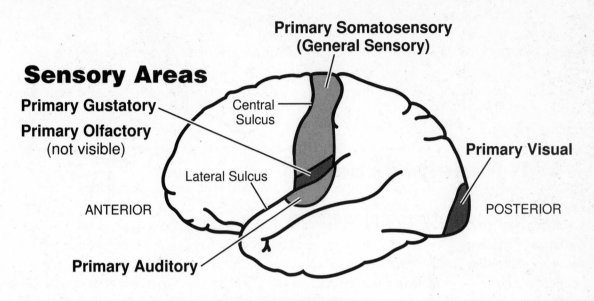

Sensory Areas

Primary Somatosensory
(General Sensory)

Primary Gustatory

Primary Olfactory
(not visible)

Central
Sulcus

Primary Visual

Lateral Sulcus

ANTERIOR

POSTERIOR

Primary Auditory

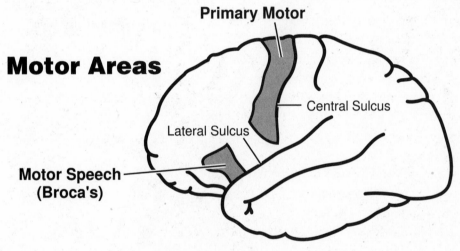

Motor Areas

Primary Motor

Central Sulcus

Lateral Sulcus

Motor Speech
(Broca's)

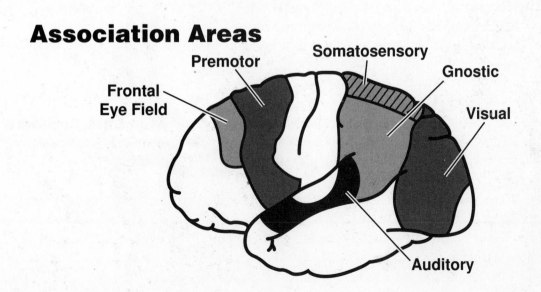

Association Areas

Premotor

Somatosensory

Gnostic

Frontal
Eye Field

Visual

Auditory

SENSORY CORTEX

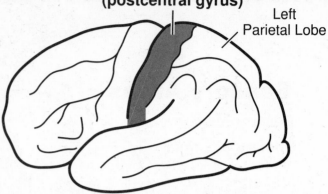

Primary Somatosensory Area
or General Sensory Area
(postcentral gyrus)

Left
Parietal Lobe

Left Parietal Lobe
frontal section
through primary somatosensory area

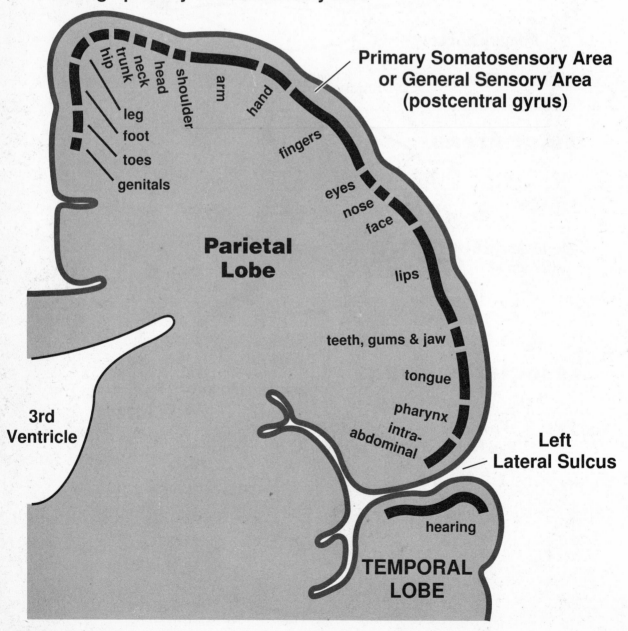

Primary Somatosensory Area
or General Sensory Area
(postcentral gyrus)

hip
trunk
neck
head
shoulder
arm
hand

leg
foot
toes
genitals

fingers

eyes
nose
face

lips

teeth, gums & jaw

tongue

pharynx
intra-
abdominal

**Parietal
Lobe**

**3rd
Ventricle**

**Left
Lateral Sulcus**

hearing

**TEMPORAL
LOBE**

MOTOR CORTEX

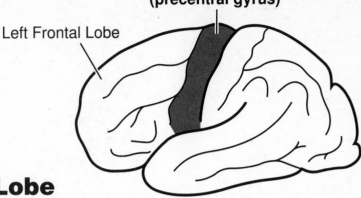

Left Frontal Lobe

Primary Motor Area
(precentral gyrus)

Left Frontal Lobe
frontal section
through primary motor area

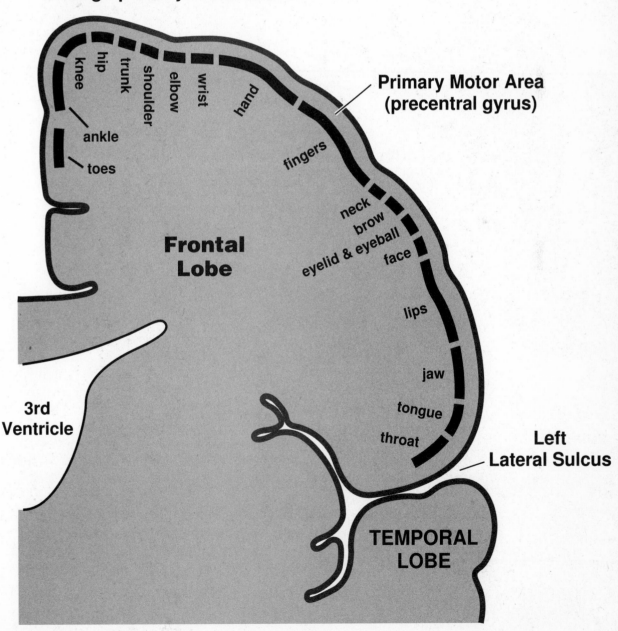

Primary Motor Area
(precentral gyrus)

knee
hip
trunk
shoulder
elbow
wrist
hand
ankle
toes
fingers

neck
brow
eyelid & eyeball
face

**Frontal
Lobe**

lips

jaw

tongue

throat

**3rd
Ventricle**

**Left
Lateral Sulcus**

**TEMPORAL
LOBE**

The Spinal Cord

Protective Coverings *88*
1. Meninges
2. Cerebrospinal Fluid
3. Epidural Space
4. Vertebral Column

Anatomy *92*
1. Cross Section :
   2 halves
   gray matter (anterior, lateral, & posterior gray horns)
   white matter (anterior, lateral, & posterior white columns)
2. Longitudinal Section :
   length
   dural sac
   cervical & lumbar enlargements
   conus medullaris
   filum terminale
   cauda equina
   central & denticulate ligaments

Columns, Tracts, & Pathways *94*
1. Definitions : column, tract, & pathway
2. Major Tracts (arranged by pathways)
   Sensory (Ascending) Pathways
   Motor (Descending) Pathways

Spinal Reflexes *98*
1. Definitions
   reflex
   visceral & somatic reflexes
   types of somatic reflexes
   reciprocal innervation
2. Examples of Somatic Spinal Reflexes
   stretch reflex (contraction)
   tendon reflex (relaxation)
   flexor reflex (withdrawal, flexion)
   crossed extensor reflex (synchronized extension & flexion)

SPINAL CORD / Protective Coverings

The spinal cord is a continuation of the brain stem; it extends from the large opening (foramen magnum) in the base of the cranium down to the upper region of the lower back (the 1st lumbar vertebra). It is a cylindrically shaped structure about 17 inches long and about 1 inch in diameter. The soft nervous tissue of the spinal cord is surrounded and protected by 3 layers of membrane (the meninges), the cerebrospinal fluid, a layer of fatty tissue (in the epidural space), and the vertebrae.

MENINGES (membranes)

The meninges (singlular : *meninx*) are three membranes that envelop the spinal cord and brain.

Pia Mater   The inner membrane. It is separated from the surface of the spinal cord by a thin layer of neuroglial processes; it contains many blood vessels.

Arachnoid   The middle membrane. It has 2 components: an outer layer next to the dura mater and a network of fibrous extensions called trabeculae, which connect with the pia mater.

> *Subarachnoid Space*   A fluid-filled space between the arachnoid and the pia mater.
> *Spinal Nerve Roots*   The roots of the spinal nerves are located in the subarachnoid space.
>> *Anterior Root (Ventral Root)*
>> The anterior root contains motor (efferent) fibers that carry impulses <u>out</u> of the CNS.
>> *Posterior Root (Dorsal Root)*
>> The posterior root contains sensory (afferent) fibers that carry impulses <u>into</u> the CNS. The posterior root contains cell bodies of sensory neurons in the *posterior root ganglion*.

Dura Mater   The outer membrane. It extends from the foramen magnum, where it adheres to the cranium, to the the 2nd sacral vertebra, where it fuses with the filum terminale.

CEREBROSPINAL FLUID

The subarachnoid space is continuous with the ventricles of the brain and is filled with cerebrospinal fluid (CSF). The CSF is produced by special capillary beds called *choroid plexuses* located in the ventricles. It circulates through the subarachnoid space around the brain and spinal cord and through the ventricles of the brain; it is an excellent shock absorber for the delicate nerve tissues.

EPIDURAL SPACE

The epidural space (*epi* = outside) is the region outside the dura mater between the dura mater and the bony walls of the vertebrae; it is filled with fat tissue which cushions the cord.

VERTEBRAL COLUMN
Regions

The vertebral column (also called spinal column) consists of 33 vertebrae, but since the 5 sacral vertebrae are fused and the 4 coccygeal vertebrae are fused, it consists of just 26 separate bones. The vertebrae are named according to the region of the back where they are located; in each region the vertebrae are numbered from top to bottom.

7 cervical vertebrae (L. *cervix* = neck) : located in the neck.

12 thoracic vertebrae (G. *thorax* = chest) : located in the chest.

5 lumbar vertebrae (L. *lumbus* = loin) : located in the lower back.

5 sacral vertebrae (L. *os sacrum* = sacred bone) : fused to form the sacrum.

4 coccygeal vertebrae (L. *coccyx* = shaped like the cuckoo's beak) : fused to form the tailbone.

Curvatures

The vertebral column has 3 main curvatures :

thoracic curvature : present at birth (fetal position).

cervical curvature : develops in infancy from the elevation of the head.

lumbar curvature : develops when the child stands erect to walk.

MENINGES & EPIDURAL SPACE

Spinal Cord
cross section inside a vertebra

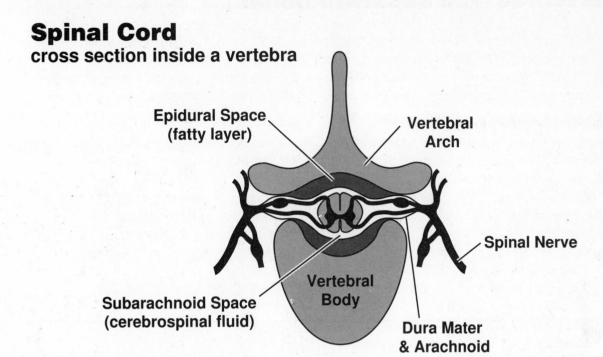

Epidural Space (fatty layer)

Vertebral Arch

Spinal Nerve

Subarachnoid Space (cerebrospinal fluid)

Vertebral Body

Dura Mater & Arachnoid

Spinal Cord
cross section showing meninges

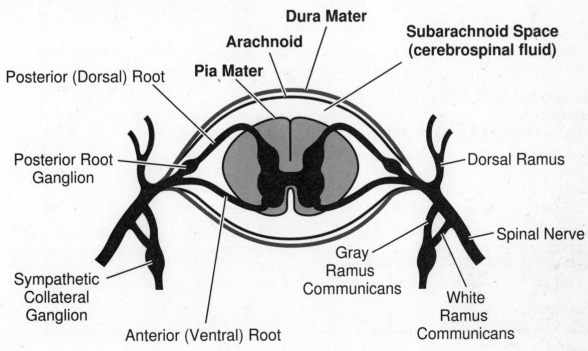

Dura Mater

Arachnoid

Subarachnoid Space (cerebrospinal fluid)

Pia Mater

Posterior (Dorsal) Root

Posterior Root Ganglion

Dorsal Ramus

Spinal Nerve

Gray Ramus Communicans

Sympathetic Collateral Ganglion

Anterior (Ventral) Root

White Ramus Communicans

VERTEBRAL COLUMN
33 vertebrae (26 separate bones)

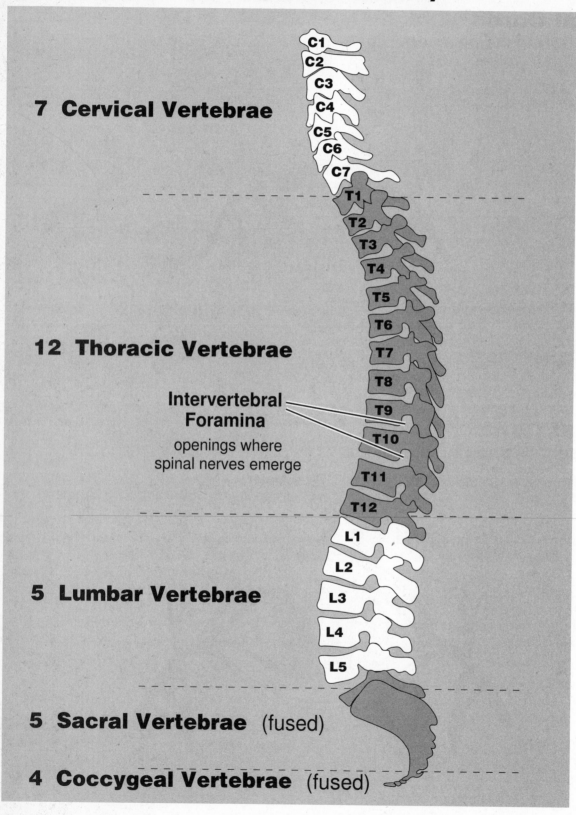

7 Cervical Vertebrae

C1
C2
C3
C4
C5
C6
C7

12 Thoracic Vertebrae

T1
T2
T3
T4
T5
T6
T7
T8
T9
T10
T11
T12

Intervertebral Foramina

openings where
spinal nerves emerge

5 Lumbar Vertebrae

L1
L2
L3
L4
L5

5 Sacral Vertebrae (fused)

4 Coccygeal Vertebrae (fused)

SPINAL CORD DIVISIONS

There are 31 pairs of spinal nerves.
They are named and numbered according to where they emerge
from the vertebral column.

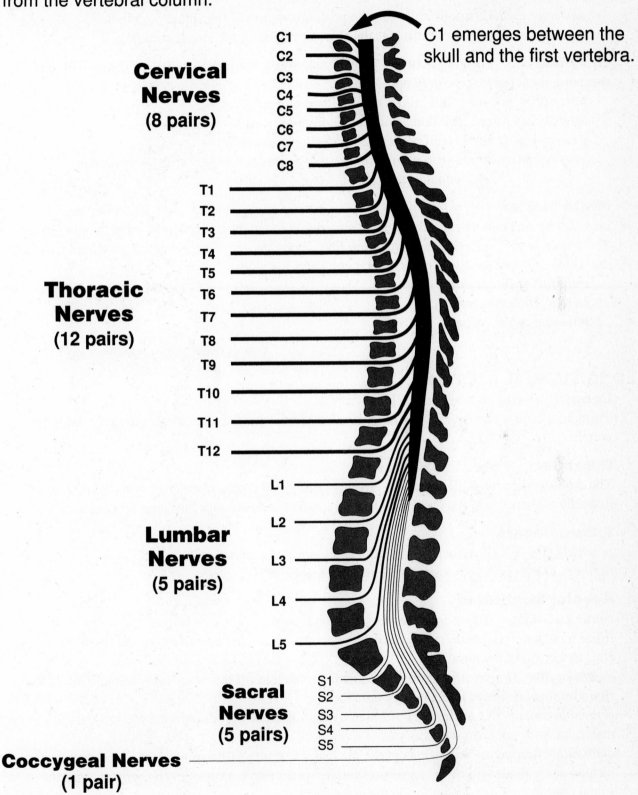

C1 emerges between the
skull and the first vertebra.

Cervical Nerves (8 pairs)

C1
C2
C3
C4
C5
C6
C7
C8

Thoracic Nerves (12 pairs)

T1
T2
T3
T4
T5
T6
T7
T8
T9
T10
T11
T12

Lumbar Nerves (5 pairs)

L1
L2
L3
L4
L5

Sacral Nerves (5 pairs)

S1
S2
S3
S4
S5

Coccygeal Nerves (1 pair)

SPINAL CORD / Anatomy

CROSS SECTION
2 Halves
posterior median sulcus : divides the posterior region of the spinal cord in half.
anterior median fissure : divides the anterior region of the spinal cord in half.

Gray Matter
The gray matter is butterfly-shaped and consists mostly of neuron cell bodies; the dense nuclei give it the gray appearance.
anterior gray horn : cell bodies of somatic motor neurons.
lateral gray horn : cell bodies of preganglionic sympathetic neurons.
posterior gray horn : cell bodies of association neurons.
gray commissure : a strip of gray matter that connects the two lateral gray masses;
contains the *central canal.*

White Matter
The white matter consists mostly of myelinated nerve fibers that carry impulses up and down the cord; the fatty material in the myelin gives it the whitish appearance. The posterior gray horns and an imaginary line extending out from the lateral gray horns divide the white matter in each half of the spinal cord into 3 regions :
anterior white column;
lateral white column;
posterior white column.

LONGITUDINAL SECTION
Length   (Foramen Magnum to L1)
The spinal cord is about 17 inches long; it extends from the foramen magnum to the 1st lumbar vertebra.

Dural Sac   (Foramen Magnum to S2)
The dural sac is a fluid-filled sac that envelops the spinal cord and extends from the foramen magnum to the level of the 2nd sacral vertebra, where it fuses with the filum terminale.

Enlargements
cervical (C3 to T2) associated with the emergence of arm nerves.
lumbar (T9 to T12) associated with the emergence of leg nerves.

Special Structures
conus medullaris (L1) tapered end of the spinal cord.
filum terminale (L1 to S2) thread of non-nervous tissue that extends from the tip of the spinal cord to the end of the dural sac.
cauda equina (horsetail) lumbar and sacral nerves that fill the dural sac on either side of the filum terminale; shaped like a horse's tail.
central ligament (S2 to Coccyx) formed by the fusion of the filum terminale and the dura mater; anchors spinal cord to coccyx.
denticulate ligaments extensions of the pia mater that attach the spinal cord to the dura mater; located along the length of the cord between the spinal nerve roots of each segment; hold the spinal cord in a fixed position inside the dural sac.

SPINAL CORD ANATOMY

Cross Section

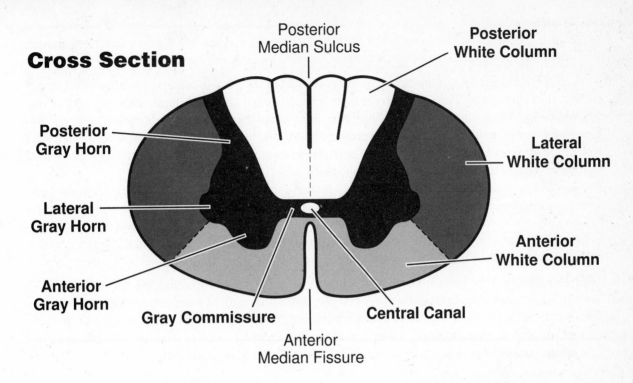

Posterior
Median Sulcus

Posterior
White Column

Posterior
Gray Horn

Lateral
White Column

Lateral
Gray Horn

Anterior
Gray Horn

Anterior
White Column

Gray Commissure

Central Canal

Anterior
Median Fissure

Longitudinal Section

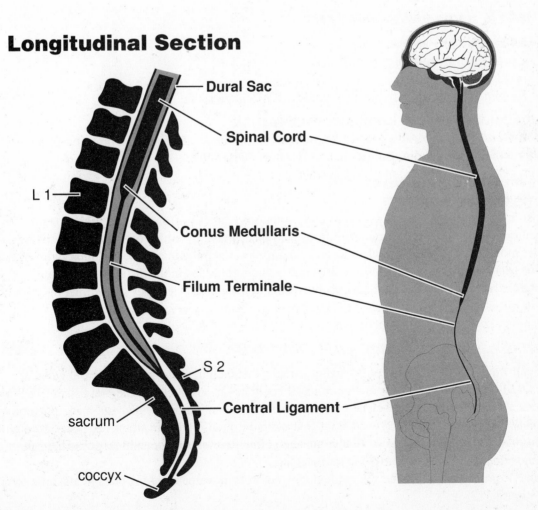

Dural Sac

Spinal Cord

L 1

Conus Medullaris

Filum Terminale

S 2

Central Ligament

sacrum

coccyx

SPINAL CORD / Columns, Tracts, & Pathways

DEFINITIONS

White Column   The white matter in each half of the spinal cord is divided into 3 areas: anterior column, lateral column, and posterior column. Each column contains a number of spinal cord tracts.

Tract   A tract is a bundle of myelinated nerve fibers located in the CNS (brain and spinal cord). Sensory (ascending) tracts consist of fibers that carry impulses up the spinal cord to different regions of the brain; motor (descending) tracts consist of nerve fibers that carry impulses down the spinal cord.

   Crossing Over   The fibers of most tracts cross over. As a result, sensory nerve impulses from the left side of the body end in the right side of the brain, and motor nerve impulses originating in the right side of the brain control muscles in the left side of the body, and vice versa.

   Decussation of Pyramids   Decussation usually refers to the crossing of most of the fibers in the large motor tracts to opposite sides of the pyramids (just above the junction of the medulla and spinal cord).

   Naming Tracts   A tract is usually named by its origin, termination, and the white column in which it is located. For example, the fibers of the **anterior spinothalamic tract** are located in the anterior white column; the fibers start somewhere in the spinal cord and end in the thalamus.

Pathway   A pathway is the route followed by a nerve impulse as it travels through the nervous system. In a sensory pathway an impulse starts at a sensory receptor, travels by way of a sensory neuron into the spinal cord, travels up the spinal cord by way of a sensory (ascending) tract, and ends in the brain. In a motor pathway an impulse starts in the brain, travels down the spinal cord by way of a motor (descending) tract, exits the spinal cord by way of a motor neuron, and ends at a muscle or gland cell.

MAJOR TRACTS   (arranged by pathways)

Sensory (Ascending) Pathways
Anterolateral (Spinothalamic) Pathways
Lateral Spinothalamic Tract : pain & temperature.
Anterior Spinothalamic Tract : tickle, itch, crude touch, and pressure.

Posterior Column – Medial Lemniscus Pathway
Fasciculus Gracilis & Fasciculus Cuneatus : discriminative touch, stereognosis, proprioception, kinesthesia, weight discrimination, and vibratory sensations.

Motor (Descending) Pathways
Direct (Pyramidal) Pathways
The upper motor neurons of direct pathways carry impulses "directly" from the cerebral cortex to lower motor neurons; fibers of the upper motor neurons pass through the pyramids of the medulla oblongata. The lower motor neurons carry impulses to skeletal muscles, resulting in precise, voluntary movements.
Lateral Corticospinal Tract : controls precise contraction of muscles in the distal extremities.
Anterior Corticospinal Tract : coordinates movements of the axial skeleton by controlling the contraction of muscles in the neck and shoulders.
Corticobulbar Tract : controls voluntary movements of the head & neck.

Indirect (Extrapyramidal) Pathways
Indirect pathways follow complex, polysynaptic circuits that include synapses in the basal ganglia, thalamus, and cerebellum. Upper motor neurons all begin in various nuclei of the brain stem. The lower motor neurons carry impulses to skeletal muscles, resulting in semivoluntary and automatic movements.
Rubrospinal Tract (starts in the red nucleus) : controls precise, discrete movements of distal extremities.
Vestibulospinal Tract (starts in the vestibular nucleus) : regulates muscle tone in response to head movements; plays a major role in balance.
Tectospinal Tract (starts in the superior colliculus) : controls movements of the head in response to visual stimuli.

SPINAL CORD TRACTS

Sensory Tracts
sensory information carried
to the brain

Vibration
Kinesthesia
Stereognosis
Proprioception
Discriminative Touch
Weight Discrimination
Fasciculus Gracilis
Fasciculus Cuneatus

**Pain &
Temperature**
Lateral
Spinothalamic

**Crude Touch & Pressure
Tickle & Itch**
Anterior Spinothalamic

Motor Tracts
instructions from the brain
carried to muscles

Precise Movements
(in distal extremities)
Lateral Corticospinal

Precise Movements
(in distal extremities)
Rubrospinal

Balance
Vestibulospinal

Head Movements
(in response to
visual stimuli)
Tectospinal

Neck & Shoulder Muscles
(coordinates movements
of the axial skeleton)
Anterior Corticospinal

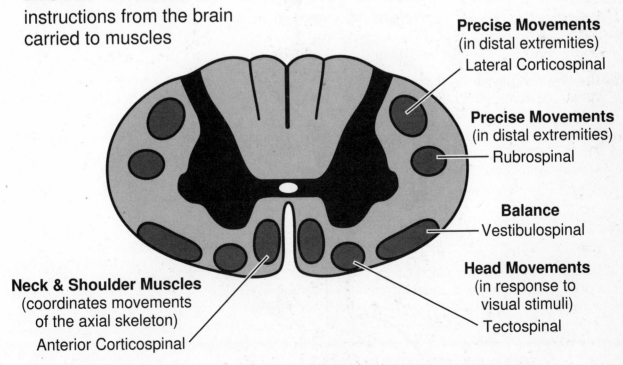

Note : The Corticobulbar Tract is not illustrated; it exits from the brain stem.

SENSORY PATHWAYS

pain & temperature

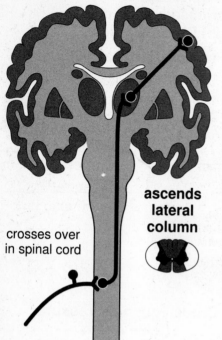

crosses over
in spinal cord

ascends
lateral
column

touch & pressure
tickle & itch

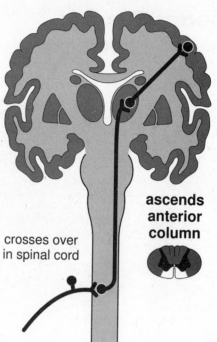

crosses over
in spinal cord

ascends
anterior
column

vibration
kinesthesia
stereognosis
proprioception
discriminative touch
weight discrimination

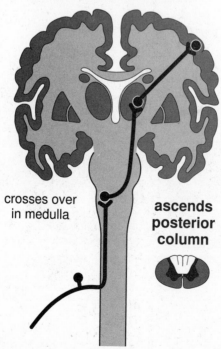

crosses over
in medulla

ascends
posterior
column

MOTOR PATHWAYS

Direct (Pyramidal) Pathways :
Voluntary Control of Skeletal Muscles

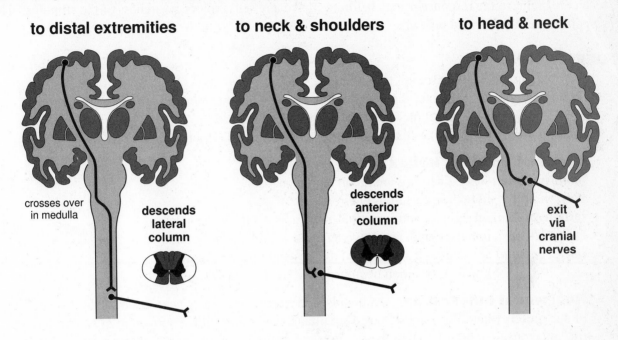

to distal extremities

crosses over
in medulla

descends
lateral
column

to neck & shoulders

descends
anterior
column

to head & neck

exit
via
cranial
nerves

Indirect (Extrapyramidal) Pathways :
Subconscious Control of Skeletal Muscles

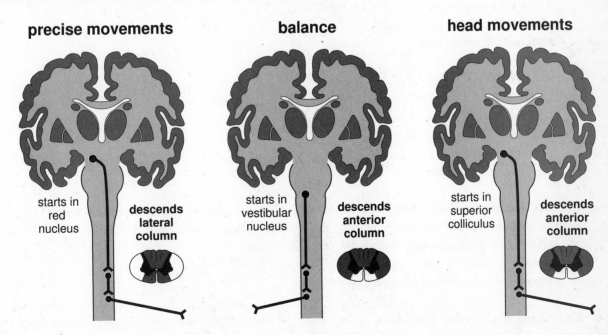

precise movements

starts in
red
nucleus

descends
lateral
column

balance

starts in
vestibular
nucleus

descends
anterior
column

head movements

starts in
superior
colliculus

descends
anterior
column

SPINAL CORD / Spinal Reflexes

Integrating Center   Besides serving as a pathway for impulses traveling between the brain and lower regions of the body, the spinal cord also acts as an integrating center.

Spinal Reflexes   The spinal cord receives sensory information and responds before any impulses reach the brain; so the response occurs before we have any sensation or awareness of the stimulus. These responses are called spinal reflexes.

DEFINITIONS

Reflex : an automatic response to a stimulus.

Visceral Reflexes : reflexes that result in the contraction of smooth or cardiac muscle or the secretion of glands (endocrine or exocrine).

Somatic Reflexes : reflexes that result in the contraction of skeletal muscles.

Types of Somatic Reflex Arcs

monosynaptic : only 2 neurons are involved (1 synapse).

polysynaptic : more than 2 neurons are involved.

ipsilateral : impulses enter and leave the spinal cord on the same side.

contralateral : impulses enter and leave on opposite sides of the spinal cord.

intersegmental : a single sensory neuron divides and forms synapses with association neurons in different segments.

Reciprocal Innervation   An impulse from a single sensory neuron stimulates the contraction of one muscle (the effector muscle) and simultaneously inhibits the contraction in another muscle (the antagonistic muscle). All of the examples of somatic reflexes that follow exhibit reciprocal innervation.

EXAMPLES OF SOMATIC REFLEXES

Stretch Reflex   When muscle <u>length</u> increases, muscle spindles are stimulated. This reflex results in the <u>contraction</u> of the muscle. An example is the knee jerk or patellar reflex.

> *reflex arc : monosynaptic, ipsilateral*
> *receptor : muscle spindles*
> *response : contraction*

Tendon Reflex   When <u>tension</u> in a tendon increases, tendon organs (Golgi tendon organs) are stimulated. This reflex results in an increased frequency of inhibitory impulses, causing <u>relaxation</u> of the attached muscle.

> *reflex arc : polysynaptic, ipsilateral*
> *receptor : tendon organ*
> *response : relaxation*

Flexor Reflex   (Pain / Withdrawal Reflex)   The stimulation of pain receptors results in the <u>flexion</u> (withdrawal) of the arm or leg that has received the painful stimulus.

> *reflex arc : polysynaptic, ipsilateral, intersegmental*
> *receptor : pain receptor*
> *response : withdrawal (flexion)*

Crossed Extensor Reflex   Often during a flexor reflex a second balance-maintaining reflex occurs. While the limb receiving a painful stimulus flexes (withdraws), the limb on the opposite side of the body extends. The extension of the limb on the opposite side helps to maintain balance.

SPINAL REFLEX

Spinal Cord Cross Section

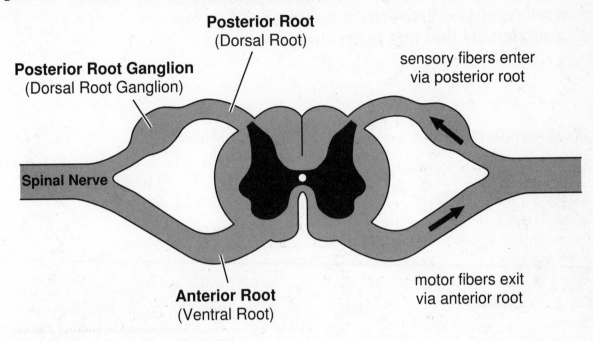

Posterior Root (Dorsal Root)

Posterior Root Ganglion (Dorsal Root Ganglion)

sensory fibers enter via posterior root

Spinal Nerve

Anterior Root (Ventral Root)

motor fibers exit via anterior root

Generalized Reflex Arc

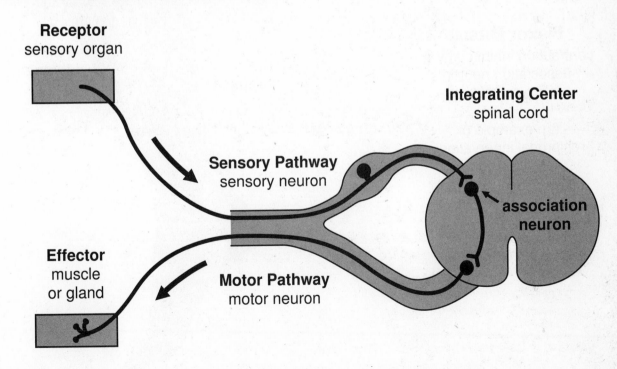

Receptor
sensory organ

Integrating Center
spinal cord

Sensory Pathway
sensory neuron

association neuron

Effector
muscle or gland

Motor Pathway
motor neuron

STRETCH REFLEX

The knee jerk reflex is an example of a stretch reflex.

When the muscle is stretched, muscle spindles are stimulated.
The stretch reflex causes contraction of
the same muscle that has been stretched.

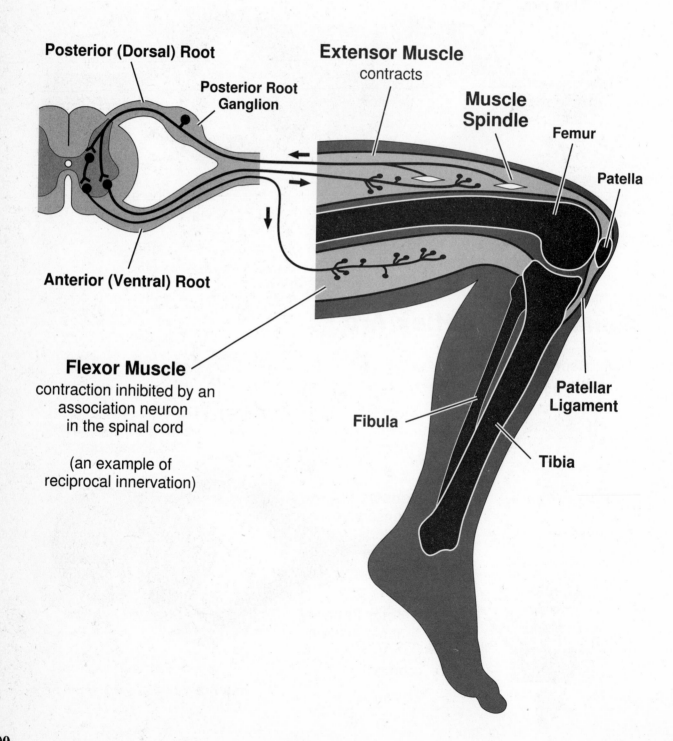

Posterior (Dorsal) Root

Posterior Root
Ganglion

Extensor Muscle
contracts

Muscle
Spindle

Femur

Patella

Anterior (Ventral) Root

Flexor Muscle
contraction inhibited by an
association neuron
in the spinal cord

(an example of
reciprocal innervation)

Fibula

Patellar
Ligament

Tibia

SPINAL REFLEX : Examples

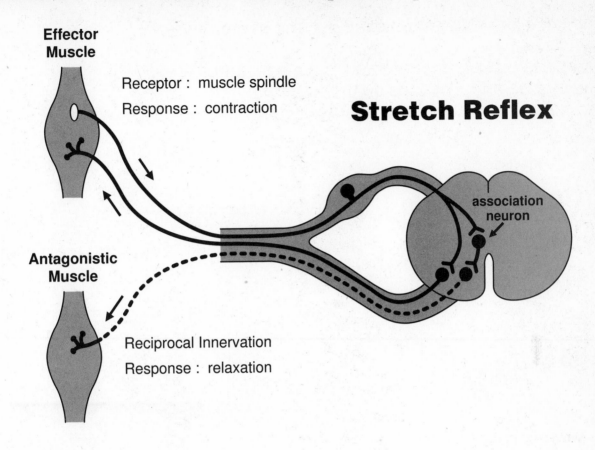

Effector Muscle

Receptor : muscle spindle

Response : contraction

Stretch Reflex

association neuron

Antagonistic Muscle

Reciprocal Innervation

Response : relaxation

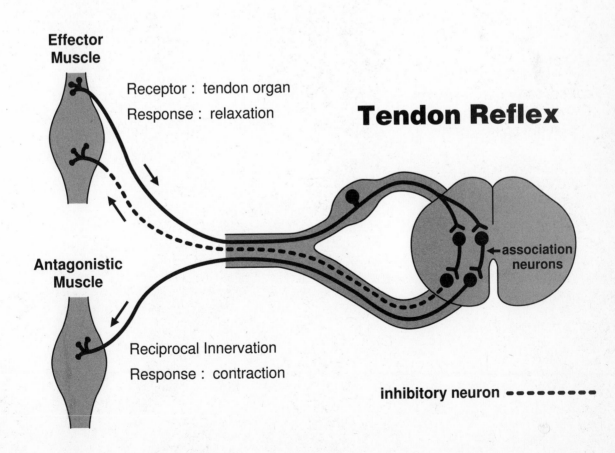

Effector Muscle

Receptor : tendon organ

Response : relaxation

Tendon Reflex

association neurons

Antagonistic Muscle

Reciprocal Innervation

Response : contraction

inhibitory neuron - - - - - - - - -

Nerves

NERVES / Composition

Fascicles

A nerve consists of bundles of nerve fibers, called fascicles, bound together by connective tissue. A small nerve may have only one fascicle, whereas a large nerve may have many separate fascicles. Fascicles are also called *fasciculi* (singular: *fasciculus*).

Connective Tissue Coverings

A fibrous sheet of connective tissue surrounds each nerve. It consists of 3 types of connective tissues:

(1) Epineurium Epineurium is the outer coat of dense connective tissue which surrounds a nerve. Epineurium also fills the space between the fascicles.

(2) Perineurium Perineurium is a sleeve formed by layers of flattened epithelium-like cells. It surrounds each fascicle within a nerve.

(3) Endoneurium Endoneurium consists of a thin layer of reticular fibers, probably produced by neurolemmocytes. It surrounds each nerve fiber within a fascicle.

Nerve Fibers

A nerve fiber is a long process (extension) of a neuron. It may be an axon of an association neuron in the CNS that carries an impulse to another neuron, an axon of a motor neuron in the PNS that carries a nerve impulse to an effector (muscle or gland), or a dendrite of a sensory neuron in the PNS that carries an impulse from a sensory receptor toward the CNS.

Sensory Fibers Nerve fibers that carry impulses from sensory receptors to association neurons in the brain or spinal cord are called sensory (or afferent) fibers; they are extensions of sensory neurons. Sensory fibers may be the dendrites of neurons in the somatic nervous system, carrying impulses from receptors for the general and special senses, or they may be the dendrites of neurons in the autonomic nervous system, carrying impulses from visceral receptors toward the CNS.

Motor Fibers Nerve fibers that carry impulses from the brain or spinal cord to effectors (muscles or glands) are called motor (or efferent) fibers; they are extensions (axons) of motor neurons. Motor fibers may be the axons of neurons in the somatic nervous system, carrying impulses to skeletal muscles, or they may be the axons of neurons in the autonomic nervous system, carrying impulses to smooth muscles, cardiac muscle, or glands.

Myelinated Fibers Each nerve fiber has many neurolemmocytes (Schwann cells) along its length that help to nourish, insulate, and support it. Myelinated fibers are surrounded by a myelin sheath, which consists of up to 100 layers of neurolemmocyte plasma membrane wrapped tightly around the fiber. The outer layer of the neurolemmocyte that contains the nucleus surrounded by cytoplasm is called the neurolemma; it facilitates regeneration of a damaged axon. Only fibers that have a neurolemma are capable of regeneration.

Unmyelinated Fibers Even an unmyelinated nerve fiber has neurolemmocytes associated with it. Unmyelinated fibers are simply embedded in their neurolemmocytes (not surrounded by a myelin sheath).

NERVE (cross section)

Bundles of nerve fibers in the PNS (outside the brain and spinal cord) are called nerves.

A typical nerve contains several bundles of nerve fibers.
A large nerve contains thousands of nerve fibers.

Fascicles
(bundles of nerve fibers)

**Myelinated
Nerve Fiber**

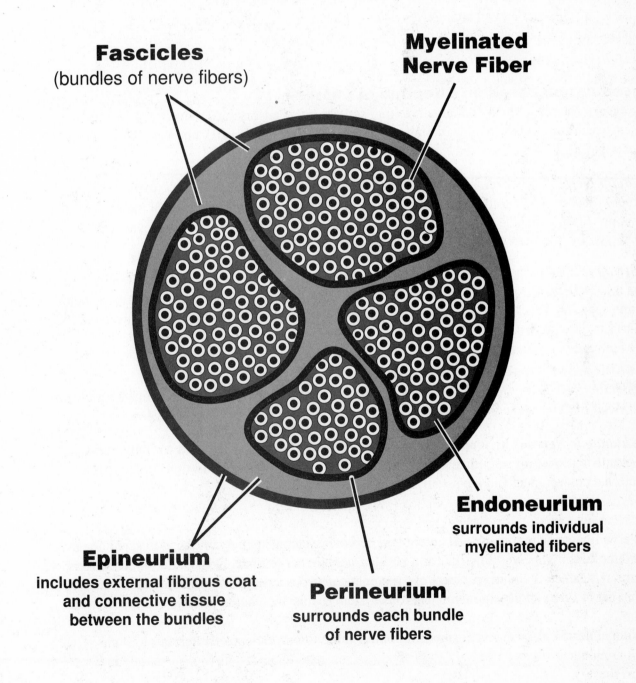

Endoneurium
surrounds individual
myelinated fibers

Epineurium
includes external fibrous coat
and connective tissue
between the bundles

Perineurium
surrounds each bundle
of nerve fibers

NERVES / Classification

Classification based on Origin

Cranial Nerves   All nerves that emerge from the *brain* are called cranial nerves. They emerge through holes in the cranium *(cranial foramina).* There are *12 pairs* of cranial nerves : 3 contain only sensory (afferent) fibers; 4 are mixed nerves (contain both sensory and motor fibers); and 5 contain only motor (efferent) fibers.

Spinal Nerves   All nerves that emerge from the spinal cord are called spinal nerves. They emerge through holes *(intervertebral foramina)* formed by the notches on adjoining vertebrae. There are *31 pairs* and all are *mixed nerves,* which means that they contain the 2 basic types of nerve fibers: sensory and motor.

Classification based on Direction of Impulse

Sensory Nerves   The 3 cranial nerves that contain only sensory (afferent) fibers are called sensory nerves. They include: the olfactory nerve (I), optic nerve (II), and vestibulocochlear nerve (VIII).

Motor Nerves   The 5 cranial nerves that contain *primarily* motor (efferent) fibers are called motor nerves. (All motor nerves contain sensory fibers from proprioceptors of the muscles they supply.) They include : the oculomotor nerve (III), trochlear nerve (IV), abducens nerve (VI), spinal accessory nerve (XI), and hypoglossal nerve (XII).

Mixed Nerves   All spinal nerves are mixed nerves; they contain both sensory (afferent) and motor (efferent) fibers. The 4 cranial nerves that contain both sensory and motor fibers include : the trigeminal nerve (V), facial nerve (VII), glossopharyngeal nerve (IX), and vagus nerve (X).

Classification based on Function

Somatic Nervous System   The somatic nervous system is concerned with voluntary actions of skeletal muscles and consciously perceived sensations that relate to the external environment.

Autonomic Nervous System   The autonomic nervous system is concerned with involuntary, automatic actions of smooth muscles, cardiac muscles, and glands; sensations relate to the internal environment and are usually not consciously perceived.

Nerve fibers of the somatic and autonomic nervous systems are not contained in separate nerves. For example, spinal nerves T1—T12 and L1—L2 contain nerve fibers of the autonomic nervous system (sympathetic) and nerve fibers of the somatic nervous system. And spinal nerves S2—S4 contain nerve fibers of the autonomic nervous system (parasympathetic) and the somatic nervous system.

Cranial nerves also consist of fibers of both the autonomic and somatic nervous systems.

PNS ORGANIZATION

Nerves :
(1) Cranial nerves emerge from the brain.
(2) Spinal nerves emerge from the spinal cord.

Neurons :
(1) Sensory (or afferent) neurons carry impulses toward the CNS.
(2) Motor (or efferent) neurons carry impulses away from the CNS.

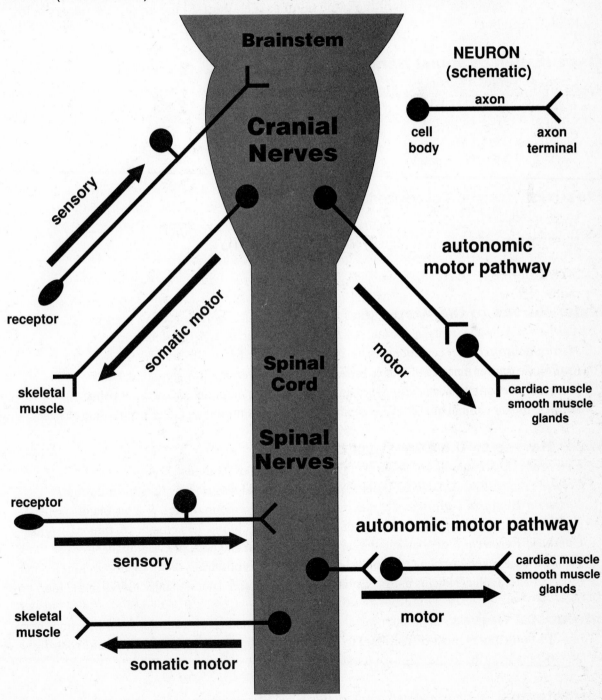

NERVES / Spinal Nerves

Naming Spinal Nerves

First 7 Spinal Nerves   The first 7 spinal nerves emerge <u>above</u> the vertebra of the same number; these include cervical nerves 1 through 7.

8th Cervical Spinal Nerve   The 8th cervical nerve emerges between the 7th cervical vertebra and the 1st thoracic vertebra. While there are only 7 cervical vertebrae, there are 8 cervical spinal nerves.

Thoracic, Lumbar & Sacral Nerves   All of the spinal nerves, starting with the 1st thoracic nerve, emerge <u>below</u> the vertebra of the same number (i.e., the 1st lumbar nerve emerges below the 1st lumbar vertebra).

Organization of Spinal Nerves

Cervical Nerves (8 pairs)
Thoracic Nerves (12 pairs)
Lumbar Nerves (5 pairs)
Sacral Nerves (5 pairs)
Coccygeal Nerves (1 pair)

Plexuses   (networks of adjacent nerves)

Cervical (C1 - C5)
Brachial (C5 - T1)
Lumbar (L1 - L4)
Sacral (L4 - S4)

Major Nerves to the Arms   (and distribution)

Axillary : deltoid & teres minor muscles; skin over deltoid & upper posterior arm.
Musculocutaneous : coracobrachialis, biceps brachii, & brachialis muscles.
Radial : extensor muscles of arm & forearm; skin of posterior arm, forearm, & hand.
Median : flexor muscles of arm & forearm (except flexor carpi ulnaris); skin of palm.
Ulnar : flexor carpi ulnaris & flexor digitorum profundus muscles; skin of medial side of hand.

Major Nerves to the Legs   (and distribution)

Femoral : flexor muscles of thigh; skin on medial aspect of thigh, leg, & foot.
Sciatic : consists of two nerves: tibial & common peroneal nerves; they diverge at the knee.
Posterior Femoral Cutaneous : skin over anal region, scrotum (male), & labia majora (female).
Pudendal : muscles of perineum; skin of penis, scrotum, clitoris, labia majora & minora, vagina.
Common Peroneal : divides into the superficial peroneal and deep peroneal branches.
Tibial : gastrocnemius, plantaris, soleus, popliteus, tibialis posterior, flexor digitorum longus, and
            flexor hallucis longus muscles; branches into medial & lateral plantar nerves in the foot.

Intercostal Nerves   The intercostal nerves are formed by the ventral rami of spinal nerves T1 – T11. T1 contributes most of its fibers to the brachial plexus. T12 is called the *subcostal nerve*, because it runs inferior to the 12th rib (costal).

Dermatomes   Each spinal nerve innervates a specific segment of the skin with sensory fibers. These segments are called dermatomes.

SPINAL NERVES   31 pairs of spinal nerves

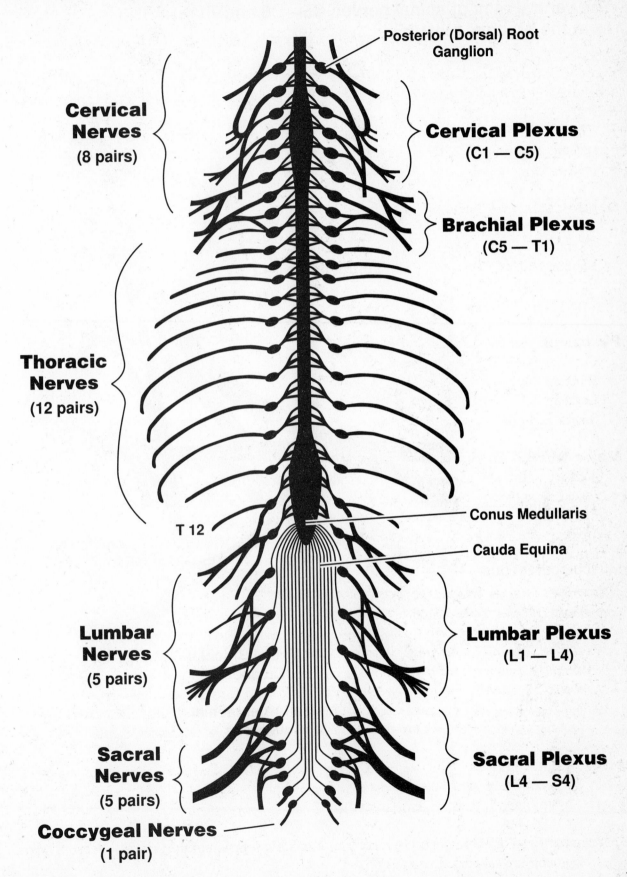

Posterior (Dorsal) Root Ganglion

Cervical Nerves (8 pairs)

Cervical Plexus (C1 — C5)

Brachial Plexus (C5 — T1)

Thoracic Nerves (12 pairs)

T 12

Conus Medullaris

Cauda Equina

Lumbar Nerves (5 pairs)

Lumbar Plexus (L1 — L4)

Sacral Nerves (5 pairs)

Sacral Plexus (L4 — S4)

Coccygeal Nerves (1 pair)

SPINAL NERVES : Brachial Plexus

The ventral rami of spinal nerves C5—C8 and T1
form the brachial plexus.

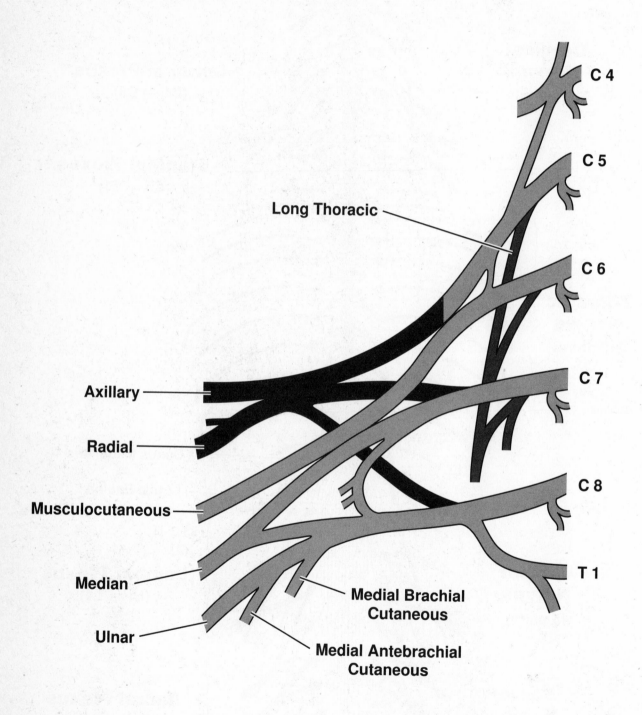

Long Thoracic

C 4

C 5

C 6

C 7

C 8

T 1

Axillary

Radial

Musculocutaneous

Median

Ulnar

Medial Brachial
Cutaneous

Medial Antebrachial
Cutaneous

SPINAL NERVES
5 Major Nerves to the Arm

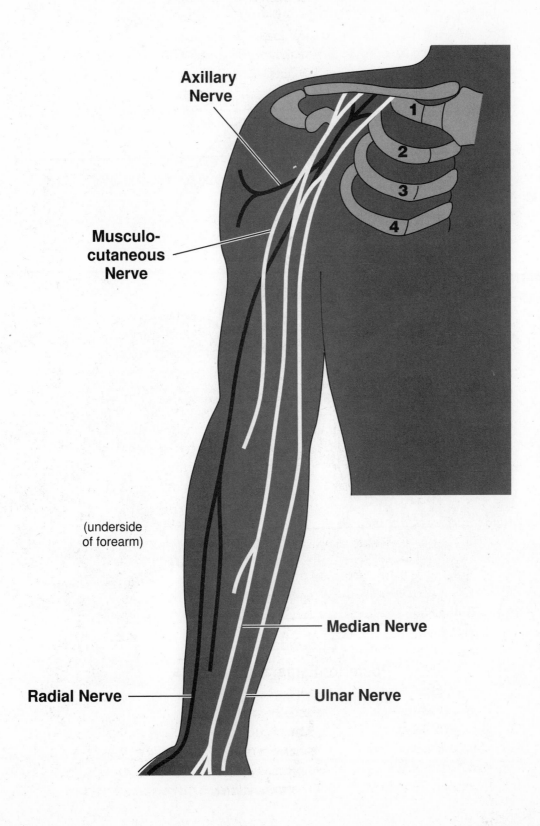

Axillary
Nerve

Musculo-
cutaneous
Nerve

1

2

3

4

(underside
of forearm)

Median Nerve

Radial Nerve

Ulnar Nerve

SPINAL NERVES : Lumbo-Sacral Plexus

The roots of the lumbosacral plexus are formed by
the ventral rami of spinal nerves L1 — S4.

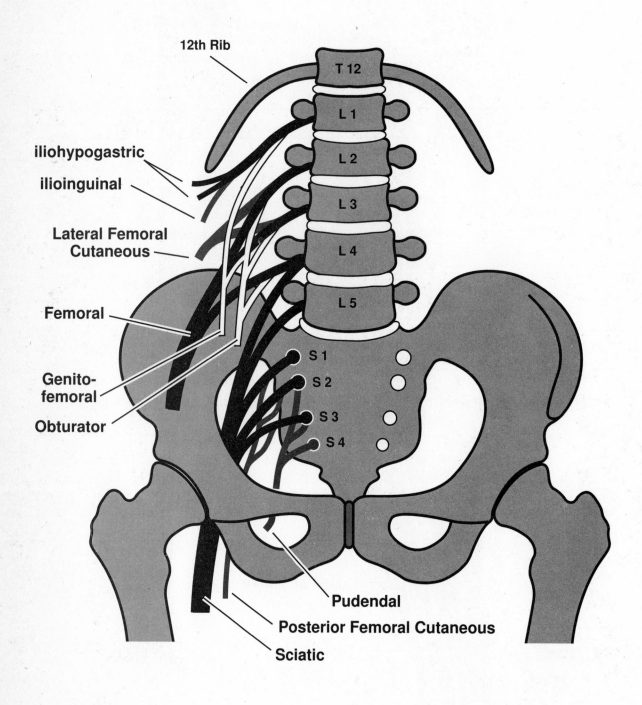

SPINAL NERVES
Sciatic Nerve

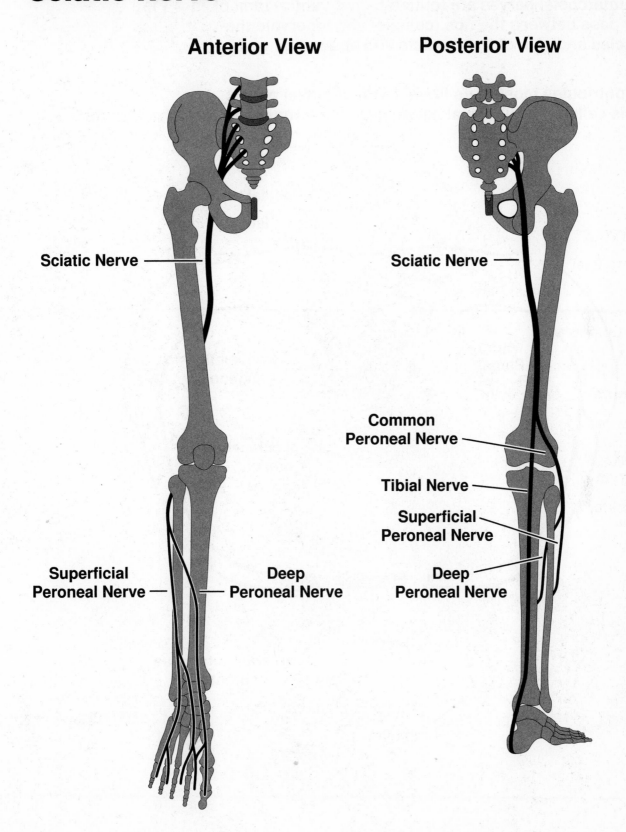

Anterior View

Posterior View

Sciatic Nerve

Sciatic Nerve

Common
Peroneal Nerve

Tibial Nerve

Superficial
Peroneal Nerve

Superficial
Peroneal Nerve

Deep
Peroneal Nerve

Deep
Peroneal Nerve

113

SPINAL NERVES : Intercostal Nerves

The intercostal nerves are formed by the ventral rami of T1 – T11; they pass between the ribs (costals) and innervate the muscles and skin of the thoracic and abdominal walls.

T1 contributes most of its fibers to the brachial plexus.
T12 is called the subcostal nerve, because it runs inferior to the 12th rib.

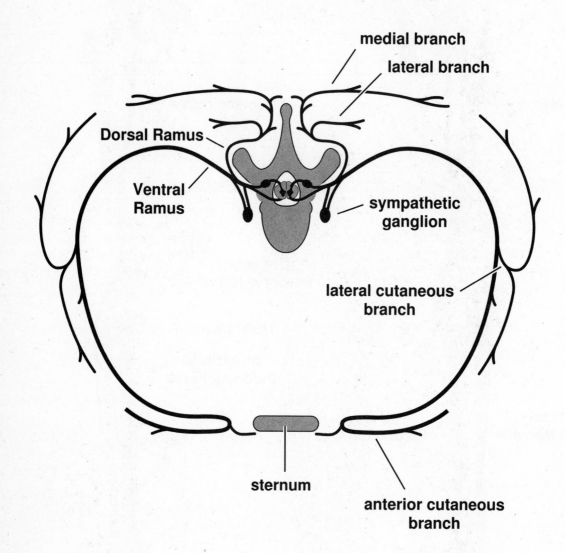

medial branch

lateral branch

Dorsal Ramus

Ventral Ramus

sympathetic ganglion

lateral cutaneous branch

sternum

anterior cutaneous branch

DERMATOMES
Segments of Skin Supplied by Spinal Nerves

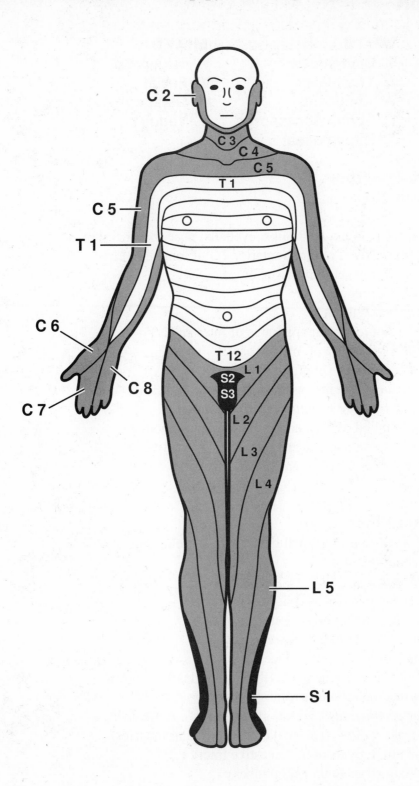

NERVES / Cranial Nerves

CLASSIFICATION

SENSORY	MOTOR	MIXED
I Olfactory	III Oculomotor	V Trigeminal
II Optic	IV Trochlear	VII Facial
VIII Vestibulo- cochlear	VI Abducens	IX Glossopharyngeal
	XI Spinal Accessory	X Vagus
	XII Hypoglossal	

Functions of Sensory Fibers

Olfactory: *smell* (olfactory bulbs)

Optic: *vision* (retina)

Trigeminal: *sensations* (face; scalp; teeth; lips; eyeballs; nose & throat lining)
general sensory from tongue (anterior 2/3 of tongue)
proprioception (muscles of mastication)

Facial: *taste* (anterior 2/3 of tongue)
proprioception (face & scalp)

Vestibulocochlear: *balance* (vestibular apparatus of internal ear)
hearing (cochlea of internal ear)

Glossopharyngeal: *taste* (posterior 1/3 of tongue)
proprioception for swallowing (throat muscles)
blood pressure receptors (carotid sinuses)

Vagus: *chemoreceptors* (blood oxygen concentration; aortic bodies)
pain receptors (respiratory & digestive tracts)
sensations (external ear, larynx, & pharynx)
taste (tongue)

Functions of Motor Fibers

Oculomotor: *eyeball movement* (4 eyeball muscles & 1 eyelid muscle)
lens accommodation
pupil constriction

Trochlear: *eyeball movement* (superior oblique muscles)

Trigeminal: *chewing* (muscles of mastication)

Abducens: *eyeball movement* (lateral rectus muscles)

Facial: *facial expressions* (muscles of the face)

Glossopharyngeal: *swallowing & gag reflex* (throat muscles)
saliva production (parotid glands)
tear production (lacrimal glands)

Vagus: *heart rate & stroke volume* (pacemaker & ventricular muscles)
peristalsis (smooth muscles of the digestive tract)
airflow (smooth muscles in bronchial tubes)
speech & swallowing (muscles of larynx & pharynx)

Spinal Accessory: *head rotation* (trapezius & sternocleidomastoid muscles)

Hypoglossal: *speech & swallowing* (tongue & throat muscles)

CRANIAL NERVES

Embryo (6 weeks old)

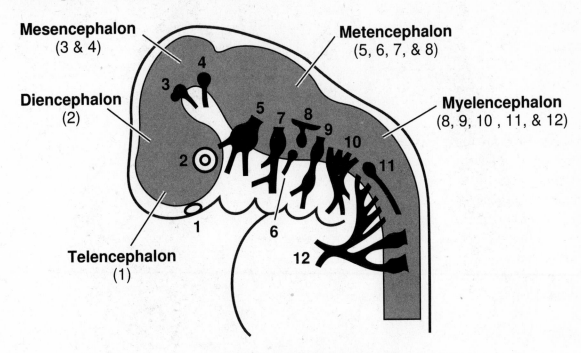

Mesencephalon (3 & 4)

Diencephalon (2)

Telencephalon (1)

Metencephalon (5, 6, 7, & 8)

Myelencephalon (8, 9, 10, 11, & 12)

Mature Brain

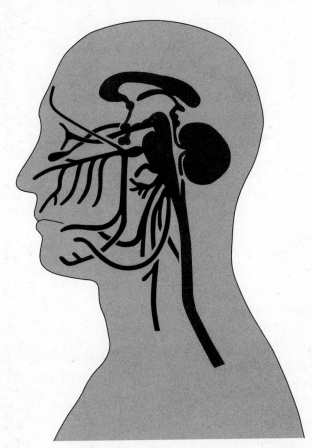

CRANIAL NERVES
ventral view

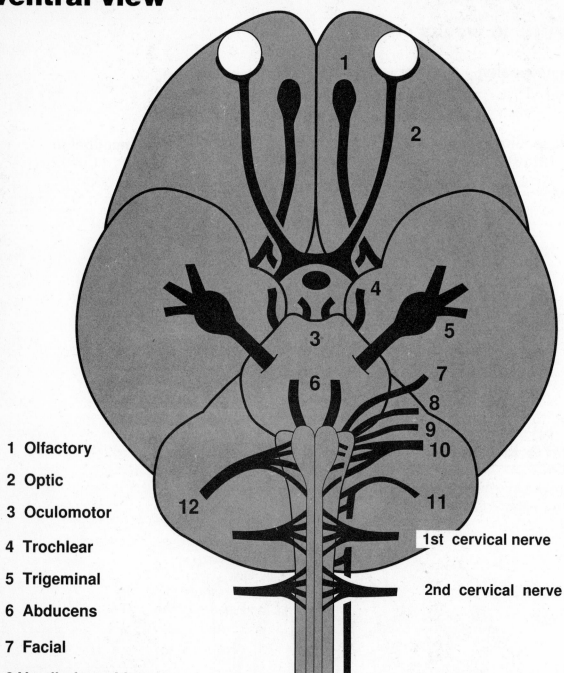

1 Olfactory

2 Optic

3 Oculomotor

4 Trochlear

5 Trigeminal

6 Abducens

7 Facial

8 Vestibulocochlear

9 Glossopharyngeal

10 Vagus

11 Spinal Accessory

12 Hypoglossal

1st cervical nerve

2nd cervical nerve

Note :
There are 12 pairs of cranial nerves.
For clarity only one nerve is shown
for cranial nerves 7 - 12.

PURELY SENSORY CRANIAL NERVES 1, 2, & 8

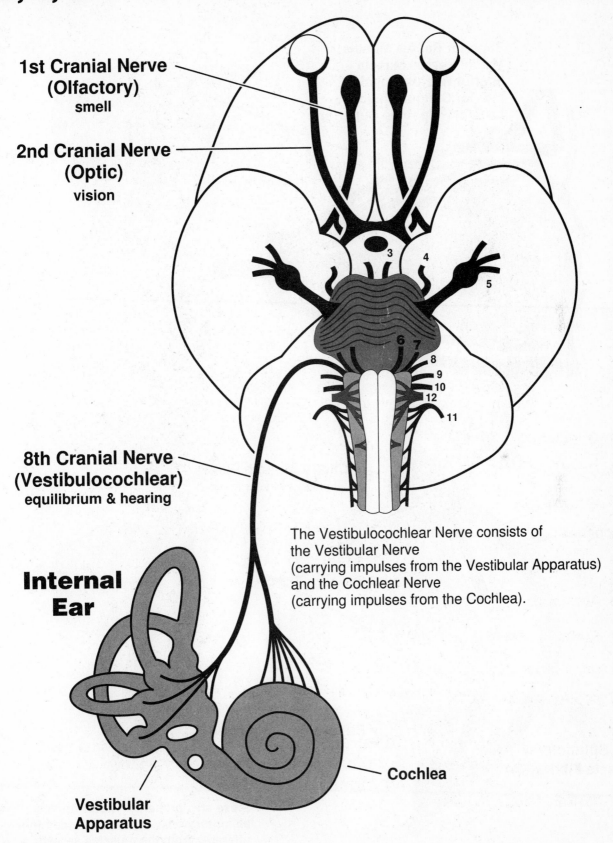

1st Cranial Nerve (Olfactory) smell

2nd Cranial Nerve (Optic) vision

8th Cranial Nerve (Vestibulocochlear) equilibrium & hearing

The Vestibulocochlear Nerve consists of the Vestibular Nerve (carrying impulses from the Vestibular Apparatus) and the Cochlear Nerve (carrying impulses from the Cochlea).

Internal Ear

Cochlea

Vestibular Apparatus

PRIMARILY MOTOR CRANIAL NERVES
3rd Cranial Nerve (Oculomotor)

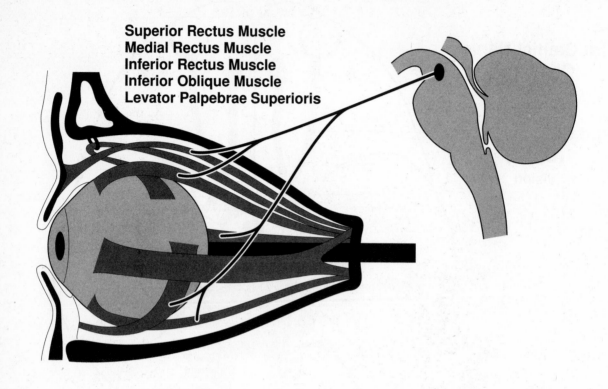

Superior Rectus Muscle
Medial Rectus Muscle
Inferior Rectus Muscle
Inferior Oblique Muscle
Levator Palpebrae Superioris

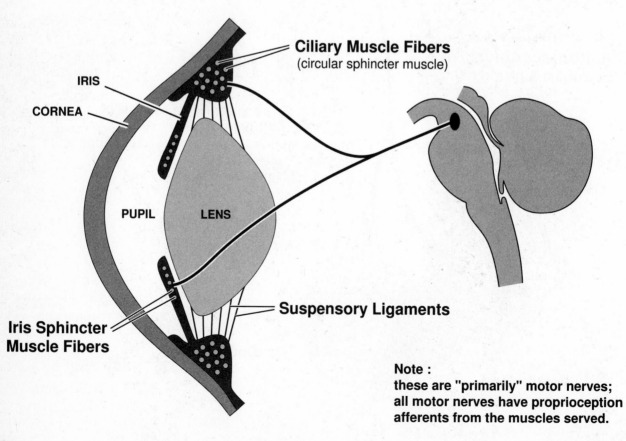

Ciliary Muscle Fibers
(circular sphincter muscle)

IRIS

CORNEA

PUPIL   LENS

Suspensory Ligaments

Iris Sphincter
Muscle Fibers

Note :
these are "primarily" motor nerves;
all motor nerves have proprioception
afferents from the muscles served.

120

PRIMARILY MOTOR CRANIAL NERVES
4, 6, 11, & 12

4th
Trochlear
Superior Oblique Muscle

6th
Abducens
Lateral Rectus Muscle

Optic Nerve

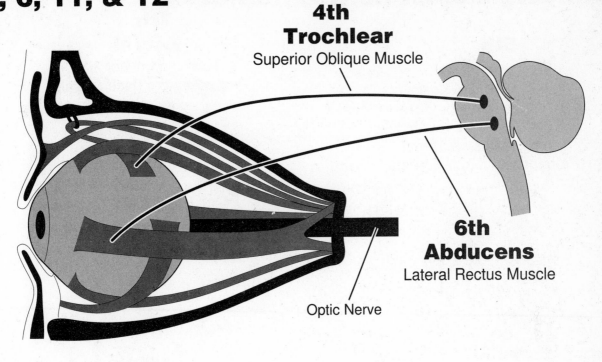

11th
Spinal Accessory
Sternocleidomastoid
& Trapezius Muscles

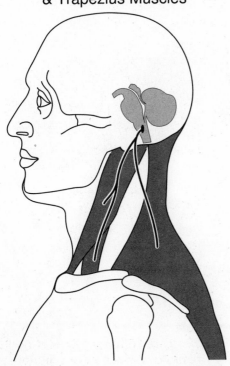

12th
Hypoglossal
Tongue Muscles
Strap Muscles

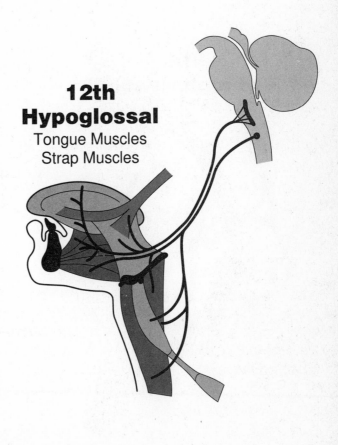

MIXED CRANIAL NERVES : 5, 7, 9, & 10
Sensory Components

5th
Trigeminal
Skin of Face & Scalp
Tongue (anterior 2/3)
Teeth, Lips, & Eyeballs
Lining of Nose & Throat
Proprioceptors (mastication)

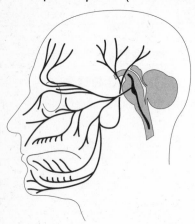

7th
Facial
Tongue (anterior 2/3)
Proprioceptors (face & scalp)

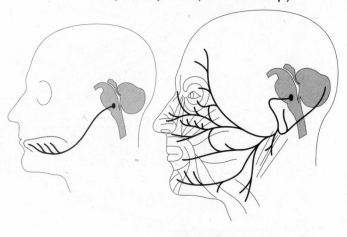

9th
Glossopharyngeal
Tongue (posterior 1/3)
Proprioceptors (swallowing)
Pressure Receptors (carotid sinus)

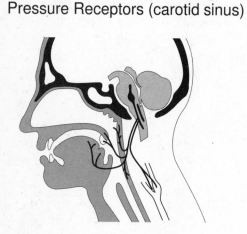

10th
Vagus
External Ear
Pharynx & Larynx
Stretch Receptors (lungs)
Chemoreceptors (aortic bodies)
Pain Receptors (Respiratory & GI Tracts)

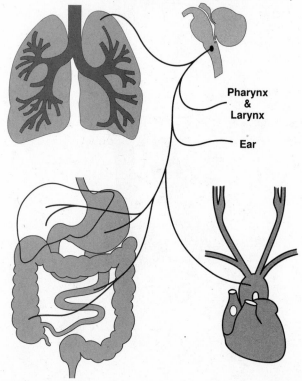

Pharynx
&
Larynx

Ear

MIXED CRANIAL NERVES : 5, 7, 9, & 10
Motor Components

5th
Trigeminal
Muscles of Mastication

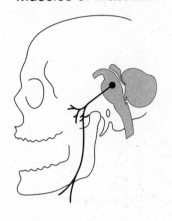

7th
Facial
Muscles of Facial Expression
Salivary & Lacrimal Glands

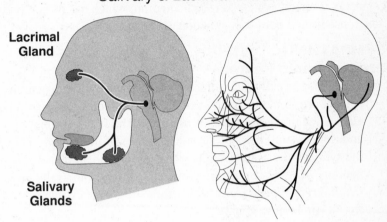

Lacrimal Gland

Salivary Glands

9th
Glossopharyngeal
Muscles for Swallowing
Parotid Gland for Saliva

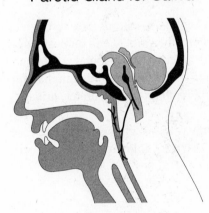

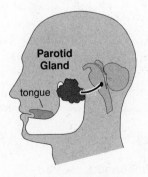

Parotid Gland

tongue

10th
Vagus
Smooth Muscle of GI & Respiratory Tracts
Pacemaker & Heart Muscle of Atria
Pharynx & Larynx

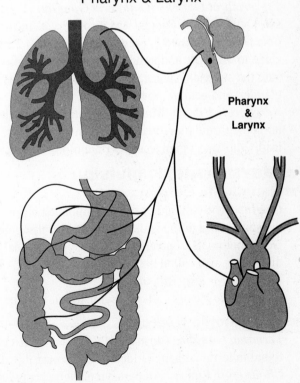

Pharynx & Larynx

NERVES / Autonomic Nervous System

The autonomic nervous system includes all motor neurons that transmit impulses to smooth muscle, cardiac muscle, and glands; and all sensory neurons that transmit impulses from the internal organs (the viscera) into the CNS.

Autonomic Motor Neurons   The motor (efferent) portion of the autonomic nervous system has 2 principal divisions: sympathetic and parasympathetic. Most internal organs are innervated by both sympathetic and parasympathetic fibers; this is referred to as *dual innervation*. Motor (outgoing) autonomic pathways consist of 2 neurons: a preganglionic neuron, which has its cell body in the CNS and a postganglionic neuron, which has its cell body in a ganglion outside the CNS.

SYMPATHETIC DIVISION
Preganglionic Neurons

Origins   The cell bodies of sympathetic preganglionic neurons are located in the lateral gray horns of the spinal cord from the 1st thoracic to the 2nd lumbar segment. For this reason, the sympathetic division is also called the *thoracolumbar division*. The fibers (axons) of these neurons leave the spinal cord in the anterior (ventral) roots of the spinal nerves of this region. They pass via the white rami communicantes to the sympathetic trunk ganglia, where most of them end at synapses with the cell bodies of postganglionic neurons. These preganglionic fibers are referred to as the *thoracolumbar outflow*.

Cholinergic Fibers   All preganglionic fibers are cholinergic, which means they release acetylcholine from their axon terminals.

Postganglionic Neurons

Sympathetic Trunk Ganglia (Paravertebral Ganglia)   The sympathetic trunk ganglia are a series of ganglia that lie in a vertical row on either side of the vertebral column. The cell bodies of many sympathetic postganglionic neurons are located in these ganglia. Postganglionic fibers from the thoracic portion of the sympathetic trunk innervate the heart, lungs, bronchi, and other thoracic viscera; they also innervate sweat glands, arrector pili muscles, and blood vessels in the skin. Postganglionic fibers from the lumbar and sacral sympathetic chain ganglia enter the gray ramus and then merge with a spinal nerve or join the hypogastric plexus in the pelvis.

Prevertebral Ganglia (Collateral Ganglia)   Some sympathetic preganglionic neurons pass through the sympathetic trunk ganglia and form nerves known as *splanchnic nerves*; their fibers end on postganglionic neurons located in prevertebral ganglia. Prevertebral ganglia lie anterior to the spinal column and close to the large abdominal arteries. Postganglionic fibers originating in the prevertebral ganglia innervate the stomach, spleen, liver, kidney, small intestine, colon, rectum, renal arterioles, ureter, urinary bladder, and genital organs.

Adrenergic Fibers   Most sympathetic postganglionic fibers are adrenergic, which means they release norepinephrine (noradrenaline) from their axon terminals. The few that are cholinergic include fibers leading to sweat glands and certain blood vessels.

PARASYMPATHETIC DIVISION
Preganglionic Neurons

Origins   The cell bodies of parasympathetic preganglionic neurons are located in the lateral gray horns of the spinal cord in the 2nd, 3rd, & 4th sacral segments; or in the nuclei of the following cranial nerves: Oculomotor (III), Facial (VII), Glossopharyngeal (IX), and Vagus (X). For this reason, the sympathetic division is also called the *craniosacral division*. These parasympathetic preganglionic fibers are referred to as the *craniosacral outflow*.

Cholinergic Fibers   All parasympathetic preganglionic fibers are cholinergic (release acetylcholine).

Postganglionic Neurons

Terminal Ganglia (Intramural Ganglia)   The cell bodies of parasympathetic postganglionic neurons are found in terminal ganglia located on or near the effector organs.

Cholinergic Fibers   All parasympathetic postganglionic fibers are cholinergic.

AUTONOMIC NERVOUS SYSTEM
origins and outgoing pathways

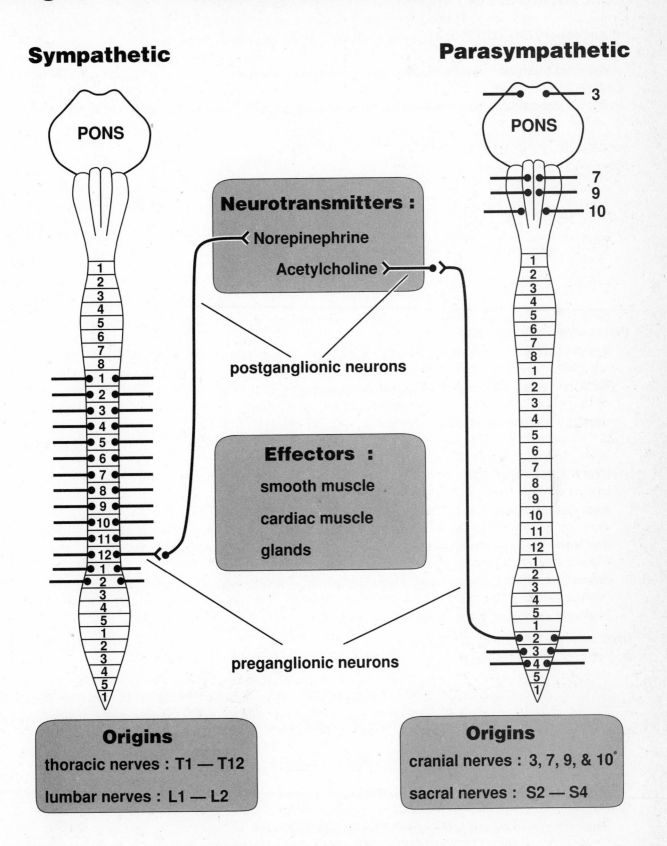

Sympathetic

Parasympathetic

PONS

PONS

Neurotransmitters :

Norepinephrine

Acetylcholine

postganglionic neurons

Effectors :

smooth muscle

cardiac muscle

glands

preganglionic neurons

Origins

thoracic nerves : T1 — T12

lumbar nerves : L1 — L2

Origins

cranial nerves : 3, 7, 9, & 10

sacral nerves : S2 — S4

NERVES / Sympathetic Nerves

STIMULATING EFFECTS

Accessory Sex Glands : secretion of alkaline fluid containing fructose.

Adrenal Medulla : secretion of epinephrine and norepinephrine.

Blood Vessels : dilation of arterioles leading to skeletal muscles.

Eye : contraction of radial muscles of iris (pupil dilates).

Heart : increased heart rate and stroke volume.

Juxtaglomerular Apparatus : secretion of the enzyme renin.

Liver : release of glucose into the bloodstream.

Lungs : dilation of bronchioles (increased airflow).

Skin : contraction of arrector pili muscles (goose pimples); secretion of sweat by sweat glands.

Sperm Ducts : peristaltic contractions propel sperm into urethra.

Spleen : release of stored blood into bloodstream.

Uterus : contractions during labor.

INHIBITING EFFECTS

Ascending Colon : peristalsis (motility) inhibited.

Bladder : internal sphincter contracts; muscular wall relaxes (inhibits urination).

Blood Vessels : arterioles to most organs constrict (inhibit bloodflow).

Descending Colon : peristalsis (motility) inhibited.

Duodenum : peristalsis (motility) inhibited; digestive enzyme secretion inhibited.

Gall Bladder : bile secretion inhibited.

Kidneys : bloodflow to kidneys inhibited (decreased urine formation).

Pancreas : digestive enzyme secretion inhibited.

Skin : bloodflow to skin decreased (pale skin).

Stomach : motility and gastric juice secretion inhibited.

SYMPATHETIC NERVE PATHWAYS

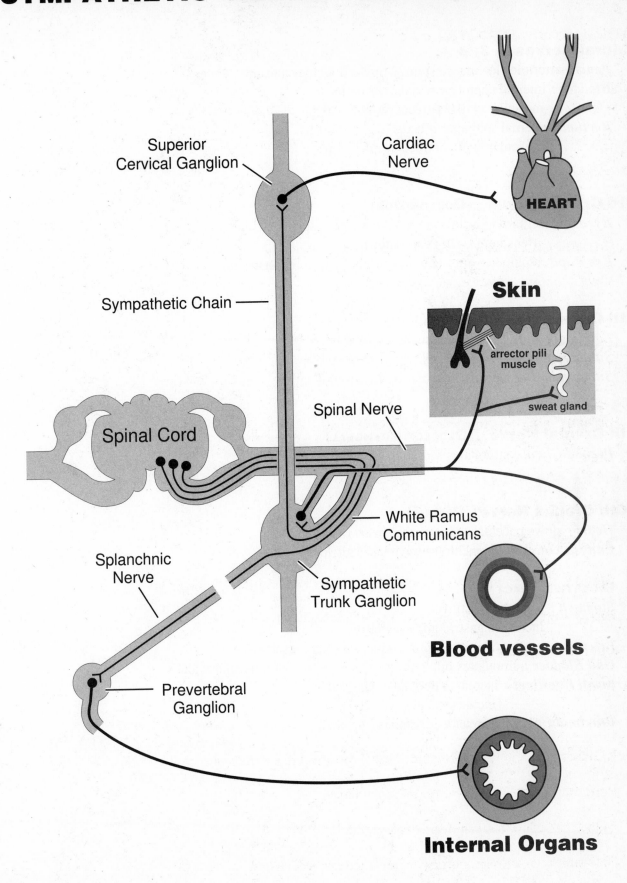

Superior Cervical Ganglion

Cardiac Nerve

HEART

Sympathetic Chain

Skin

arrector pili muscle

sweat gland

Spinal Nerve

Spinal Cord

White Ramus Communicans

Splanchnic Nerve

Sympathetic Trunk Ganglion

Blood vessels

Prevertebral Ganglion

Internal Organs

NERVES / Parasympathetic Nerves

Sacral Nerves 2, 3, & 4

Penis : arterioles leading to spongy tissue dilate (erection).
Bladder : internal sphincter relaxes (urination).
            muscular wall contracts (urination).
Rectum : internal sphincter relaxes (defecation).
            muscular wall contracts (defecation).

3rd Cranial Nerve (OCULOMOTOR)

Eye Lens : ciliary muscle contracts, relaxing suspensory ligaments
            (lens bulges for near vision).
Eye Pupil : sphincter muscle in iris contracts (pupil constricts).

7th Cranial Nerve (FACIAL)

Lacrimal Gland : stimulates secretion of tears.
Sublingual Gland : stimulates secretion of saliva.
Submandibular Gland : stimulates secretion of saliva.

9th Cranial Nerve (GLOSSOPHARYNGEAL)

Parotid Gland : stimulates secretion of saliva.

10th Cranial Nerve (VAGUS)

Heart : slows pacemaker (decreases heart rate).
Lungs : constricts bronchioles (decreases airflow).

DIGESTIVE TRACT

Stomach : increases motility.
            increases gastric juice secretion.
Liver : increases glucose storage (converted to glycogen).
Gall Bladder : stimulates bile secretion (contraction of muscular wall).
Small Intestines : increases peristalsis (motility).
            increases digestive secretions.
Proximal Colon : increases peristalsis (motility).

PARASYMPATHETIC SPINAL NERVES
Sacral Nerves 2, 3, and 4

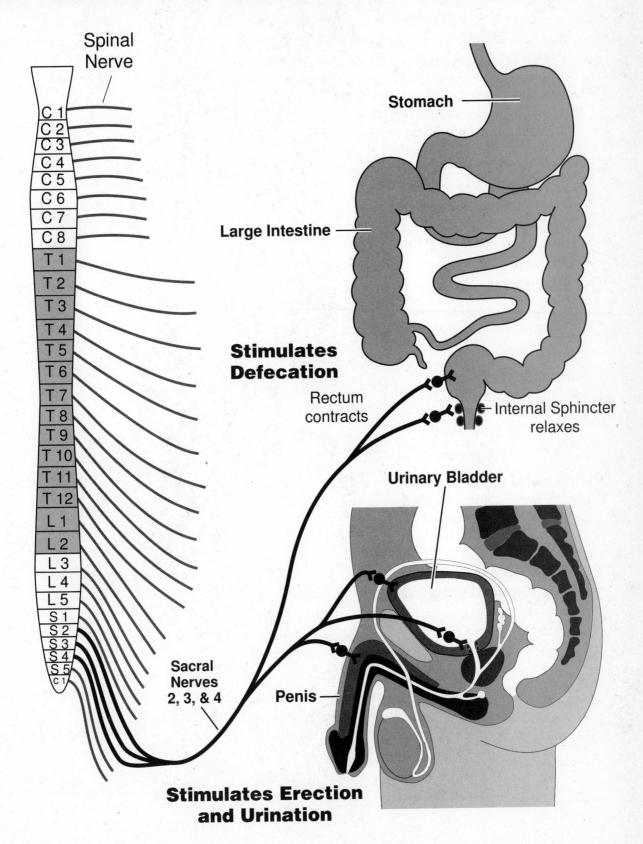

Spinal Nerve

Stomach

Large Intestine

Stimulates Defecation

Rectum contracts

Internal Sphincter relaxes

Urinary Bladder

Sacral Nerves 2, 3, & 4

Penis

Stimulates Erection and Urination

PARASYMPATHETIC CRANIAL NERVES
Cranial Nerves 3, 7, & 9

3rd
Oculomotor

Lens: ciliary muscle contracts
relaxing suspensory ligaments
lens bulges for near vision

Iris: sphincter muscle contracts
constricts pupil

7th
Facial

Lacrimal Gland:
tears

Sublingual Gland &
Submandibular Gland:
saliva secretion

Sublingual Gland

Submandibular Gland

9th
Glossopharyngeal

Parotid Gland:
saliva secretion

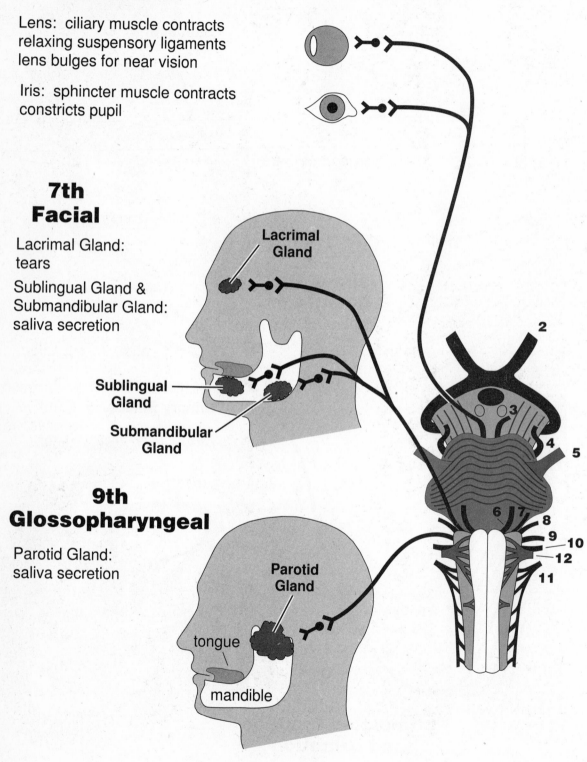

Lacrimal Gland

Parotid Gland

tongue

mandible

2

3

4

5

6 7

8

9 10

12

11

PARASYMPATHETIC CRANIAL NERVES
10th Cranial Nerve (Vagus Nerve)

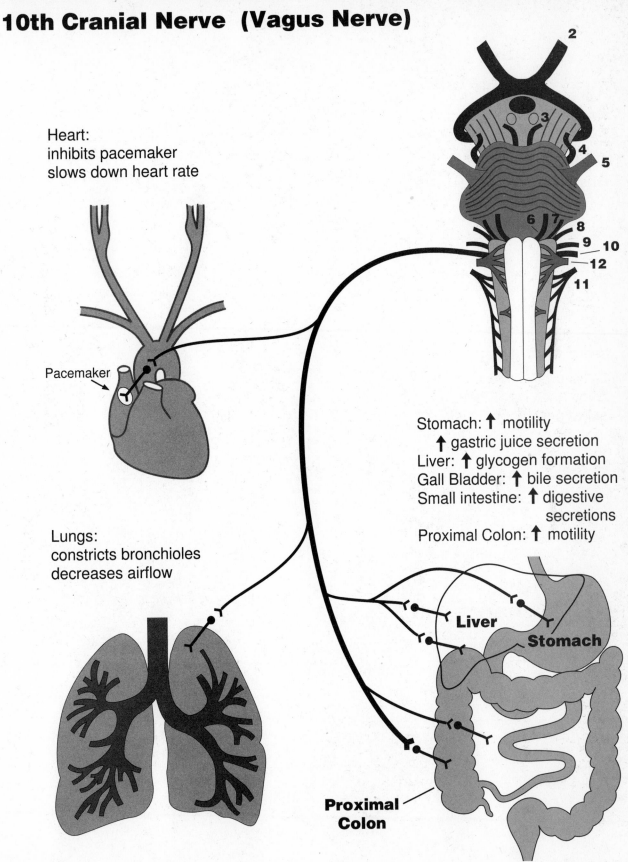

Heart:
inhibits pacemaker
slows down heart rate

Pacemaker

Lungs:
constricts bronchioles
decreases airflow

Stomach: ↑ motility
↑ gastric juice secretion
Liver: ↑ glycogen formation
Gall Bladder: ↑ bile secretion
Small intestine: ↑ digestive
secretions
Proximal Colon: ↑ motility

Liver

Stomach

Proximal
Colon

2
3
4
5
6 7
8
9 10
12
11

Sensory Receptors

SENSORY SYSTEM / Sensory Receptors

When changes occur in the external and internal environments, sensory receptors are stimulated. Activated sensory receptors trigger nerve impulses that travel on sensory pathways into the central nervous system where they are processed and interpreted. When the impulses reach the appropriate region of the cerebral cortex, a particular type of sensation is perceived.

Structurally, sensory receptors are either the peripheral ends of sensory neurons or a separate adjacent cell. They are grouped into 2 major categories: those associated with the general senses and those associated with the special senses.

GENERAL SENSES
Somatic
(1) Tactile: touch, pressure, vibration, itch, & tickle
(2) Thermal : hot & cold
(3) Pain : acute & chronic
(4) Proprioceptive : muscle, tendon, & joint position

General Somatic Sensory (Afferent) Neurons transmit impulses from the receptors into the CNS.

Visceral
(1) Distention of Viscera (internal organs)
(2) Chemical Composition of the ECF (extracellular fluid)

General Visceral Sensory (Afferent) Neurons transmit impulses from the receptors into the CNS.

SPECIAL SENSES
Somatic
(1) Visual (sight)
(2) Auditory (hearing)
(3) Equilibrium (balance) : static equilibrium & dynamic equilibrium

Special Somatic Sensory (Afferent) Neurons transmit impulses from the receptors into the CNS.

Visceral
(1) Olfactory (smell)
(2) Gustatory (taste)

Special Visceral Sensory (Afferent) Neurons transmit impulses from the receptors into the CNS.

SENSORY MODALITIES

There are 11 main types of sensory information, which have been outlined above. Most types of sensory information reach consciousness; however, there are also types of sensory information of which we are not consciously aware, such as changes in body fluids (blood pressure, blood glucose, plasma oxygen concentration, plasma osmotic pressure, pH of the CSF).

Each specific type of sensation is called a sensory modality. A given sensory neuron carries only one modality. Each sensory modality is monitored by a specific type of sensory receptor.

SENSORY RECEPTORS

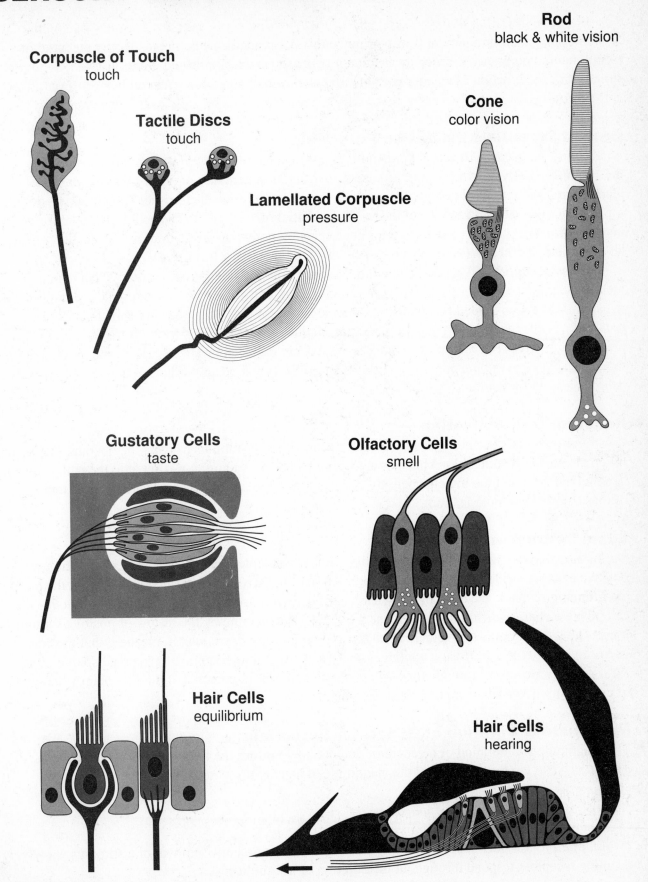

Corpuscle of Touch
touch

Tactile Discs
touch

Lamellated Corpuscle
pressure

Rod
black & white vision

Cone
color vision

Gustatory Cells
taste

Olfactory Cells
smell

Hair Cells
equilibrium

Hair Cells
hearing

SENSORY SYSTEM / Generator Potentials

defined : A generator potential (receptor potential) is a graded change in the electric potential of a receptor cell membrane. *Graded* means that it may vary in amplitude and duration.
function : The function of a generator potential is to trigger an action potential in a sensory (afferent) neuron.

Graded Potentials vs. Action Potentials

Action Potentials   An action potential is an all-or-none response; it does not matter how intense the stimulus or how long the stimulus persists. An action potential will occur on a section of cell membrane if the threshold potential is reached; for motor neurons the threshold potential is − 55 millivolts (a change of 15 mV from the resting potential of − 70 mV). The action potential for a given neuron is always the same: a motor neuron action potential has a duration of 1 millisecond and an amplitude of 100 mV (− 70 mV up to + 30 mV, and then back to − 70 mV).

Graded Potentials   A graded potential, like an action potential, is a temporary change in a membrane potential. But it is a graded or variable change; it varies with the strength and duration of the stimulus. When graded potentials occur on sensory receptor cells, they are called *generator potentials*. Other examples of graded potentials include the *end-plate potentials* that occur at neuro-muscular junctions, the *pacemaker potentials* that occur on the specialized cells of the pacemaker in the heart, and *postsynaptic potentials* (EPSP's and IPSP's) that occur on the cell bodies of association neurons and motor neurons.

Receptor Cell Activation

Generator potentials occur on sensory receptor cells. First, a stimulus triggers the opening or closing of ion channels. If sodium ion channels are opened, positive sodium ions flow into the cell, causing *de*polarization; if sodium ion channels are closed or more potassium channels are opened, the flow of ions causes *hyper*polarization.

Local Decremental Currents

During depolarization, when sodium ions diffuse into a receptor cell, there is an accumulation of positive charges inside the cell and an accumulation of negative charges outside the cell at the point of stimulation. Inside the cell positive charges diffuse away from the point of stimulus; outside the cell positive charges diffuse toward the negative region generated by the inflow of positive sodium ions. The local currents (movement of charges) produced are *decremental*, meaning that they decrease in magnitude as diffusion continues and the positive ions become more spread apart. If the local currents are strong enough, they will generate a threshold potential at the first neurofibral node of the sensory nerve fiber and trigger an action potential.

Magnitude & Duration of Generator Potentials

The magnitude and duration of a generator potential determines the frequency of nerve impulses generated. The factors that control the magnitude of a generator potential include:
(1) *Stimulus intensity.*
(2) *Rate of change of stimulus application.*
(3) *Summation of successive generator potentials.*
(4) *Adaptation.* Rapidly adapting receptors respond at the onset and removal of a stimulus; slowly adapting receptors respond throughout the duration of a stimulus.

GENERATOR POTENTIAL

The magnitude of the generator potential is controlled by:
the stimulus intensity,
the rate of change of stimulus application,
the summation of successive generator potentials,
and adaptation.

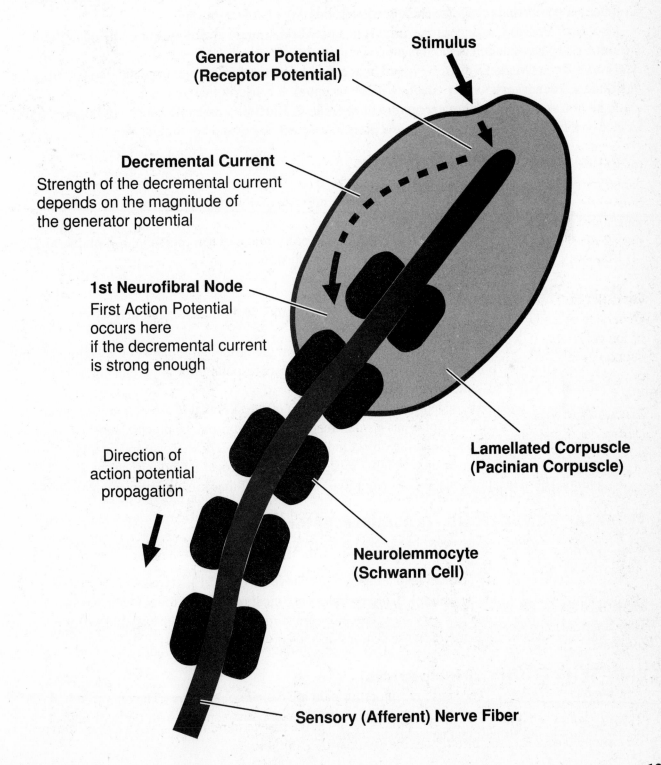

Stimulus

**Generator Potential
(Receptor Potential)**

Decremental Current
Strength of the decremental current
depends on the magnitude of
the generator potential

1st Neurofibral Node
First Action Potential
occurs here
if the decremental current
is strong enough

Direction of
action potential
propagation

**Lamellated Corpuscle
(Pacinian Corpuscle)**

**Neurolemmocyte
(Schwann Cell)**

Sensory (Afferent) Nerve Fiber

Receptors in the skin monitor 3 basic types of cutaneous sensations : tactile, thermal, and pain.

TACTILE SENSATIONS
Touch Receptors

Corpuscles of Touch (Meissner's corpuscles) : encapsulated nerve endings; rapidly adapting touch receptors that recognize exactly what point of the body is touched.

Root Hair Plexuses : dendrites arranged in a network around hair follicles; rapidly adapting touch receptors that detect movement when hairs are disturbed.

Tactile Discs (Merkel's discs / Type I Cutaneous Mechanoreceptor) : expanded nerve endings (flattened dendrites); slowly adapting touch receptors for discriminative touch.

Type II Cutaneous Mechanoreceptors (end organ of Ruffini) : expanded nerve endings embedded in the dermis; slowly adapting receptors that detect heavy and continuous touch.

Pressure & Vibration Receptors

Lamellated Corpuscles (Pacinian corpuscles) : oval structures composed of a connective tissue capsule, layered like an onion, that enclose a dendrite; rapidly adapting receptors that respond to pressure and high frequency vibrations.

Corpuscles of Touch (Meissner's corpuscles) : rapidly adapting receptors that respond to low frequency vibrations, as well as to pressure and touch stimuli.

Itch & Tickle Receptors

Free Nerve Endings Free nerve endings are the receptors for both tickle and itch sensations.

Adaptation *Rapidly adapting* receptors respond at the onset and removal of a stimulus with a burst of action potentials. *Slowly adapting* receptors respond throughout the duration of a stimulus with a sustained discharge.

Receptive Fields The receptive field is the region of the skin that is monitored by a given sensory receptor. If a receptor has a small receptive field it provides precise information about the shape and texture of the object indenting the skin. These receptors are highly concentrated at the finger tips. A large receptive field can cover a whole finger or part of the palm. These receptors respond to vibrations, stretching of the skin, and movement of joints.

THERMAL SENSATIONS   (Thermoreceptors)

Free Nerve Endings The sense receptors for cold and warm are called thermoreceptors. They are free (naked) nerve endings.

Warm receptors are most sensitive to temperatures above 25 C (77 F); above 45 C pain receptors are stimulated (burning sensation). Cold receptors are most responsive to temperatures between 10 C & 20 C (50 — 68 F); below 10 C pain receptors are stimulated (freezing sensation). Both warm and cold receptors adapt rapidly; sensations disappear within minutes.

PAIN SENSATIONS   (Nociceptors)

Free Nerve Endings The sense receptors for pain are called nociceptors. They are free (naked) nerve endings located between cells of the epidermis. Nociceptors respond to all types of high intensity stimuli and stimuli that cause tissue damage.

SKIN RECEPTORS
Touch, Temperature, Pain, & Pressure

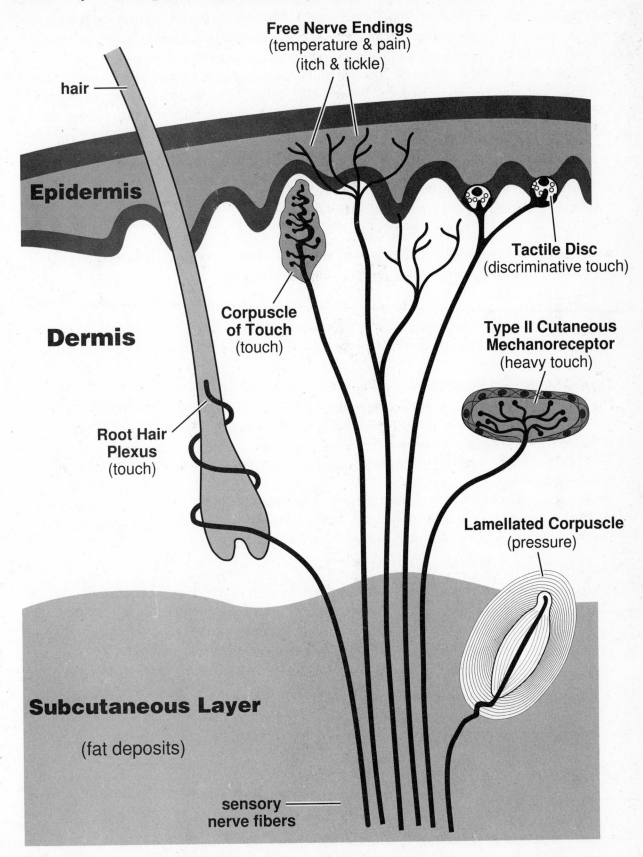

Free Nerve Endings
(temperature & pain)
(itch & tickle)

hair

Epidermis

Dermis

Corpuscle of Touch
(touch)

Tactile Disc
(discriminative touch)

Type II Cutaneous Mechanoreceptor
(heavy touch)

Root Hair Plexus
(touch)

Lamellated Corpuscle
(pressure)

Subcutaneous Layer

(fat deposits)

sensory nerve fibers

SENSORY SYSTEM / Smell

Anatomy

Olfactory Epithelium (also called *Olfactory Mucosa*) The olfactory epithelium is a small patch (about 1 square inch) of mucous membrane in the superior portion of the nasal cavity, the middle nasal conchae, and the upper portion of the nasal septum. It consists of 3 cell types:

(1) Olfactory Receptors There are 10 - 100 million receptor cells in the olfactory epithelium. Each has a life span of about 30 days. Several cilia, called olfactory hairs, project from each receptor cell. The axons of receptor cells extend through holes in the cribriform plate of the ethmoid bone into the olfactory bulb, which lies below the frontal lobes.

(2) Supporting Cells (also called Sustentacular Cells) Supporting cells are columnar epithelial cells that surround and support the olfactory receptors.

(3) Basal Cells Basal cells lie between the bases of supporting cells. They produce new olfactory cells, replacing the cells that die after about 30 days.

Olfactory Glands (also called Bowman's glands)
Olfactory glands are located within the connective tissue that supports the olfactory epithelium. They produce mucus that is needed to dissolve odorant molecules.

Physiology

Primary Sensations There are probably hundreds of different primary scents. One classification system includes just seven: floral, pungent, musky, pepperminty, putrid, camphoraceous, and etheral.

Transduction An olfactory cell is a neuron specialized to be sensitive to specific chemicals. Chemical interaction with receptor sites in the membranes of olfactory hairs, causes sodium channels to open. This leads to depolarization. A generator potential occurs that triggers an action potential in the axon leading to the olfactory bulb.

Threshold Olfaction has a low threshold. Only a few molecules of a substance stimulate the olfactory receptors.

Adaptation Olfactory receptors undergo sensory adaptation rapidly, but even though they have adapted to one odor, their sensitivity to other odors remains unchanged. They adapt about 50% in the first second after stimulation; thereafter they adapt very slowly.

Olfactory Pathway

(1) Olfactory Receptors : the bipolar neurons that are activated by specific chemicals.

(2) Olfactory Nerves : unmyelinated axons of the olfactory receptor cells. They pass through holes (foramina) in the cribriform plate of the ethmoid bone and end in the olfactory bulbs.

(3) Olfactory Bulbs : paired masses of gray matter which lie beneath the frontal lobes of the cerebrum on either side of the crista galli of the ethmoid bone. The axons of olfactory nerves synapse with olfactory bulb neurons.

(4) Olfactory Tract : the axons of olfactory bulb neurons. They extend posteriorly and divide into 2 pathways before entering the cerebrum.

(5) Prepyriform Cortex & Limbic System : One pathway leads to primitive regions of the cerebral cortex on the inferior surface of the brain. Nerve impulses transmitted to the prepyriform cortex give rise to sensations of smell; nerve impulses to the limbic system give rise to emotions and memories associated with a particular scent.

(6) Frontal Lobes : The second pathway transmits impulses via the thalamus to the cortex of the frontal lobes. Impulses reaching the frontal lobes give rise to sensations of smell.

OLFACTORY BULB

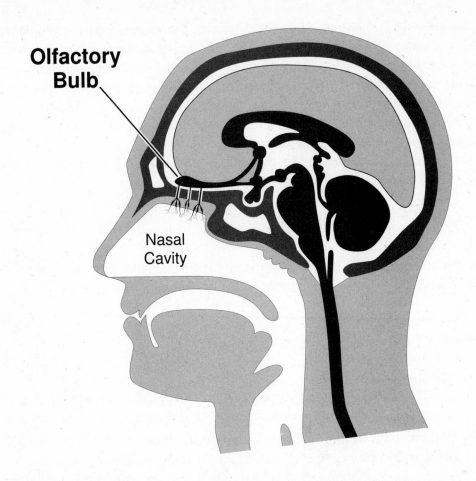

Olfactory
Bulb

Nasal
Cavity

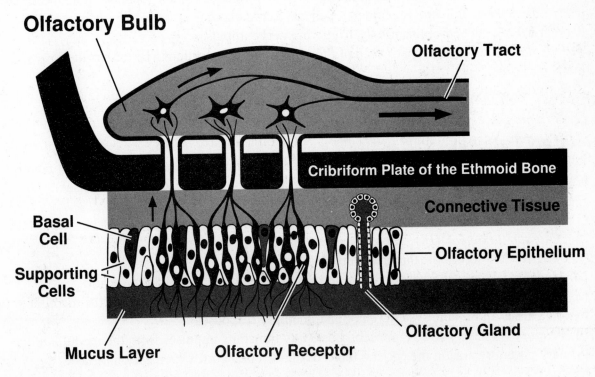

Olfactory Bulb

Olfactory Tract

Cribriform Plate of the Ethmoid Bone

Connective Tissue

Basal
Cell

Olfactory Epithelium

Supporting
Cells

Olfactory Gland

Mucus Layer

Olfactory Receptor

SENSORY SYSTEM / Taste

Anatomy

Taste Buds   There are about 10,000 taste buds on the surface of the tongue, throat, and epiglottis. On the tongue they occur in tiny elevations called papillae. Each taste bud consists of 3 cell types:

(1) Gustatory Receptor Cells   There are about 50 receptor cells per taste bud. Each has a life span of about 10 days. A single microvillus, called a *gustatory hair*, projects from each receptor cell through an opening in the taste bud called a *taste pore*.

(2) Supporting Cells (also called Sustentacular Cells)   Supporting cells are columnar epithelial cells that surround and support the gustatory receptors.

(3) Basal Cells   Basal cells lie between the bases of supporting cells. They produce new gustatory cells, replacing the cells that die after about 10 days.

Papillae (location of taste buds)   There are 3 types of papillae:

(1) Circumvallate (circular shape)   These are the largest of the papillae. They form a row at the posterior portion of the tongue.

(2) Fungiform (mushroom-shaped)   They are found on the tip and sides of the tongue.

(3) Filiform (threadlike)   They cover the anterior 2/3 of the tongue; contain no taste buds.

Physiology

Primary Sensations   There are 4 primary taste sensations:

(1) Sour (HCl)   Lateral edges of the tongue are highly sensitive to sour stimuli.

(2) Salty (NaCl)   Anterior portions of the tongue are highly sensitive to salty stimuli.

(3) Bitter (quinine)   Posterior portions of the tongue are highly sensitive to bitter stimuli.

(4) Sweet (sucrose)   Anterior portions of the tongue are highly sensitive to sweet stimuli.

All other tastes are combinations of these four, modified by accompanying olfactory sensations.

Transduction   A gustatory receptor cell is separate from the sensory neuron. Chemical interaction with receptor sites in the membranes of the receptor cells causes generator potentials that trigger the release of neurotransmitters. Sensory nerve endings close to the receptor cells are depolarized by the neurotransmitters, triggering nerve impulses.

Threshold   Thresholds vary for each of the primary taste sensations. Bitter has the lowest threshold.

Adaptation   Gustatory receptors undergo sensory adaptation rapidly. Complete adaptation can occur after 1 to 5 minutes of continuous stimulation.

Gustatory Pathway

(1) Gustatory Receptors : Receptor cells release neurotransmitter, activating sensory neurons.

(2) Sensory Fibers : Sensory nerve fibers generate action potentials (nerve impulses).

(3) Cranial Nerves : Sensory nerve fibers become part of 3 cranial nerves.

   Facial (VII) serves the anterior 2/3 of the tongue.

   Glossopharyngeal (IX) serves the posterior 1/3 of the tongue.

   Vagus (X) serves the throat and epiglottis.

(4) Medulla : Cranial nerves carry gustatory impulses to the medulla oblongata.

(5) Hypothalamus & Limbic System : One pathway transmits impulses from the medulla to the hypothalamus and limbic system (emotional memory responses).

(6) Primary Gustatory Area : A second pathway transmits impulses from the medulla to the primary gustatory area in the parietal lobes of the cerebral cortex (perception of taste).

TASTE RECEPTORS

Tongue

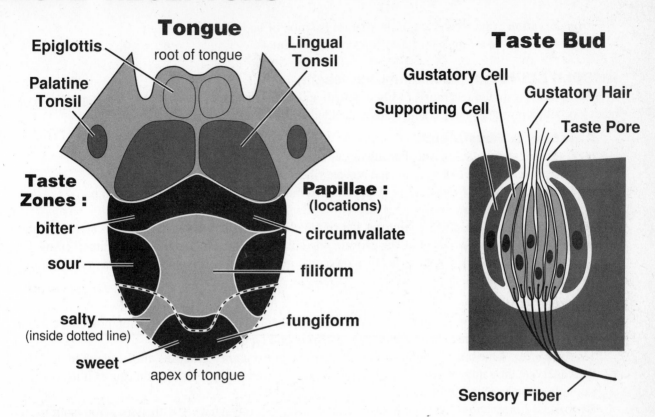

Epiglottis
root of tongue
Lingual Tonsil
Palatine Tonsil

Taste Zones :
- bitter
- sour
- salty (inside dotted line)
- sweet

apex of tongue

Papillae : (locations)
- circumvallate
- filiform
- fungiform

Taste Bud

Gustatory Cell
Supporting Cell
Gustatory Hair
Taste Pore

Sensory Fiber

Circumvallate Papilla

upper surface of tongue

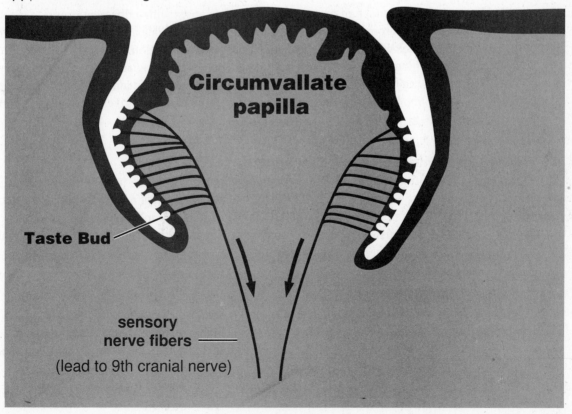

Circumvallate papilla

Taste Bud

sensory nerve fibers

(lead to 9th cranial nerve)

SENSORY SYSTEM / Proprioceptive Sensations

Proprioception : the awareness of the precise position of body parts.
Kinesthesia : the awareness of directions of movement.

MUSCLE SPINDLES (monitor muscle length)

Muscle Spindles (stretch receptors) Muscle length and changes in muscle length are monitored by stretch receptors called muscle spindles, which are embedded within skeletal muscle.

Anatomy & Physiology

(1) Capsule : a spindle-shaped connective tissue capsule.
(2) Extrafusal Muscle Fibers : normal muscle fibers surrounding the capsule.
(3) Intrafusal Muscle Fibers : 3 to 10 specialized muscle fibers enclosed in the capsule.
The intrafusal fibers are of two types: *nuclear chain fibers* and *nuclear bag fibers*.
Passive stretch of a muscle also stretches the spindle fibers within that muscle, and this activates the sensory nerve fibers that penetrate the capsule; the greater the stretch, the greater the rate of firing. Contraction of a muscle decreases the tension on the muscle spindles, which decreases the rate of firing by the sensory neurons.

Nerve Pathways

When a sensory fiber from a muscle spindle enters the central nervous system (brain or spinal cord), it divides into branches that synapse with four different cell types.
Stretch Reflex One branch of the sensory neuron forms excitatory synapses directly with motor neurons that innervate the same muscle. So, when the muscle is stretched, a reflex action causes it to contract. An example is the knee jerk reflex.
Reciprocal Innervation Another branch of the sensory neuron synapses with association neurons; the association neurons then release neurotransmitter that inhibits motor neurons that control antagonistic muscles. The excitation of one muscle and the simultaneous inhibition of its antagonistic muscle is called reciprocal innervation.
Synergistic Muscles A third branch of the sensory neuron synapses with a different group of association neurons; these association neurons release a neurotransmitter that activates motor neurons that control synergistic muscles (muscles whose contractions assist the intended motion.)
Motor Cortex A fourth branch of the sensory neuron synapses with association neurons that carry signals to the motor cortex of the cerebrum. The information about muscle length is integrated with input from receptors in the joints, ligaments, and skin; the combined information gives an awareness of limb and joint position.

TENDON ORGANS (monitor muscle tension)

Tendon organs (also called Golgi tendon organs) are located in tendons near the junction with its muscle. These receptors are made up of sensory nerve endings wrapped around collagen bundles of the tendon. When the attached muscle contracts, it straightens the normally bowed collagen bundles; the change in shape of the collagen bundles stimulates the sensory nerve endings to fire. The greater the muscle tension, the greater the frequency of firing.

JOINT KINESTHETIC RECEPTORS

There are 3 types of receptors located within and around articular capsules of synovial joints:
(1) Encapsulated receptors (similar to type II cutaneous mechanoreceptors) respond to pressure.
(2) Small lamellated corpuscles (Pacinian corpuscles) respond to acceleration and deceleration of joint movement.
(3) Receptors similar to tendon organs adjust reflex inhibition of adjacent muscles when excessive strain is placed on a joint.

144

TENDON ORGAN & MUSCLE SPINDLE

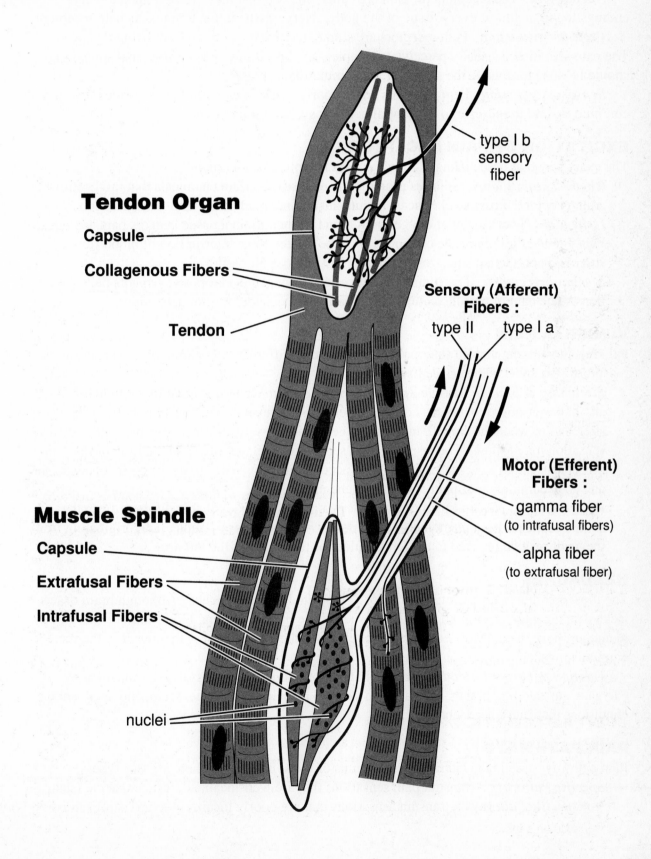

Tendon Organ

Capsule

Collagenous Fibers

Tendon

type I b
sensory
fiber

Sensory (Afferent)
Fibers :

type II   type I a

Motor (Efferent)
Fibers :

gamma fiber
(to intrafusal fibers)

alpha fiber
(to extrafusal fiber)

Muscle Spindle

Capsule

Extrafusal Fibers

Intrafusal Fibers

nuclei

SENSORY SYSTEM / Pain

Nociceptors   The receptors for pain are called nociceptors; they are free (naked) nerve endings found in almost every tissue of the body. Nerve tissue in the brain lacks pain receptors.

Protective Function   Pain receptors are stimulated whenever tissues are being damaged. The pain sensation is usually perceived as unpleasant, and it serves as a signal that something should be done to remove the source of the stimulation.

Sensory Adaptation   Pain receptors adapt poorly. Once a receptor has been activated, it may continue to send impulses into the central nervous system for some time.

EXCITATION OF PAIN RECEPTORS

The exact way that tissue damage activates pain receptors is unknown.

Chemical Stimulants   Injuries promote the release of certain chemicals that might stimulate pain receptors. Possible chemicals include histamine, bradykinin, and potassium ions.

Ischemia   A deficiency of oxygen-rich blood (ischemia) in a tissue triggers pain sensations. Pain elicited during muscle cramp seems to be related to an interruption of blood flow; sustained contraction squeezes capillaries and reduces blood flow.

Mechanoreceptors   The stimulation of certain mechanoreceptors also triggers pain sensations. The pain of muscle cramps is due partly to mechanoreceptor activation.

VISCERAL PAIN

Pain receptors in the viscera (internal organs) respond differently to stimulation than sensory receptors associated with surface tissues.

Stretching & Smooth Muscle Spasms   Localized damage to intestinal tissue may not elicit any pain sensations, even in a conscious person. However, when intestinal tissues are stretched or when the smooth muscles in the intestinal walls undergo spasms, a strong pain sensation may follow. The resulting pain seems to be related to the stimulation of mechanoreceptors and to a decreased blood flow accompanied by lower tissue oxygen concentration and an accumulation of pain-stimulating chemicals.

Referred Pain   Visceral pain is often felt in a part of the body that is different from the source of the pain—a phenomenon called *referred pain*. For example, pain originating from the heart may be referred to the left shoulder or the inside of the left arm.

HEADACHES

The most common pain sensations are those associated with headaches. Although brain tissue lacks pain receptors, nearly all the other tissues of the head, including blood vessel walls and meninges, have them. Most headaches are related to the types of stress that result in fatigue, emotional tension, anxiety, or frustration.

Dilation of Cranial Blood Vessels   Dilations of cranial blood vessels, accompanied by edema in surrounding tissues, or spasms in skeletal muscles of the face, scalp, and neck are the conditions that cause headaches.

PAIN PATHWAYS

Pain pathways ascend the lateral white columns of the spinal cord. There are two types:

Specific Pathways : transmit pain sensations that are well-localized, fast, and acute (sharp).

Nonspecific Pathways : transmit sensations that are poorly localized, long-lasting, and dull.

REFERRED PAIN
Areas of the skin to which visceral pain is referred.

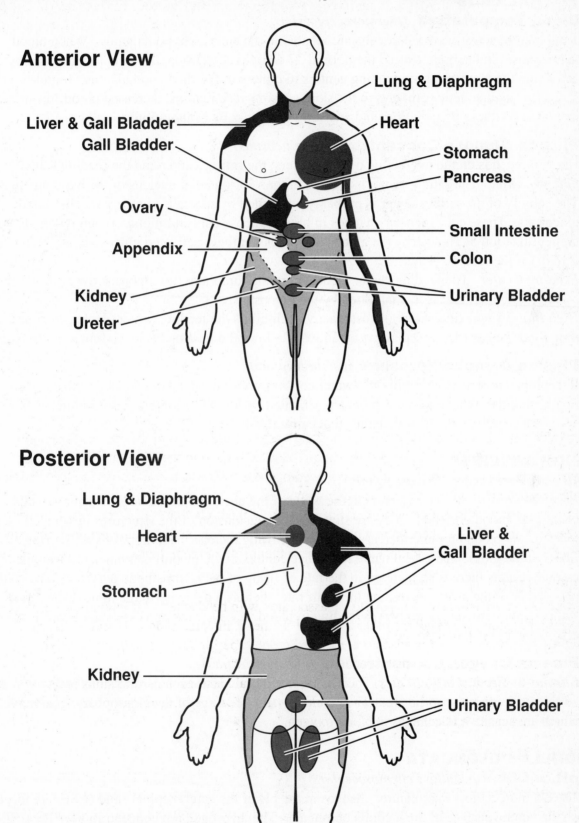

Anterior View

Lung & Diaphragm

Liver & Gall Bladder

Gall Bladder

Heart

Stomach

Pancreas

Ovary

Small Intestine

Appendix

Colon

Kidney

Urinary Bladder

Ureter

Posterior View

Lung & Diaphragm

Heart

Liver & Gall Bladder

Stomach

Kidney

Urinary Bladder

SENSORY SYSTEM / Internal Environment Receptors

HYPOTHALAMUS

Blood Temperature *(thermoreceptors)*

Temperature-sensitive receptor cells are located in the anterior hypothalamus. When blood temperatures in the brain exceed the normal 37 degrees centigrade, the receptors respond by activating the temperature-regulating centers in other parts of the hypothalamus. Impulses are sent along sympathetic pathways to the skin, causing vasodilation (increased bloodflow and increased heat loss by radiation) and sweating (heat loss by evaporation).

Plasma Glucose Concentration *(glucostats)*

Hunger depends on the interaction of two centers: the satiety center and the feeding center.
Satiety Center The satiety center is located in the ventromedial nucleus of the hypothalamus. The activity of the satiety center is probably controlled by specialized receptor cells called glucostats. These cells monitor changes in blood glucose concentrations. When blood glucose is high, utilization of glucose by the glucostats increases; these activated glucostats inhibit the activity of the feeding center.
Feeding Center The feeding center is located in the forebrain. It remains active, causing the feeling of hunger, unless it is inhibited by the glucostats.
High Blood Sugar (increased glucostat activity) inhibits the feeding center, decreasing hunger.
Low Blood Sugar (decreased glucostat activity) allows the feeding center to function normally.

Plasma Osmotic Pressure *(osmoreceptors)*

Receptors that sense the osmolality (water concentration) of blood are located in the anterior hypothalamus. When these receptors are activated by low ECF water concentrations, they stimulate centers in the hypothalamus that cause thirst.

MAJOR ARTERIES

Blood Pressure *(baroreceptors)*

Baroreceptors are stretch receptors in the walls of the heart and blood vessels that respond to changes in blood pressure. They are stimulated by distension of the structures in which they are located. As blood pressure increases, the rate of firing increases and impulses are carried by fibers of the glossopharyngeal nerve to cardiac centers in the medulla oblongata. From the cardiac centers there is an <u>increase</u> in the rate of firing of parasympathetic nerves leading to the pacemaker of the heart, decreasing the heart rate; there is a <u>decrease</u> in the tonic discharge of sympathetic vasoconstrictor nerves leading to blood vessels, causing vessels to dilate. Both effects lower the blood pressure.

Plasma Oxygen Concentration *(chemoreceptors)*

Carotid Bodies & Aortic Bodies There is a carotid body near each carotid sinus and two or more aortic bodies near the aortic arch. They contain nerve endings of the glossopharyngeal nerve, which are sensitive to changes in blood oxygen.

MEDULLA OBLONGATA

pH of CSF *(medullary chemoreceptors)*

The chemoreceptors that monitor changes in the pH of the cerebrospinal fluid (CSF) are located on the ventral surface of the medulla oblongata. The hydrogen ion concentration of the CSF parallels the carbon dioxide concentration of the arterial blood.

INTERNAL ENVIRONMENT RECEPTORS

Hypothalamus

contains receptors for :
blood temperature in the head
osmotic pressure of plasma (osmoreceptors)
blood glucose (glucostats)

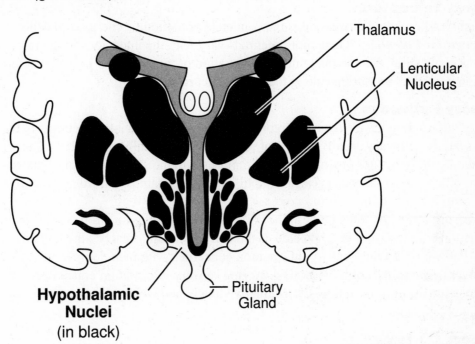

Thalamus

Lenticular Nucleus

Hypothalamic Nuclei (in black)

Pituitary Gland

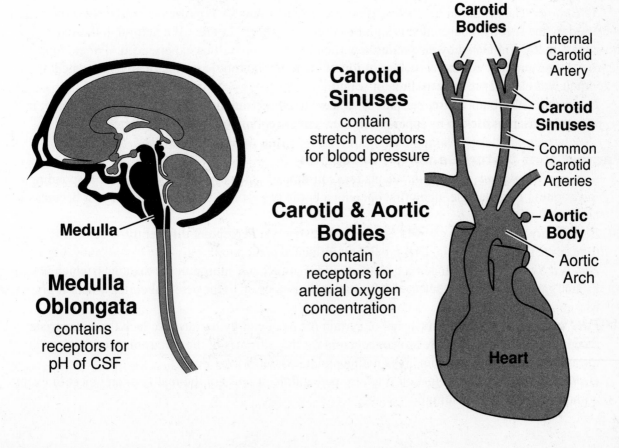

Medulla Oblongata
contains receptors for pH of CSF

Medulla

Carotid Sinuses
contain stretch receptors for blood pressure

Carotid & Aortic Bodies
contain receptors for arterial oxygen concentration

Carotid Bodies

Internal Carotid Artery

Carotid Sinuses

Common Carotid Arteries

Aortic Body

Aortic Arch

Heart

SENSORY SYSTEM / Sensory Processing

Awareness of objects and events in the world around us results from the processing of incoming sensory information. The processing of sensory information is not just a function of the brain; the stimulation of sensory receptors and the transmission of data along the sensory pathways are also important components of sensory processing.

Sensory Receptors

The first step in sensory processing is the conversion of stimulus energy into action potentials.

Generator Potentials Generator potentials vary with the intensity and the rate of change of the stimulus application; and the magnitude and duration of the generator potential determines the frequency of action potentials transmitted along the sensory neuron.

Sensory Pathways

Sensory information travels from receptors along chains of association neurons to the cerebral cortex. These sensory pathways usually consist of 3 neurons synaptically connected. The sensory neuron activated by the generator potential carries impulses into the spinal cord and synapses with an association neuron. The association neuron carries impulses to the thalamus; a third association neuron carries the impulses to a region of the sensory cortex.

Crossing Over At some point in the pathway an association neuron crosses over, so that sensory information entering from the right side of the body eventually reaches the left side of the brain and vice versa. Pathways carrying sensory information concerned with pain, temperature, touch, and pressure cross over in the spinal cord. Pathways carrying sensory information concerned with vibration, kinesthesia, stereognosis, proprioception, discriminative touch, and weight discrimination cross over in the medulla oblongata.

Sensory Cortex

Sensation The sensation or "feeling" that occurs when sensory impulses are interpreted by the brain is caused by the specific neuron that is stimulated in the cerebral cortex. If a neuron in the sensory cortex is directly stimulated by electrodes, a particular sensation will be experienced. For example, if neurons in the auditory cortex (superior portion of the temporal lobe) are electrically stimulated, the individual will experience the sensation of sound.

Projection The brain causes sensations to seem to come from the receptors being stimulated; it *projects* the sensation back to its apparent source. An exception to this rule is referred pain.

Factors that Distort Sensory Perception

Sensory Adaptation A receptor adapts to a constant stimulus by not responding (or responding at a lower rate). For example, upon first opening a bottle of perfume the scent is intense; it becomes less noticeable with time.

Personality Two people can witness the same event, yet perceive it differently. Personality, emotions, experience, and social background all influence perception.

Blocked Sensory Input Incoming sensory information passes through the thalamus, which is known as the "gatekeeper." Only selected information continues on to the cerebral cortex where it gives rise to a conscious sensation.

Lack of Receptors We are unaware of certain forms of energy because we lack the appropriate receptors. For example, there are no receptors for the extremes of the electromagnetic spectrum: ultraviolet light, x-rays, gamma rays, radio, and television waves.

Hallucinations An hallucination is a false perception; a sense of the reality of an object or event without the appropriate stimuli.

SENSORY PATHWAYS

pain / temperature

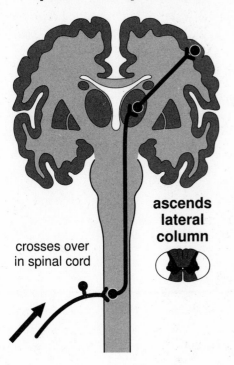

ascends lateral column

crosses over in spinal cord

touch / pressure

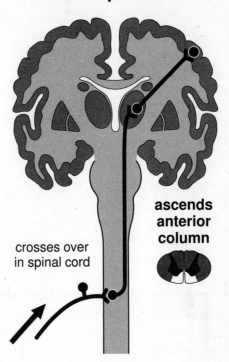

ascends anterior column

crosses over in spinal cord

vibration
kinesthesia
stereognosis
proprioception
discriminative touch
weight discrimination

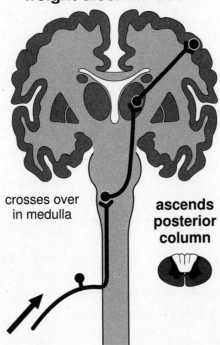

crosses over in medulla

ascends posterior column

The Eye

EYE / Nature of Light

ELECTROMAGNETIC SPECTRUM

The electromagnetic spectrum includes all the different forms of electromagnetic radiation. The types of electromagnetic radiation are determined by wavelength. In order of increasing wavelength they include: gamma rays, x-rays, ultraviolet rays, visible light rays, infrared rays, microwaves, radio, and television waves. The wavelengths range in length from a small fraction of a millimeter to several kilometers. A wavelength is the distance between two successive peaks of electromagnetic radiation.

Visible Light   Visible light rays include all electromagnetic wavelengths between 400 and 700 nanometers (nm). One nanometer is one-billionth of a meter. The receptors in the retina of the eye are sensitive only to wavelengths in this range; for this reason it is *visible* light, we can perceive it.

Colors   When visible light is split into its component wavelengths, the result is all the colors of the rainbow. As wavelengths increase from 400 nm to 700 nm, there is a gradual change in the color perceived from violet to red; in order of increasing wavelengths the colors we perceive are violet, blue, green, yellow, orange, and red. Wavelengths slightly shorter than violet are called ultraviolet; wavelengths slightly longer than red are called infrared.

OPTICS

Light Rays   The paths that light waves follow are called light rays, and for convenience are indicated as straight lines. In reality the light reflected from an object radiates out in all directions. Light waves behave more like the ripples on the surface of water than like the straight trajectory of a bullet fired from a gun.

Refraction

Light rays bend (are refracted) as they pass from one transparent medium into another of a different density. They bend because the velocity of light varies with the density of the medium; one edge of the light wave enters the second medium before the other edge, and thus changes its velocity earlier. The result is that the light wave rotates.

The degree of rotation depends upon two factors: the difference in the densities of the two media and the angle that the light ray strikes the interface between the two media. The greater the difference in densities and the more acute the angle of incidence, the greater the degree of rotation. When the light ray strikes the interface at right angles there is no refraction, because both edges of the light wave enter the second medium at the same time.

Biconvex Lenses

Focal Distance   Light rays from an object more than 20 feet away are considered to be parallel. Parallel rays striking a biconvex lens are refracted to a point behind the lens called the principal focus. The distance between the lens and the principal focus is called the principal focal distance. Light rays from an object closer than 20 feet are diverging, so the focal point is farther back.

Refractive Power of a Lens   (diopters)   The greater the curvature of a lens, the greater the refractive power (measured in diopters). A diopter is the reciprocal of the focal distance measured in meters. At rest, the lens in a human eye has a principal focal length of 15 mm (.015 meters), therefore its refractive power is 66.7 diopters (1 / .015 = 66.7).

Inverted and Reversed Image   The image projected behind a convex lens is both inverted (upside down) and reversed from left to right.

OPTICS

Refraction of Light

light rays bend as they enter obliquely
into a medium of a different density

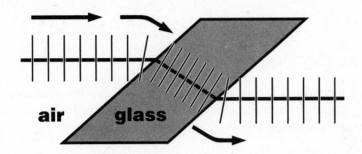

air   glass

Diffraction of Light

a beam of light passed through a glass prism
breaks up into the colors of the spectrum

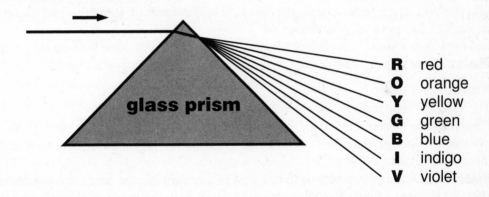

glass prism

R red
O orange
Y yellow
G green
B blue
I indigo
V violet

Inverted Image

an image passed through a lens
is turned upside down

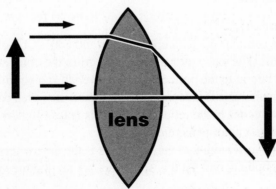

lens

EYE / Anatomy of the Eyeball

CAVITIES

There are 2 cavities in the eyeball, which are separated by the lens.

Anterior Cavity

The anterior cavity is between the lens and the cornea and is filled with a watery fluid called the *aqueous humor*; it is divided into the *anterior chamber* (anterior to the iris) and the *posterior chamber* (posterior to the iris).

Posterior Cavity

The posterior cavity (also called the *vitreous chamber*) is between the lens and the retina and is filled with a jellylike substance called the *vitreous body*.

Lens   The lens is an elastic, transparent, biconvex structure that separates the anterior and posterior cavities of the eyeball. It is suspended from the ciliary body by suspensory ligaments. Tension in the suspensory ligaments controls the shape of the lens.

TUNICS   (Layers)

The eyeball has 3 distinct tunics : an outer fibrous tunic, a middle vascular tunic, and an inner nervous tunic.

Fibrous Tunic

The outer or fibrous tunic has two parts: the tough, opaque sclera, and the transparent cornea.

Sclera   The posterior 5/6 of the fibrous tunic is called the sclera. It is a tough, opaque layer of collagenous and elastic fibers. It protects the delicate structures of the eyeball and serves as a point of attachment for the extrinsic muscles that control movements of the eyeball.

Cornea   The anterior 1/6 of the fibrous tunic is called the cornea. It is a transparent structure consisting of an orderly arrangement of collagen fibers. It bulges forward, forming a convex surface that bends (refracts) light rays as they enter the eye.

Scleral Venous Sinus   (canal of Schlemm) At the junction of the sclera and the cornea there is a sinus that drains the aqueous humor from the anterior chamber of the eyeball into the blood.

Vascular Tunic

The vascular tunic includes the choroid, the ciliary body, and the iris.

Choroid   The posterior 5/6 of the vascular tunic is called the choroid. It contains blood vessels and melanin-producing cells called melanocytes. Melanin is a pigment that absorbs light after it passes through the retina.

Ciliary Body   The ciliary body is the thickest part of the vascular tunic. It extends forward from the choroid, forming a ring in the anterior part of the eyeball. Radiating folds called ciliary processes secrete aqueous humor into the anterior cavity.

Iris   The iris is a structure extending out from the ciliary body; it is anterior to the lens. The opening in the center of the iris is called the *pupil*. Reflexes control the size of the pupil, and thus regulate how much light enters the eyeball.

Retina (Inner Nervous Tunic)

Cell Types   The retina contains photoreceptors (rods and cones), bipolar cells, horizontal cells, amacrine cells, and ganglion cells. The axons of ganglion cells form the optic nerve.

Fovea Centralis   Just lateral to the optic axis of the eyeball is a yellowish spot called the *macula lutea*. In the center of the macula lutea is a depressed area called the fovea centralis. The fovea centralis has the highest concentration of cones in the retina, and for this reason light that strikes this area produces the sharpest vision and the best color perception.

Optic Disc (blind spot) Just medial to the optic axis is the area where the fibers of the ganglion cells exit the eyeball to form the optic nerve. At this spot there are no photoreceptors, so light striking this area produces no image.

EYEBALL ANATOMY
right eyeball viewed from above

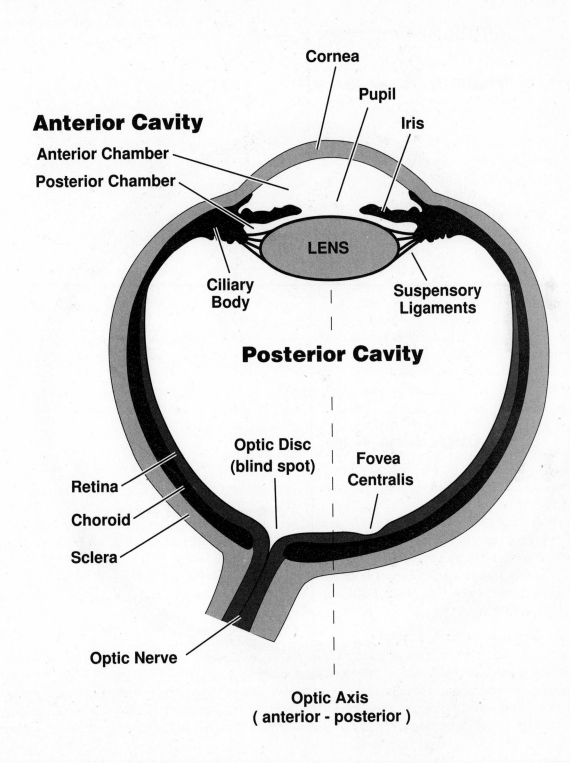

Cornea

Pupil

Iris

Anterior Cavity

Anterior Chamber

Posterior Chamber

LENS

Ciliary Body

Suspensory Ligaments

Posterior Cavity

Optic Disc (blind spot)

Fovea Centralis

Retina

Choroid

Sclera

Optic Nerve

Optic Axis (anterior - posterior)

RIGHT EYEBALL
viewed from above

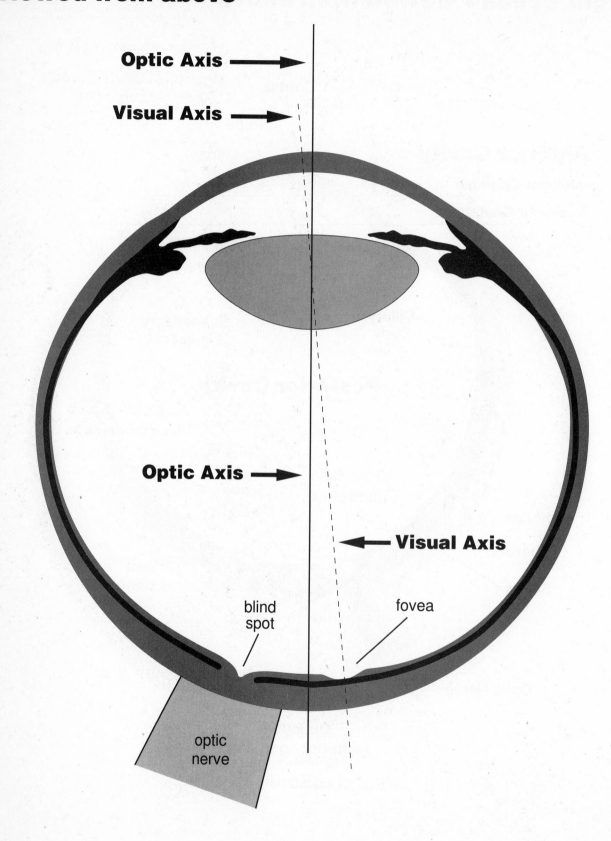

Optic Axis ➝

Visual Axis ➝

Optic Axis ➝

← Visual Axis

blind
spot

fovea

optic
nerve

RETINA
left eyeball as seen through an ophthalmoscope

Optic Disc
(blind spot)
blood vessels & optic nerve
enter and exit here

Fovea Centralis
concentration of cones
for color vision &
high visual acuity

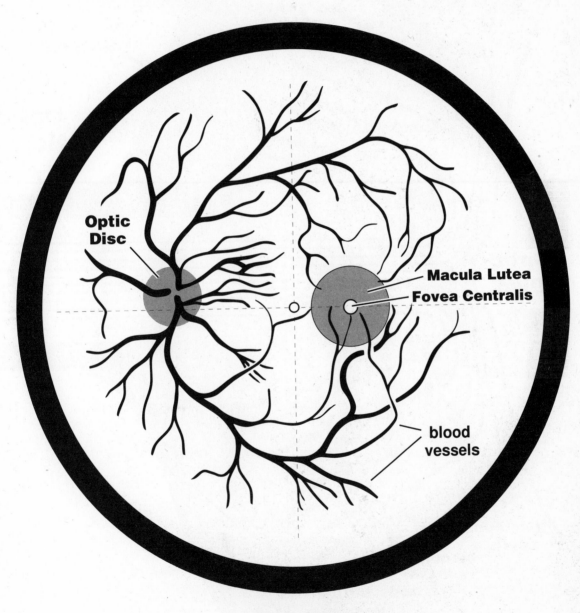

Optic
Disc

Macula Lutea
Fovea Centralis

blood
vessels

Optic Axis
(at center of crossed dashed lines)

RETINA AND OPTIC NERVE

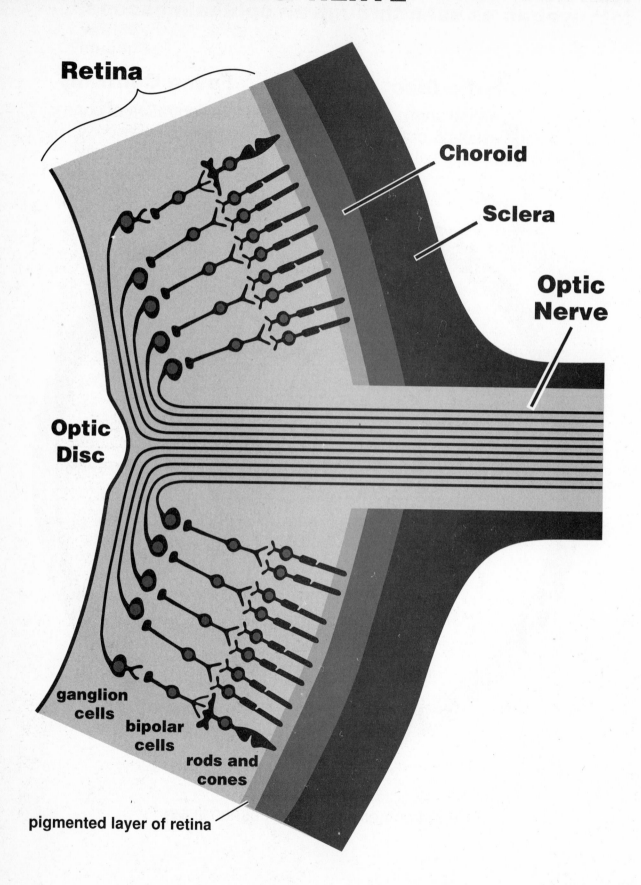

Retina

Choroid

Sclera

Optic Nerve

Optic Disc

ganglion cells

bipolar cells

rods and cones

pigmented layer of retina

160

RETINA ULTRASTRUCTURE

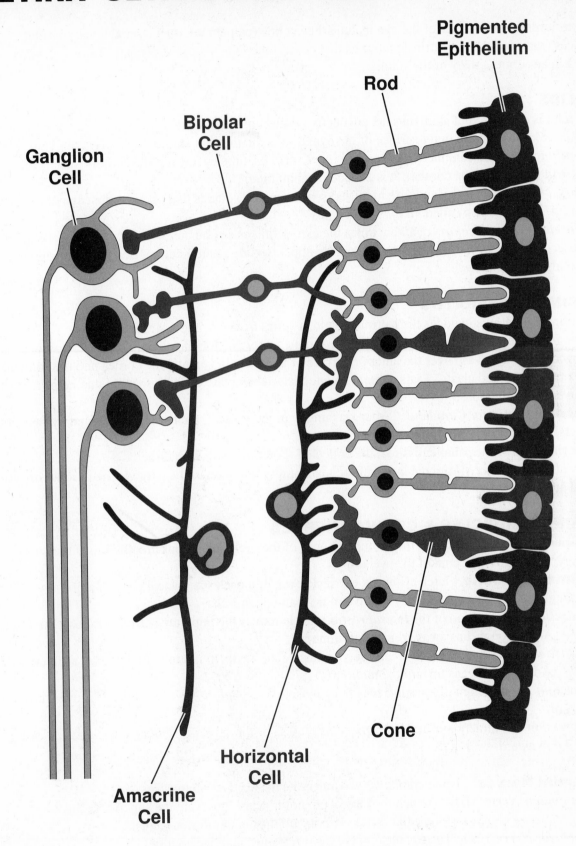

Ganglion
Cell

Bipolar
Cell

Rod

Pigmented
Epithelium

Amacrine
Cell

Horizontal
Cell

Cone

EYE / Accessory Structures

The accessory structures of the eye include the eyelids (palpebrae), the lacrimal apparatus that produces tears, and the six extrinsic muscles that control movements of the eyeball. Each eyeball is housed in an *orbital cavity* of the skull.

EYELIDS

The eyelid is composed of skin, muscle, connective tissue, and conjunctiva.

Skin   Skin covers the outer surface of the eyelid; it is the thinnest skin of the body.

Conjunctiva   The conjunctiva covers the inner surface of the eyelid and the anterior surface of the eyeball (except for the cornea); it is a mucous membrane.

Tarsal Glands   Tarsal glands are modified sebaceous (oil) glands that open on the edge of each eyelid. They are also called *Meibomian glands*.

Muscles   The *orbicularis oculi* encircles the eye, acting as a sphincter; when it contracts, the eyelids close. The *levator palpebrae* is located in the upper eyelid; when it contracts, it raises the upper eyelid, opening the eye.

LACRIMAL APPARATUS

The lacrimal apparatus includes the lacrimal gland, a series of ducts, and a lacrimal sac.

Lacrimal Gland   A lacrimal gland is located in the upper portion of each orbit. It secretes a constant flow of tears that wash over the anterior surface of the eyeball, keeping the cornea and the conjunctiva moistened and clean. Tears contain an antibacterial enzyme called lysozyme that helps to prevent eye infections.

Superior & Inferior Canaliculi   After washing over the eyeball, the tears are collected by two small ducts, the superior and inferior canaliculi.

Lacrimal Sac   The canaliculi direct the collected tears into the lacrimal sac.

Nasolacrimal Duct   From the lacrimal sac tears empty into the nasal cavity via the nasolacrimal duct and are swallowed.

EXTRINSIC MUSCLES & CRANIAL NERVES

The extrinsic muscles of the eye arise from the bones of the orbit and are inserted by broad tendons on the sclera, the tough outer coat of the eyeball.

Primary Actions   Each of the six extrinsic eyeball muscles is associated with a primary action, although any eye movement may involve more than one muscle.

Abduction   Contraction of the *lateral rectus* muscle moves the pupil away from the nose, out to the side. (Abduction means away from the midline)

Adduction   Contraction of the *medial rectus* muscle moves the pupil toward the nose, as in crossed eyes. (Adduction means toward the midline)

Elevation   Contraction of the *superior rectus* muscle or the *inferior oblique* muscle moves the pupil upward.

Depression   Contraction of the *inferior rectus* muscle or the *superior oblique* muscle moves the pupil downward.

Cranial Nerves   Three cranial nerves innervate the six eyeball muscles.

Oculomotor Nerve (III)   Branches of the oculomotor nerve innervate the superior rectus, medial rectus, inferior oblique, and inferior rectus.

Trochlear Nerve (IV)   The trochlear nerve innervates the superior oblique.

Abducens Nerve (VI)   The abducens nerve innervates the lateral rectus.

EYE : Accessory Structures
Eyelid & Conjunctiva

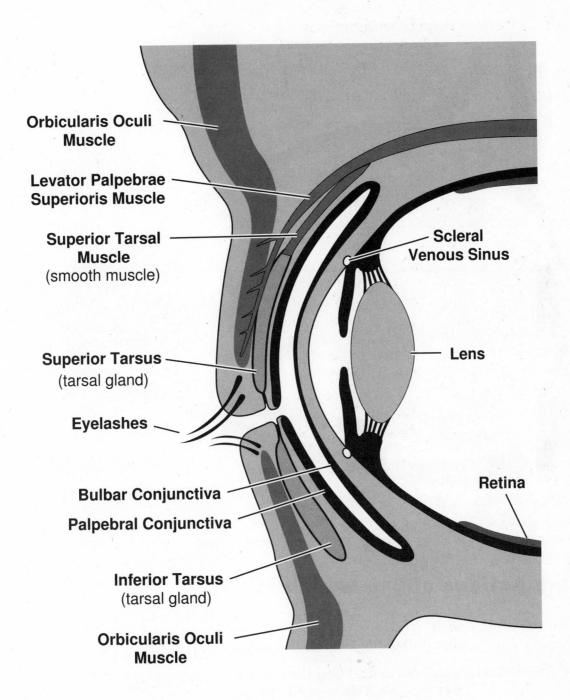

Orbicularis Oculi Muscle

Levator Palpebrae Superioris Muscle

Superior Tarsal Muscle (smooth muscle)

Scleral Venous Sinus

Superior Tarsus (tarsal gland)

Lens

Eyelashes

Bulbar Conjunctiva

Palpebral Conjunctiva

Retina

Inferior Tarsus (tarsal gland)

Orbicularis Oculi Muscle

EYE MUSCLES
6 muscles that move the eyeball
(and the levator palpebrae superioris, which raises the upper eyelid)

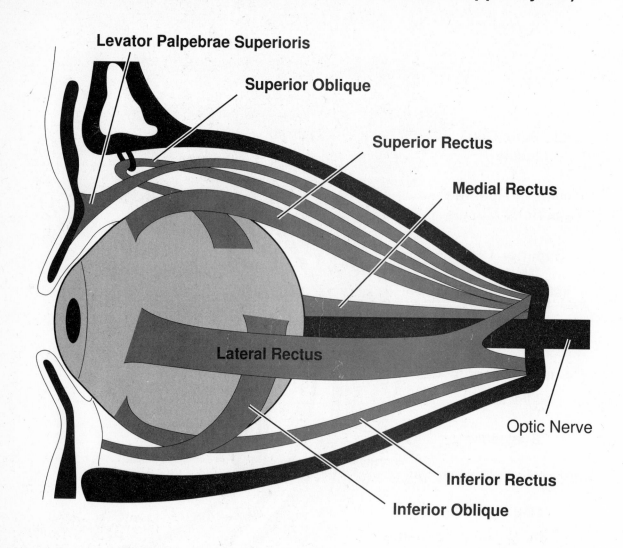

Levator Palpebrae Superioris

Superior Oblique

Superior Rectus

Medial Rectus

Lateral Rectus

Optic Nerve

Inferior Rectus

Inferior Oblique

Primary Actions of Eye Muscles:

Abduction   pupil moves away from the midline
eye muscle : Lateral Rectus

Adduction   pupil moves toward the midline
eye muscle : Medial Rectus

Elevation   pupil moves upward
eye muscles : Superior Rectus & Inferior Oblique

Depression   pupil moves downward
eye muscles : Inferior Rectus & Superior Oblique

LACRIMAL APPARATUS

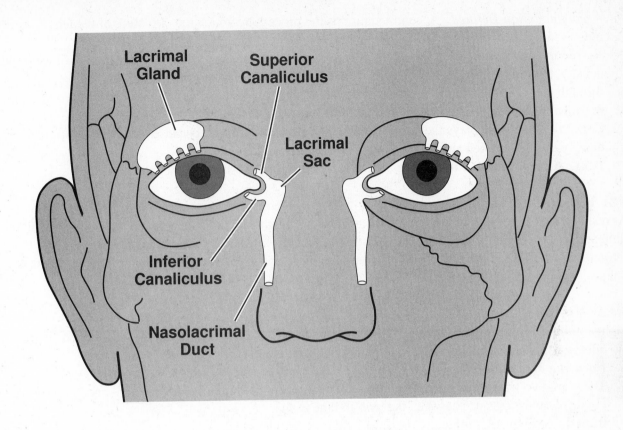

Lacrimal Gland

Superior Canaliculus

Lacrimal Sac

Inferior Canaliculus

Nasolacrimal Duct

Cranial Nerves to the Eye Muscles

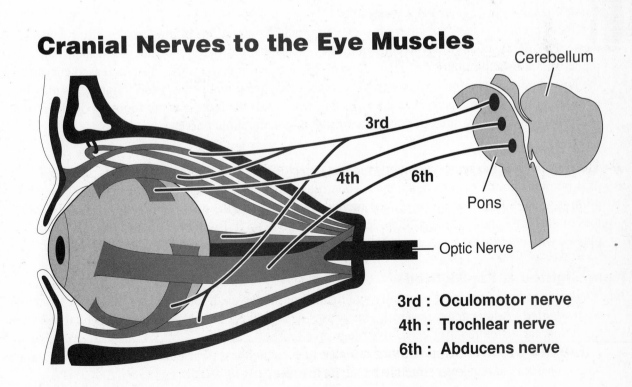

Cerebellum

3rd

4th

6th

Pons

Optic Nerve

3rd : Oculomotor nerve

4th : Trochlear nerve

6th : Abducens nerve

EYE / Lens Accommodation

Accommodation Defined Accommodation is the process by which the curvature of the lens is increased for near vision.

Refraction of Light Rays When light rays pass from one transparent medium to another of different density, they bend (refract) and change direction. This happens four times as a light ray passes through the eye to the retina. It occurs at the interfaces between the air and the cornea, the cornea and the aqueous humor, the aqueous humor and the lens, and the lens and the vitreous body.

Cornea The cornea plays the largest role in the refraction of light, because the greatest difference in density occurs between air and the tissues of the cornea.

Lens All adjustments for distance are made by changing the shape of the lens.

Far Vision

At rest, the lens is held under tension by the suspensory ligaments; the tension pulls the elastic lens into a flattened shape. Light coming from an object over 20 feet away strikes the eye in parallel rays, and the refractory power of the eye is sufficient to bring the light rays to focus on the retina, producing a sharp image.

Near Vision

Light coming from near objects (closer that 20 feet) strikes the eye as diverging rays. If the lens is flat, the light rays focus behind the retina, producing a blurred image.

Focusing Mechanisms

There are two ways to bring diverging rays to a focus on the retina:

(1) Increase the distance between the lens and the retina.

Bony fish achieve this effect by increasing their eyeball length.

Cameras are focused on near objects by moving the lens farther away from the film.

(2) Increase the curvature of the lens. This is called accommodation.

Ciliary Muscles & Suspensory Ligaments

To focus on near objects the ciliary muscles contract. Contractions of the *circular* ciliary muscles cause the ringlike ciliary body to constrict; this relaxes the tension on the attached suspensory ligaments and allows the anterior surface of the elastic lens to bulge forward. The increased curvature of the lens increases its refractory power. The degree of tension on the suspensory ligaments may be adjusted until the image perceived is sharp; this means that the light rays are focusing on the retina. The ciliary muscles are smooth muscles controlled by autonomic nerves.

Near Point

The near point is the nearest point at which an object can be brought into clear focus. At age 10 the near point is about 10 cm from the eye. The distance becomes greater with age; at age 60 the near point is about 80 cm from the eye. The increasing distance of the near point is due primarily to the loss of elasticity and hardening of the lens. By age 40 to 45 it usually becomes necessary to use glasses with convex lenses to assist in the refraction of the diverging light rays of near objects.

Near-Sighted & Far-Sighted

Inherited near or far-sightedness is usually due to an abnormal eyeball length.

Near-sighted A long anteroposterior axis causes near-sightedness. Near objects can be focused on the retina; far vision requires corrective biconcave lenses.

Far-sighted A short anteroposterior axis causes far-sightedness. Far objects can be focused on the retina; near vision requires corrective biconvex lenses.

LENS ACCOMMODATION

When the eye focuses on near objects, ciliary muscles contract,
relaxing the tension on the suspensory ligaments of the lens.
This allows the elastic lens to contract and bulge, becoming more rounded.

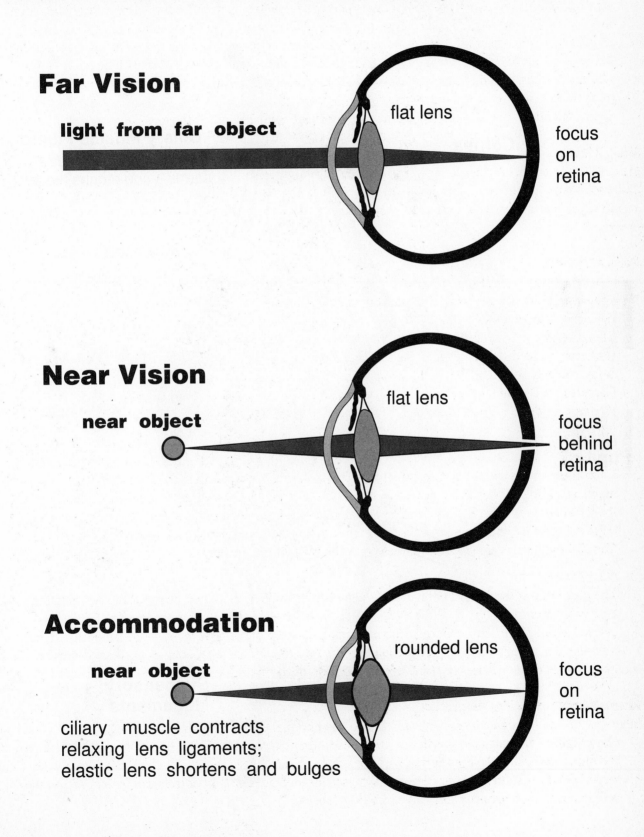

Far Vision

light from far object

flat lens

focus
on
retina

Near Vision

near object

flat lens

focus
behind
retina

Accommodation

near object

rounded lens

focus
on
retina

ciliary muscle contracts
relaxing lens ligaments;
elastic lens shortens and bulges

CILIARY MUSCLES

For near vision, the ciliary muscles contract.
This decreases the tension on the suspensory ligaments;
the elastic lens bulges, becoming more rounded.

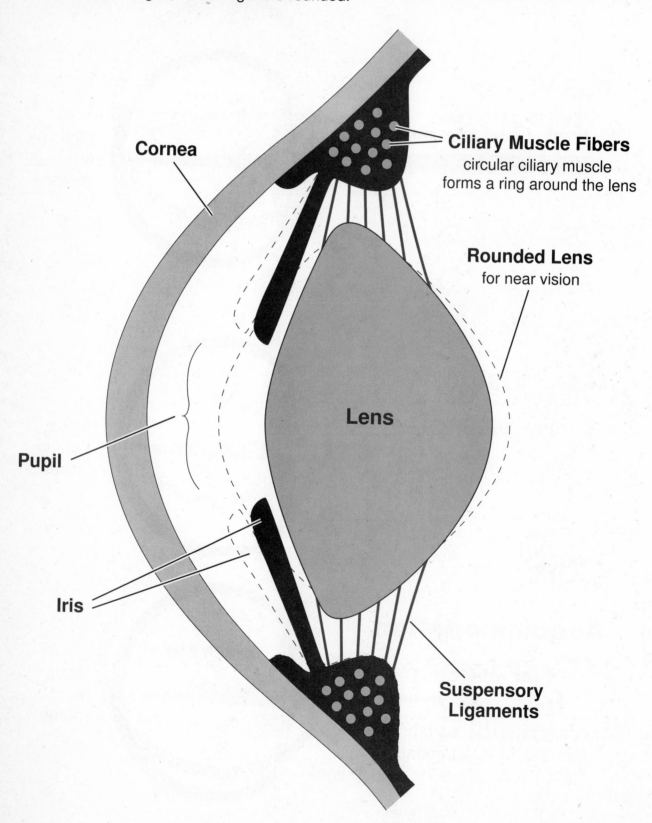

Cornea

Ciliary Muscle Fibers
circular ciliary muscle
forms a ring around the lens

Rounded Lens
for near vision

Lens

Pupil

Iris

Suspensory Ligaments

EYEBALL SHAPES

The focus of light rays on the retina is affected by the length of the optic axis.

Normal Eye

(Emmetropic Eye)

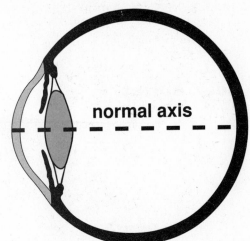

normal axis

Farsighted Eye

(Hypermetropic Eye)

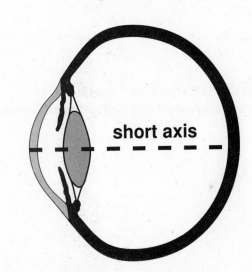

short axis

Nearsighted Eye

(Myopic Eye)

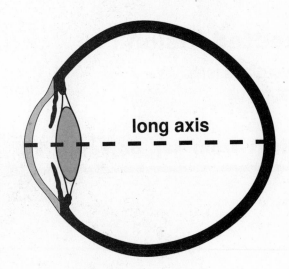

long axis

NEARSIGHTED EYE (Myopic Eye)
far objects unclear

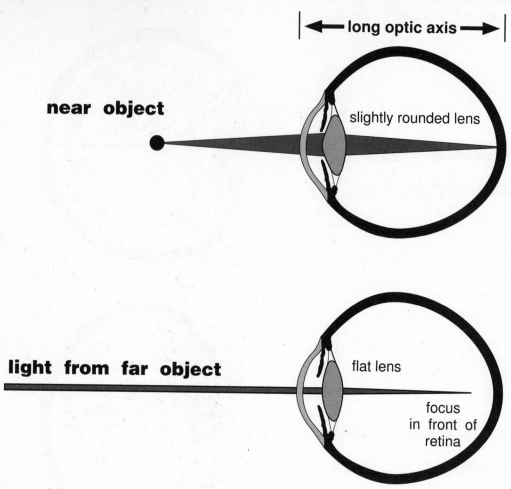

long optic axis

near object

slightly rounded lens

light from far object

flat lens

focus
in front of
retina

Corrected Vision :

concave glass lens
corrects focus

light from far object

flat lens

FARSIGHTED EYE (Hypermetropic Eye)
near objects unclear

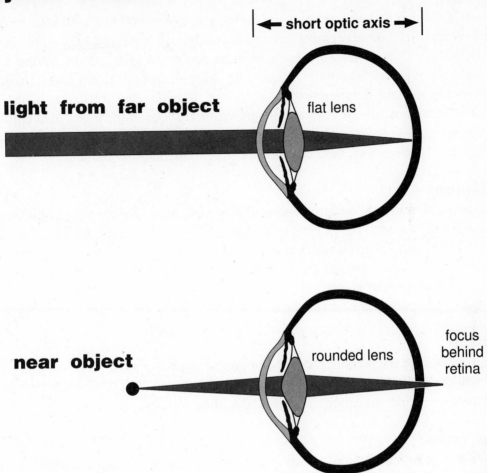

short optic axis

light from far object

flat lens

near object

rounded lens

focus
behind
retina

Corrected Vision :

convex glass lens
corrects focus

near object

rounded lens

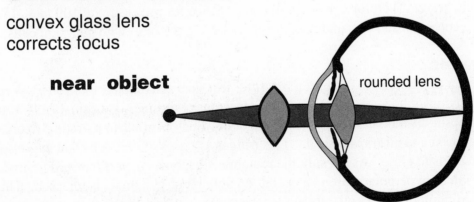

EYE / Photoreceptors : Rods

Structures

Each rod cell is divided into an outer and an inner segment.

Outer Segment The outer segment has a thin, rod-shaped appearance. It contains many flattened saccules or discs called *lamellae*, which are composed of membrane and arranged parallel to the light-receiving surface of the retina. The photosensitive pigment called rhodopsin is an integral part of the lamellar membrane. New discs (lamellae) are constantly being formed at the inner edge, and old worn-out discs are phagocytized by cells of the pigmented epithelium.

Inner Segment The inner segment contains many mitochondria, the cell nucleus, and the synaptic base. The synaptic base contains the neurotransmitter *glutamate*.

Photopigment

Photopigments The light-sensitive molecules in rods and cones are called photopigments. There are four different types of photopigments present in the retina; each is made up of a protein bound to Vitamin A (more accurately, the aldehyde of vitamin A). The aldehyde of vitamin A is called *retinal* or *retinene* and it is the same in all four photopigments. The protein or *opsin* differs in each of the four types.

Rhodopsin The photopigment in rods is called rhodopsin. Its protein is called *scotopsin*.

Distribution

Location Rods are the predominant type of photoreceptor in all areas of the retina except the fovea centralis. The fovea centralis contains only cone cells.

Concentration There are approximately 120 million rods in each eye.

Types of Vision

Night Vision (Scotopic Vision) Rods are extremely sensitive to light. In the dim light of night they are the only photoreceptors that are stimulated.

Black & White Vision Rods do not distinguish between different colors; at night all images are black, white, and shades of gray.

Low Visual Acuity The image produced by the stimulation of rods is not sharp. The brain cannot know precisely where a given ray of light has struck the retina, because many rods converge on the same ganglion cell. Thus, the information transmitted by the ganglion cell is vague and the image produced is fuzzy. There are 120 million rods in each eye and 1.2 million nerve fibers in each optic nerve. Therefore, the overall convergence for rods is about 100 to 1. (There are only 6 million cones in each eye, and many of them have a 1:1 ratio with ganglion cells).

Receptor Activation

In the dark there is a steady release of neurotransmitter from the synaptic base of rods. When light is absorbed by rhodopsin it causes a change in the structure of retinal: scotopsin-11-cis- retinal is converted into scotopsin-all-trans-retinal, which is unstable. Scotopsin-all-trans-retinal spontaneously breaks into scotopsin and all-trans-retinal. This triggers a series of reactions that cause some of the sodium ion channels to <u>close</u>. As a result, the membrane becomes *hyper*polarized (a graded potential). As the result of hyperpolarization, a decreased amount of glutamate is released. This change activates the adjoining bipolar cell, which then activates an adjacent ganglion cell, producing a nerve impulse that is transmitted to the brain.

RODS : Rhodopsin Cycle

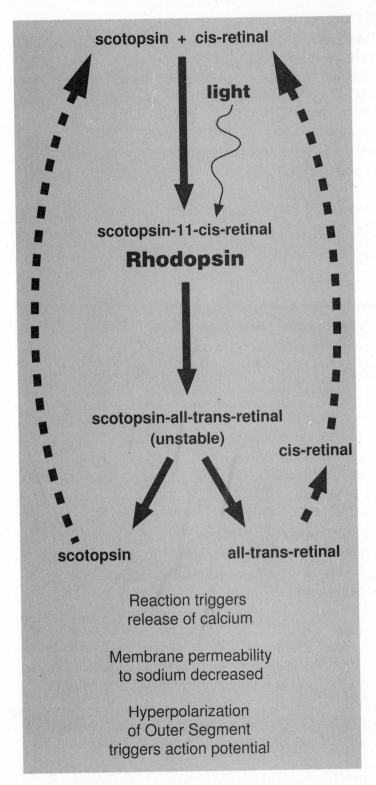

scotopsin + cis-retinal

light

scotopsin-11-cis-retinal
Rhodopsin

scotopsin-all-trans-retinal
(unstable)

cis-retinal

scotopsin   all-trans-retinal

Reaction triggers
release of calcium

Membrane permeability
to sodium decreased

Hyperpolarization
of Outer Segment
triggers action potential

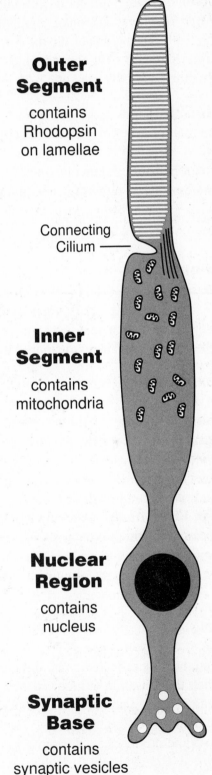

Outer Segment

contains
Rhodopsin
on lamellae

Connecting
Cilium

Inner Segment

contains
mitochondria

Nuclear Region

contains
nucleus

Synaptic Base

contains
synaptic vesicles

EYE / Photoreceptors : Cones

Structure
Each cone is divided into an outer and an inner segment.

Outer Segment The outer segment has a conical shape. It contains pigment-containing saccules formed by infoldings of the the cell membrane.

Inner Segment The inner segment contains many mitochondria, the cell nucleus, and a large synaptic base. The synaptic base contains neurotransmitter (probably glutamate).

Photopigments
There are three types of cones; each contains a pigment that is sensitive to a specific range of color.

Blue-Sensitive Pigments (maximal response: 440 nm)

Green-Sensitive Pigments (maximal response: 535 nm)

Red-Sensitive Pigments (maximal response: 565 nm)

Genetics chromosome 7 : gene for blue-sensitive pigment
X chromosome : genes for red-sensitive and green-sensitive pigments

Distribution
Fovea Centralis The fovea centralis contains a high concentration of cones (and no rods). In the fovea centralis other retinal layers and retinal blood vessels are displaced to one side, creating a slight depression, and increasing the exposure of the cones to incoming light rays.

Concentration There are approximately 6 million cones in each eye.

Types of Vision
Daytime Vision (bright light sensitivity) High levels of light are needed to activate the visual pathways that begin with the cones; cones do not respond to low intensity light. In bright light rods have reached their maximal levels of response, so they have little or no function.

Color Vision Each of the three types of cones is maximally sensitive to a particular frequency (color) of light. The sensation of color produced in the brain results from comparing the degrees of stimulation of the three types of cones.

High Visual Acuity (sharp images) Most cone cells in the fovea centralis synapse with one bipolar cell, which synapses with one ganglion cell; thus, there is no convergence. Each foveal cone is connected to a single fiber in the optic nerve, and, consequently, the brain knows precisely where the light stimulus is striking the retina.

Color
A *pigment* is a substance that reflects certain wavelengths of light and absorbs other wavelengths. If an object appears green, it contains pigments that reflect green light and absorb all other wavelengths. The reflected green light enters the eye and is absorbed by green-sensitive cones, producing the sensation of green in the brain. Each type of cone responds maximally to one specific wavelength, but it also responds to other wavelengths. So, for any given wavelength, all three cones are stimulated to different degrees. The brain adds up the degrees of stimulation of the three cone cell types and produces a color sensation.

White & Black Light from the sun is perceived as white when reflected from an object that contains no pigment. It is a mixture of all the wavelengths of the visible spectrum, so all the cones are maximally stimulated. Black is the absence of all light. When an object contains a pigment that absorbs all wavelengths of light, no cones are activated and we see black.

CONES : Color Perception

Electromagnetic Spectrum

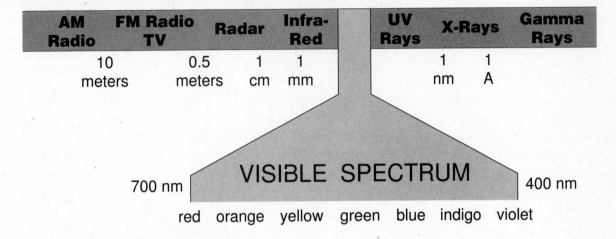

AM Radio	FM Radio TV	Radar	Infra-Red		UV Rays	X-Rays	Gamma Rays
10 meters	0.5 meters	1 cm	1 mm		1 nm	1 A	

VISIBLE SPECTRUM

700 nm   400 nm

red   orange   yellow   green   blue   indigo   violet

Absorption of Light by 3 Types of Cones

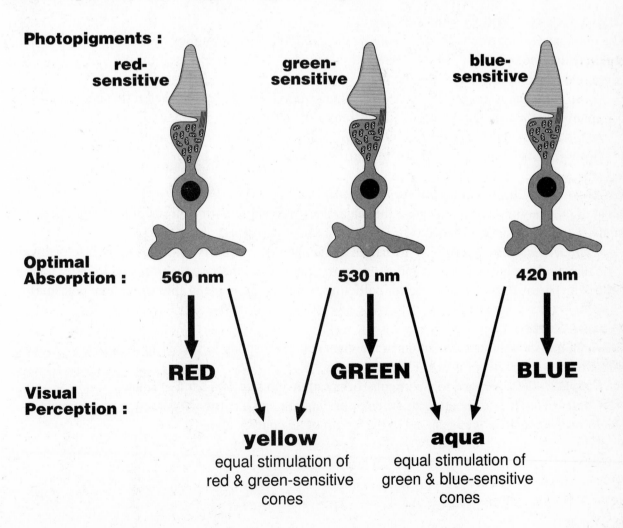

Photopigments :

red-sensitive   green-sensitive   blue-sensitive

Optimal Absorption :   560 nm   530 nm   420 nm

RED   GREEN   BLUE

Visual Perception :

yellow   aqua

equal stimulation of red & green-sensitive cones

equal stimulation of green & blue-sensitive cones

EYE / Visual Pathway

The visual pathway begins in the retina, travels via the optic nerve to the lateral geniculate nucleus in the thalamus, and ends in various regions of the brain (especially in the visual cortex of the occipital lobe). The processing of visual information occurs along the entire pathway, not just in the brain.

Retina

The visual pathway begins in the photoreceptors of the retina. Rods are stimulated by low intensity light, and the three types of cones are stimulated by high intensity light of different colors (wavelengths). Rods and cones synapse with bipolar cells, which in turn synapse with ganglion cells. Horizontal cells allow visual information to flow between rods and cones; amacrine cells transfer visual information horizontally between bipolar cells and ganglion cells.

Receptive Field   A receptive field is an area of the retina that, when stimulated by light, can influence the activity of a particular neuron in the visual pathway.

On-Center Ganglion Cell   An on-center ganglion cell increases its rate of firing when light stimulates a spot in the center of its receptive field.

Off-Center Ganglion Cell   An off-center ganglion cell increases its rate of firing when light stimulates a ring in the periphery of its receptive field.

Optic Nerve   (2nd Cranial Nerve)

The optic nerves are formed by the axons of the ganglion cells. Ganglion cells exit the eyeball in the region called the optic disc, which is located just medial to the optic axis of the eyeball. The optic nerves carry visual information to the brain.

Optic Chiasma (crossing over)   Nerve fibers from the *nasal* half of each retina cross over just anterior to the pituitary gland. This portion of the optic nerves is called the optic chiasma.   As a result of crossing over, fibers from the right half of each retina carry impulses to the right brain; fibers from the left half of each retina carry impulses to the left brain.

Thalamus   (Lateral Geniculate Nucleus)

Most of the ganglion cell axons enter the thalamus and synapse with neurons in the lateral geniculate nucleus, which is located in the posterior portion of the thalamus.

Optic Radiations   Neurons in the lateral geniculate nucleus carry impulses in diverse pathways called optic radiations. Optic radiations carry impulses to the visual cortex and to other non-cortical areas of the brain (superior colliculus, cerebellum, nucleus above the optic chiasma).

Visual Cortex

Research has shown that the neurons in the visual cortex respond to slits of light or edges. There are three basic types of neurons in the visual cortex:

Simple Cells :   respond to a particular orientation and size of a band of light.

Complex Cells :   respond to a particular orientation and a particular direction of an edge.

Hypercomplex Cells :   respond to the length of an edge or line.

VISUAL PATHWAY

Visual information received by the right side of each retina travels to the right occipital lobe of the brain.

Visual information received by the left side of each retina travels to the left occipital lobe of the brain.

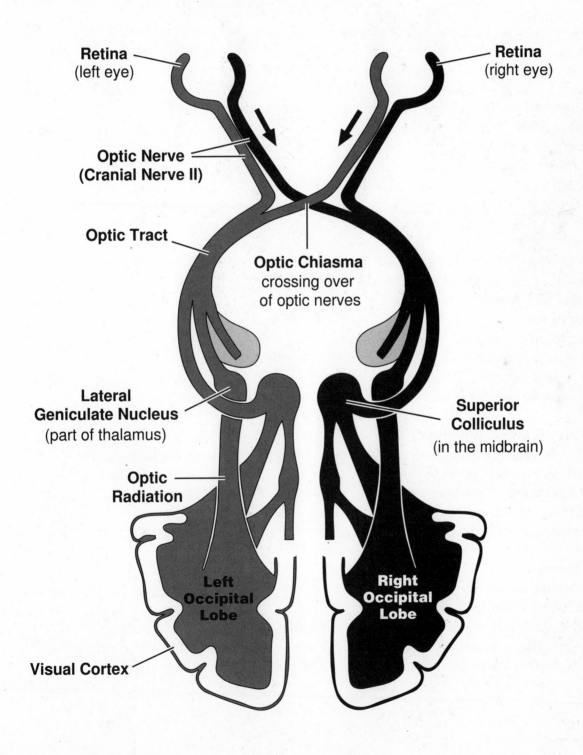

Retina
(left eye)

Retina
(right eye)

Optic Nerve
(Cranial Nerve II)

Optic Tract

Optic Chiasma
crossing over
of optic nerves

Lateral
Geniculate Nucleus
(part of thalamus)

Superior
Colliculus
(in the midbrain)

Optic
Radiation

Left
Occipital
Lobe

Right
Occipital
Lobe

Visual Cortex

The Ear

EAR / The Nature of Sound

Sound Waves

Sound sensations heard by the ear are caused by vibrations transmitted through the air. When an object vibrates, it generates waves in the gas or liquid that surrounds it. This can be observed when an object vibrates in water: how close together the waves are depends on the frequency of the vibrations; how high the waves are depends on the amplitude of the vibrations.

Regions of Compression & Rarefaction When an object (such as a tuning fork) vibrates in air, it generates regions of compression and rarefaction. As the arms of the tuning fork move outward, they push air molecules ahead of them, creating a zone of compression (high density molecules). When the arms of the tuning fork move back, they leave a partial vacuum with few air molecules — the zone of rarefaction. A chain reaction occurs: the molecules in the zone of compression collide with the molecules ahead of them, creating a new zone of compression, and so on. These self-generating zones of dense and rarefied air molecules are the sound waves. They travel through the air and into the external auditory canal, where they cause the eardrum to vibrate.

Pitch

Frequency The frequency of vibrations of the sound source determines the pitch. The higher the frequency of vibrations, the higher the pitch (in music, the higher the note). In the human voice, the pitch is determined by the vibrations of the vocal cords that are located in the voice box (larynx). In stringed instruments, thicker and longer strings vibrate at lower frequencies. The same is true of vocal cords; relaxing the tension on a vocal cord lowers its frequency of vibrations, producing a lower note.

Pure Tones A tuning fork for a particular note vibrates at a single fixed frequency, so the regions of compression and rarefaction are evenly spaced, producing a pure tone.

Timbre Most sounds are complex waves made up of many frequencies. The *timbre* is the quality of a sound that makes it possible to determine the sources of two different sounds of the same pitch. For example, the note C played on the piano and on the flute: although each note has the same pitch (frequency), it is easy to distinguish the sources because of the *overtones* (secondary frequencies that mix with the fundamental frequency).

Hertz (Hz) The unit for measuring the frequency of sound waves is the hertz.

One hertz is equal to one cycle per second.

Loudness

Loudness is determined by the amplitude of the sound waves.

Amplitude Amplitude is the difference between the molecular density in the zones of compression and rarefaction.

Decibels The unit for measuring the loudness of a sound (wave magnitude) is the decibel. Human conversation must be at about 40 decibels to be heard.

Damage to Receptors The receptor cells (hair cells) of the internal ear are damaged by excessively loud noises. High-intensity noise, such as that produced by amplified music, jet planes, and power equipment, causes the receptor cells to become malformed and nonfunctional. Long term exposure to loud sounds (less intense than those mentioned above) causes receptor cells and supporting cells to degenerate with serious loss of hearing.

THE NATURE OF SOUND

Vibrations

vibrations produce areas of
rarefaction & compression

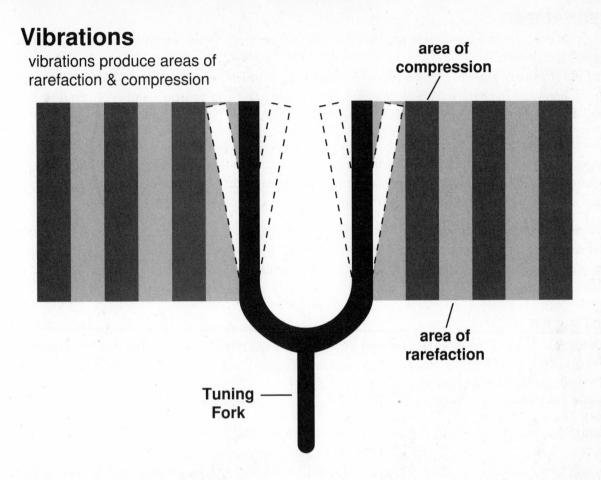

area of
compression

area of
rarefaction

Tuning
Fork

Human Audibility Curve

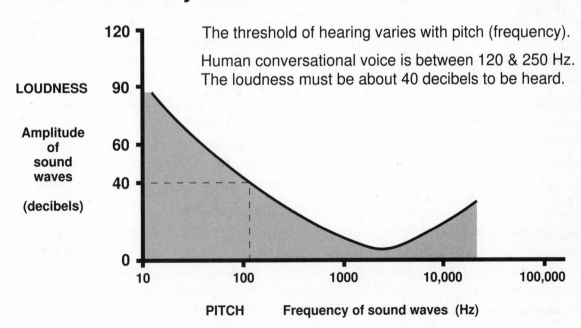

The threshold of hearing varies with pitch (frequency).

Human conversational voice is between 120 & 250 Hz.
The loudness must be about 40 decibels to be heard.

LOUDNESS

Amplitude
of
sound
waves

(decibels)

120

90

60

40

0

10   100   1000   10,000   100,000

PITCH   Frequency of sound waves (Hz)

EXTERNAL EAR

The external ear includes the auricle (pinna), the external auditory canal (meatus), and the tympanic membrane (eardrum).

Auricle (Pinna)   The auricle is a funnel-shaped structure that helps to collect sound waves and direct them into the external auditory canal. It is made of elastic cartilage and is covered by a thick layer of skin. The rim is called the *helix* and the inferior portion is the *lobule* (ear lobe).

External Auditory Canal (Meatus)   The external auditory canal is a tube about 1 inch long, extending from the pinna to the eardrum; it lies in the temporal bone of the skull. Near the exterior opening it contains *ceruminous glands* that secrete cerumen (ear wax). The ear wax and hairs in the same region help to trap foreign matter and keep the tympanic membrane clean.

Tympanic Membrane (Eardrum)   The tympanic membrane is a thin semitransparent membrane that separates the auditory canal from the middle ear. It is a cone-shaped structure with the apex directed inward. Sound waves in the auditory canal cause pressure changes that produce eardrum vibrations.

MIDDLE EAR

The middle ear is an air-filled cavity located between the eardrum and the internal ear. It contains three small bones called the auditory ossicles and is connected to the mouth cavity by a narrow tube called the auditory (Eustachian) tube.

Tympanic Cavity   The middle ear is also called the tympanic cavity.

Auditory Ossicles (Malleus, Incus, & Stapes)   Three small bones transfer vibrations from the eardrum to the oval window of the internal ear. The malleus (hammer) is attached to the internal surface of the eardrum at its apex; the incus (anvil) is the intermediate bone; the footplate of the stapes (stirrup) is attached to the membrane of the oval window.

The malleus vibrates in unison with the tympanic membrane, passes the vibrations to the incus, and the incus causes the stapes to vibrate on the oval window. As a result, the oval window is pushed in and out, causing motion in the fluid within the internal ear. The action of the fluid activates receptor cells (hair cells), which send impulses to the temporal lobe of the cerebrum and cause the sensation of sound.

Stapedius & Tensor Tympani Muscles   The ossicles are attached to the tympanic membrane and the walls of the tympanic cavity by muscles and ligaments which help regulate the tension on the tympanic membrane. Adjustments in muscle tension help to protect the delicate receptor cells of the internal ear from loud noises. The *tensor tympani muscle* prevents damage from prolonged loud noises; the *stapedius muscle* prevents damage from brief loud noises, such as a gunshot.

Auditory (Eustachian) Tube   For the tympanic membrane to function properly, the air pressure must be the same on both sides. The auditory tube connects the tympanic cavity with the mouth cavity (specifically, with the nasopharynx). So when the atmospheric pressure changes, the pressure changes in both the external auditory canal and the tympanic cavity. For this reason there is no change in the tension of the tympanic membrane, and it functions optimally. If for some reason the auditory tube is blocked (inflammation during a cold), pressure equilibrium is not maintained and hearing is impaired.

EAR ANATOMY

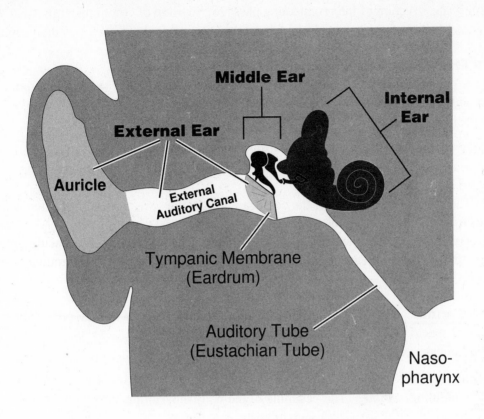

Middle Ear

External Ear

Internal Ear

Auricle

External Auditory Canal

Tympanic Membrane (Eardrum)

Auditory Tube (Eustachian Tube)

Naso-pharynx

Middle Ear
(between eardrum & internal ear)

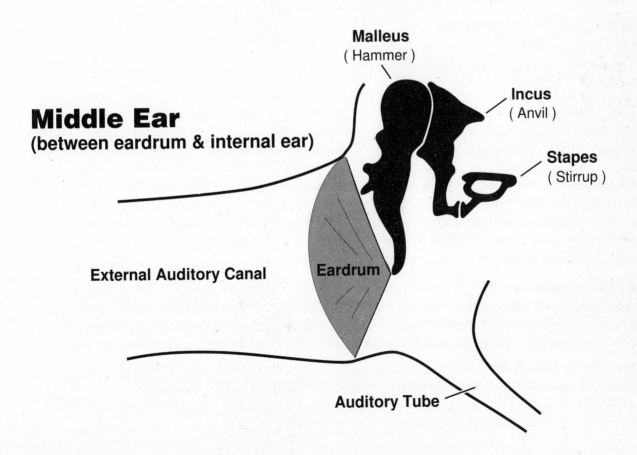

Malleus (Hammer)

Incus (Anvil)

Stapes (Stirrup)

External Auditory Canal

Eardrum

Auditory Tube

Labyrinth : an intricate structure of interconnecting passages; a group of communicating anatomical cavities. The internal (inner) ear consists of two labyrinths, one inside the other.

BONY LABYRINTH

The bony labyrinth is a group of communicating cavities in the petrous portion of the temporal bone. Its inner walls are lined with periosteum (fibrous membrane) and it contains a fluid called *perilymph*. The 3 main parts of the bony labyrinth are named according to their shapes.

Cochlea (Latin: snail shell) The cochlea is a spiral-shaped cavity resembling a snail shell. The inside of the cochlea has a bony shelf that divides the spiral cavity into 2 compartments. The cochlea is filled with a fluid called perilymph.
Scala Vestibuli The upper compartment of the cochlea is called the scala vestibuli; it extends from the oval window (fenestra vestibuli) to the tip of the spiral cavity.
Scala Tympani The lower compartment is called the scala tympani; it extends from the tip of the spiral cavity to the round window (fenestra cochlea). The two compartments are continuous with each other at the tip of the cochlea.

Semicircular Canals There are 3 semicircular canals at right angles to each other (positioned in the three planes of space).
Ampulla One end of each canal has an enlarged region called the ampulla.

Vestibule (entrance hall) A vestibule is a small entrance hall or antechamber between two doors of a house or building; a lobby. The vestibule of the bony labyrinth is the cavity between (and continuous with) the cochlea and the semicircular canals.

MEMBRANOUS LABYRINTH

The membranous labyrinth is a series of sacs and tubes that lie within the bony labyrinth. It contains a fluid called the *endolymph*. It has 3 main parts: the cochlear duct, the semicircular ducts, and the utricle & saccule.

Cochlear Duct (also called the *membranous cochlea* or *scala media*) The cochlear duct lies between the two bony compartments of the cochlea (the scala vestibuli and the scala tympani). It is separated from the scala vestibuli by the *vestibular membrane*; it is separated from the scala tympani by the *basilar membrane*.
Spiral Organ (also called the *organ of Corti*) The spiral organ is the sense organ for hearing; it is located on the upper surface of the basilar membrane within the cochlear duct. It is composed of receptor cells (hair cells) and supporting cells. The *tectorial membrane* (tectum = cover or roof) projects out from the bony shelf of the cochlea, just above the spiral organ. The tips of the processes of the hair cells are in contact with the tectorial membrane.

Semicircular Ducts (also called the *membranous semicircular canals*) The portions of the membranous labyrinth that lie within the semicircular canals are called the semicircular ducts.
Crista At one end of each semicircular duct is a dilated region called the *membranous ampulla*. A crista (sense organ for dynamic equilibrium) is located in each of the three membranous ampullae.

Utricle & Saccule The portions of the membranous labyrinth that lie within the vestibule consist of two sacs connected by a small duct; they are called the utricle and saccule.
Macula A macula (sense organ for static equilibrium) is located in each sac.

INTERNAL (INNER) EAR

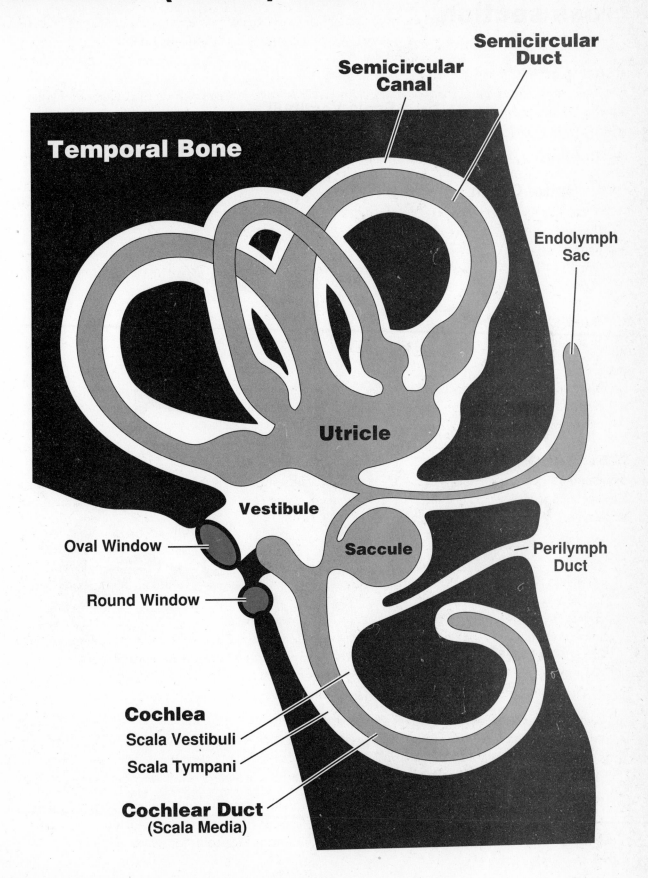

Semicircular
Canal

Semicircular
Duct

Temporal Bone

Endolymph
Sac

Utricle

Vestibule

Oval Window

Saccule

Perilymph
Duct

Round Window

Cochlea
Scala Vestibuli

Scala Tympani

Cochlear Duct
(Scala Media)

COCHLEA
cross section

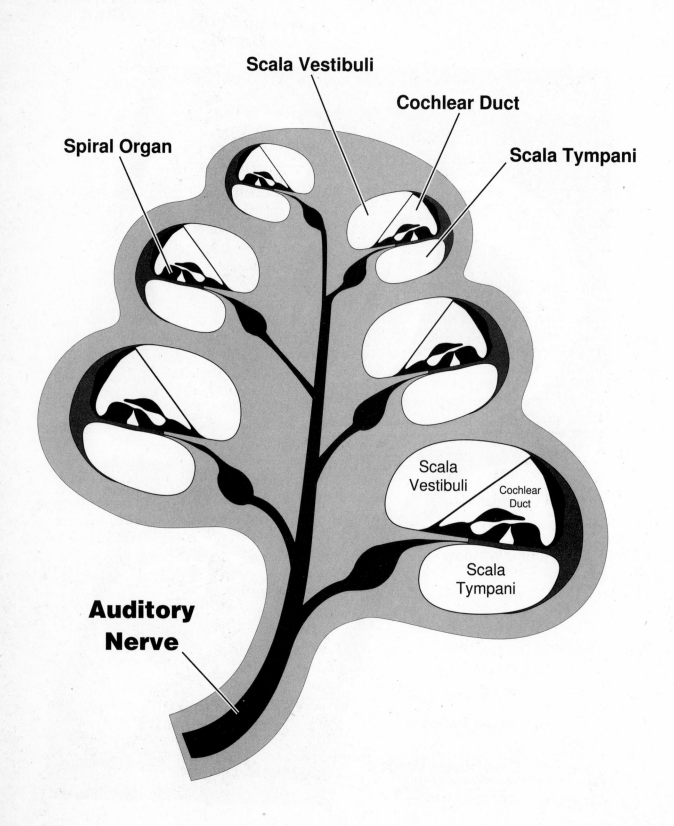

Scala Vestibuli

Cochlear Duct

Spiral Organ

Scala Tympani

Scala
Vestibuli

Cochlear
Duct

Scala
Tympani

**Auditory
Nerve**

SPIRAL ORGAN (organ of Corti)

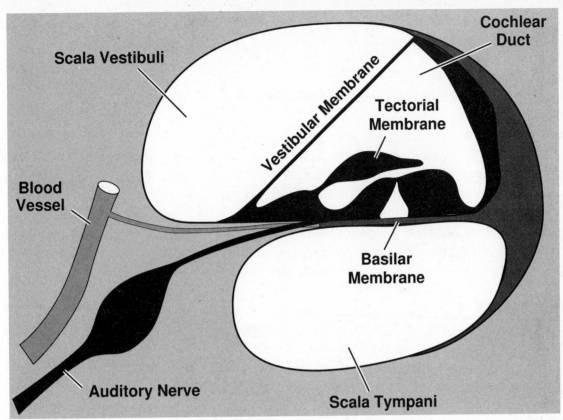

Scala Vestibuli

Cochlear Duct

Vestibular Membrane

Tectorial Membrane

Blood Vessel

Basilar Membrane

Auditory Nerve

Scala Tympani

Spiral Organ

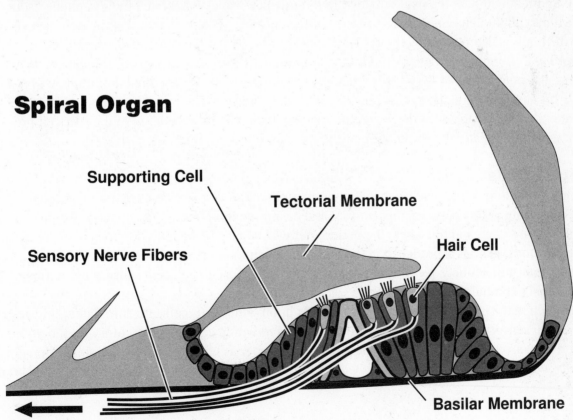

Supporting Cell

Tectorial Membrane

Sensory Nerve Fibers

Hair Cell

Basilar Membrane

EAR / Hearing

Transmission of Sound   The ear converts sound waves from the air into nerve impulses. The nerve impulses are carried by fibers of the auditory pathway to the temporal lobe of the cerebrum where they are interpreted as sound.

Tympanic Membrane

The tympanic membrane (eardrum) reproduces the vibrations of the sound source.

Auditory Ossicles

The ossicles transmit the vibrations of the tympanic membrane to the membrane that covers the oval window. As sound energy is transferred from the air to the tympanic membrane, to the ossicles, and to the oval window, energy is lost. The ossicles minimize this loss by two mechanisms: First, the malleus and incus act as a lever system that multiplies the force 1.3 times. Secondly, because the area of the tympanic membrane is 22 times greater than the area of the oval window covered by the footplate of the stapes, the pressure per unit area is increased. About 60% of the sound energy reaching the tympanic membrane is transmitted through the ossicles to the fluid in the cochlea.

Traveling Waves

The oval window bows in and out with the movements of the stapes, setting up a series of traveling waves in the perilymph of the scala vestibuli.

Pitch   As a wave moves along the length of the scala vestibuli, its amplitude increases gradually, then suddenly drops off. The location where a given wave reaches its maximum amplitude is determined by its frequency: high frequency waves (generated by high-pitched sounds) reach maximum height near the oval window; low frequency waves (generated by low-pitched sounds) reach maximum height near the apex (tip) of the cochlea. The pitch that is ultimately perceived by the brain is determined by the region of the spiral organ that is maximally stimulated.

Loudness   Loudness is determined by the amplitude of a wave at any given frequency. When a particular note is played very softly (pianissimo) on the piano, its maximal amplitude will not be as great as when the same note is played very loudly (forte). The greater the amplitude, the greater the displacement of the basilar membrane, the greater the bending of the hair cell processes, and the greater the stimulation of the receptor cells.

Receptor Cells

When a traveling wave reaches its maximum amplitude, it displaces the basilar membrane and causes a shearing action between the tectorial and basilar membranes. Consequently, the processes of a hair cell are bent, and this alters the permeability of its plasma membrane. Ion channels open and a generator potential is produced in the hair cell; calcium ions diffuse into the cell and trigger the release of neurotransmitter. Neurotransmitter molecules diffuse to adjacent sensory nerve fibers and trigger action potentials.

The pitch that is perceived in the brain depends upon which hair cells are stimulated; this determines which sensory fibers carry signals to the brain and which cells in the auditory region of the temporal lobe are stimulated. The loudness perceived depends upon the degree of stimulation of the hair cells, which determines the frequency of impulses transmitted by the sensory fibers to the brain.

SOUND TRANSMISSION (in Cochlea)

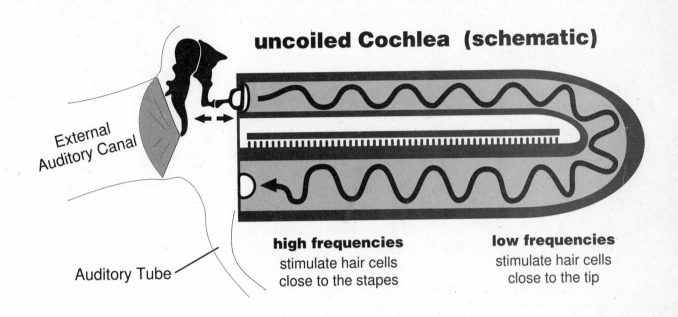

uncoiled Cochlea (schematic)

External
Auditory Canal

Auditory Tube

high frequencies
stimulate hair cells
close to the stapes

low frequencies
stimulate hair cells
close to the tip

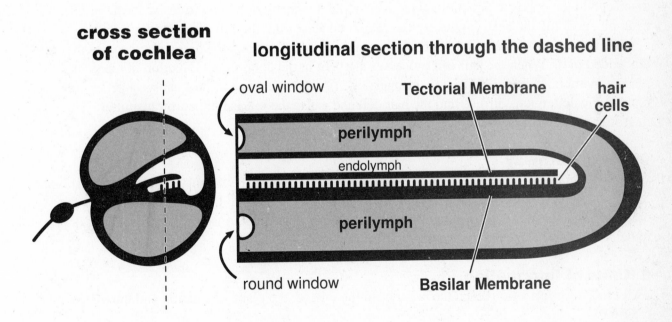

**cross section
of cochlea**

longitudinal section through the dashed line

oval window

Tectorial Membrane

**hair
cells**

perilymph

endolymph

perilymph

round window

Basilar Membrane

EAR / Dynamic Equilibrium

definition : Dynamic equilibrium is the maintenance of body position, mainly the head, in response to sudden movements such as rotation, acceleration, and deceleration.

Semicircular Ducts

There are 3 semicircular ducts positioned at right angles to one another in 3 planes:
- (1) Anterior Duct : frontal plane
- (2) Posterior Duct : sagittal plane
- (3) Lateral Duct : horizontal plane

Each semicircular duct has an enlarged portion at one end called the membranous ampulla.

Crista (sense organ of dynamic equilibrium)

A crista (plural: cristae) is located in the membranous ampulla of each semicircular duct. It is the sense organ for dynamic equilibrium (also called rotational acceleration or angular acceleration). A crista is composed of receptor cells (hair cells), supporting cells, and a mass of gelatinous material called the *cupula*. The processes of the hair cells are embedded in the gelatinous cupula, which is surrounded by the fluid called endolymph. The cupula is very sensitive to any movement of fluid in the semicircular duct.

Receptor Cell Activation

When the head moves in a particular plane, the fluid in the corresponding semicircular duct is displaced in the opposite direction due to inertia (the tendency of a body to resist acceleration). For example, nodding the head (in the sagittal plane) displaces the fluid in the posterior duct.

The movement of the endolymph pushes on the cupula, bending the hair cell processes that are embedded in it. When the hair cell processes are bent in the appropriate direction, it alters the plasma membrane permeability (ion channels open). The exchange of ions causes a generator potential; calcium ions diffuse into the hair cell and cause the release of neurotransmitter. The neurotransmitter diffuses to adjacent sensory nerve fibers and triggers action potentials.

Sensory Pathway

Nerve impulses (propagated action potentials) are carried by the sensory fibers of the vestibular branch of the vestibulocochlear nerve (cranial nerve VIII) to the brain. The brain integrates the incoming signals and sends the appropriate instructions to skeletal muscles, which contract or relax to help maintain balance in the new body position.

2 Kinds of Information

Two kinds of information reach the brain from the cristae: the plane of rotation and the direction of rotation.

Plane of Rotation Rotation causes maximal stimulation in the semicircular duct that is most nearly in the plane of rotation; in the other ducts there is less displacement of fluid and less stimulation of the cristae. The degrees of stimulation of the three cristae are integrated by the brain, so the person can perceive the exact plane of rotation.

Direction of Rotation When the cupula in the ampulla of the right superior duct is displaced in one direction, the cupula in the left superior duct is displaced in the opposite direction. Based on the input from the left and right superior ducts, the brain senses the direction of rotation.

CRISTA (ampulla organ)

Locations of the 3 cristae inside the ampullae of the membranous labyrinth

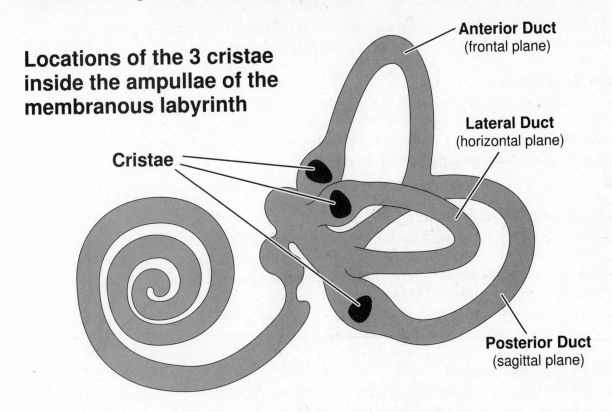

Anterior Duct (frontal plane)

Lateral Duct (horizontal plane)

Cristae

Posterior Duct (sagittal plane)

Crista

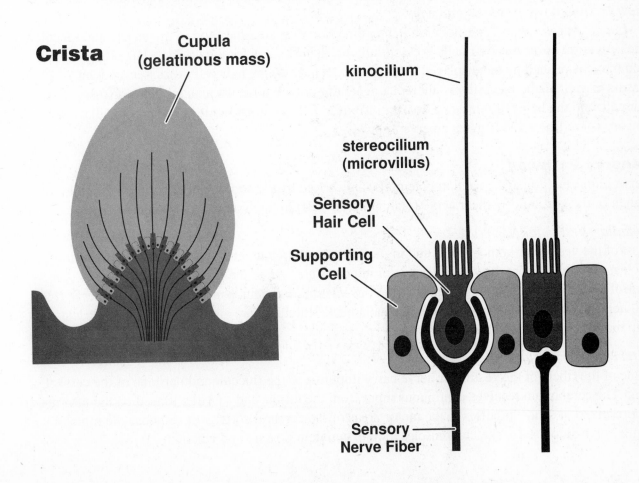

Cupula (gelatinous mass)

kinocilium

stereocilium (microvillus)

Sensory Hair Cell

Supporting Cell

Sensory Nerve Fiber

191

EAR / Static Equilibrium

definition : Static equilibrium is the maintenance of posture in response to changes in the orientation of the body, mainly the head, relative to the ground.

Utricle & Saccule

The membranous sacs, the utricle and saccule, lie within the vestibule of the bony labyrinth. They are filled with a fluid, the endolymph, that is continuous with the fluid in the semicircular ducts and the cochlear duct. A macula is attached to the inner wall of each sac. The two maculae are at right angles to each other; the macula in the utricle is horizontal and the macula in the saccule is vertical.

Macula (sense organ of static equilibrium)

Maculae (singular: macula) are the sense organs of static equilibrium (also called linear acceleration or gravity). Maculae consist of receptor cells (hair cells), supporting cells, and a gelatinous mass called the *otolithic membrane*. A layer of calcium carbonate crystals called *otoliths* (*oto* = ear, *liths* = stones) covers the surface of the otolithic membrane, giving it additional weight and making it more sensitive to gravity. The macula in the utricle responds to horizontal acceleration and the macula in the saccule responds to vertical acceleration.

Receptor Cell Activation

Gravity The two maculae discharge tonically in response to the pull of gravity on the otoliths. So, even when there is no movement, there are impulses traveling to the brain that allow the brain to know up from down (sense of gravity).

Linear Acceleration Acceleration in any direction displaces the fluid in the utricle and saccule. The activation of the receptor cells is essentially the same as it is for the cristae. The otolithic membrane is pushed by the displaced fluid, and consequently the hair cell processes are bent. Plasma membrane permeability is altered, a generator potential results; calcium ions diffuse into the hair cell, and the hair cell releases a neurotransmitter. The neurotransmitter diffuses to adjacent sensory nerve fibers and triggers a nerve impulse.

Sensory Pathway

Nerve impulses (propagated action potentials) are carried by the sensory fibers of the vestibular branch of the vestibulocochlear nerve (cranial nerve VIII) to the brain.

Medulla (Vestibular Nuclei)

Most of the vestibular branch fibers end in the medulla oblongata in a region called the vestibular nuclear complex. From the vestibular nuclei impulses are sent to the nuclei of cranial nerves that control eye movements (cranial nerves III, IV, & VI) and to the nucleus of the accessory nerve (XI) that helps to control movements of the head and neck. Impulses are also sent to skeletal muscles that help maintain posture and balance.

Cerebellum (Flocculonodular Lobe)

Some of the fibers of the vestibular nerve carry impulses to the flocculonodular lobe of the cerebellum. The cerebellum receives continuous input from the utricle and saccule. Based on the information received, it sends impulses to the motor areas of the cerebral cortex. In response the motor cortex sends impulses to skeletal muscles to help maintain posture and balance.

MACULA (utricle organ)

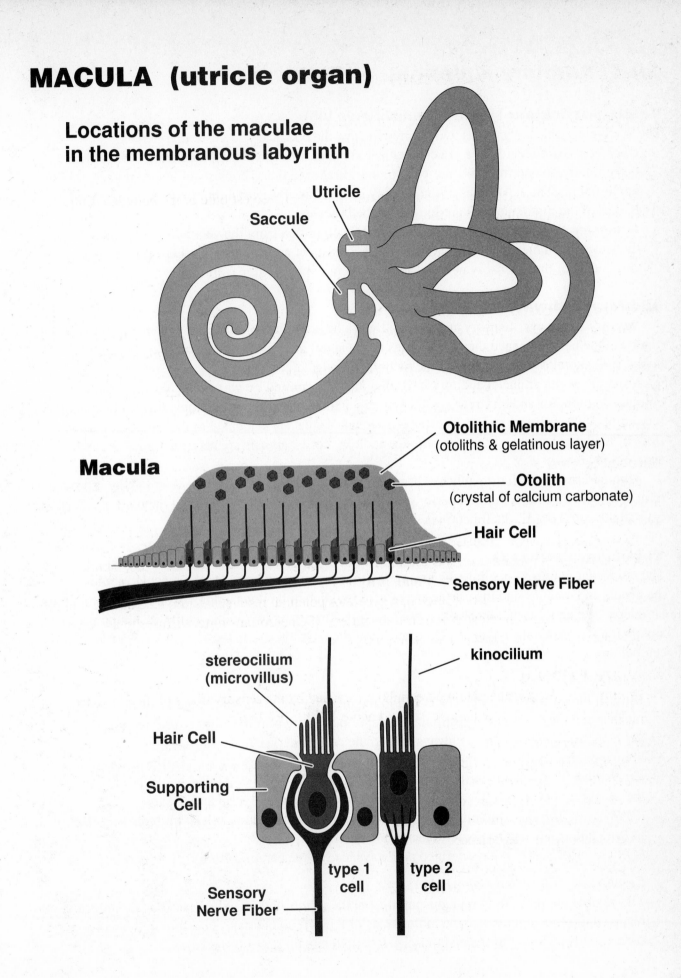

Locations of the maculae in the membranous labyrinth

Utricle

Saccule

Macula

Otolithic Membrane
(otoliths & gelatinous layer)

Otolith
(crystal of calcium carbonate)

Hair Cell

Sensory Nerve Fiber

stereocilium
(microvillus)

kinocilium

Hair Cell

Supporting
Cell

type 1
cell

type 2
cell

Sensory
Nerve Fiber

EAR / Auditory & Vestibular Pathways

Vestibulocochlear Nerve (Cranial Nerve VIII)

The vestibulocochlear nerve has two main branches: the cochlear and vestibular nerves.

Cochlear (Auditory) Nerve Each cochlear nerve carries impulses to and from the cochlea (specifically, to and from the hair cells in the spiral organ) and consists of approximately 28,000 nerve fibers. The cell bodies of the sensory neurons are located in the *spiral ganglion*. The cell bodies of the motor neurons are located in the brain stem.

Vestibular Nerve Each vestibular nerve carries impulses from the vestibule (specifically, from the hair cells in the maculae and cristae) and consists of approximately 19,000 nerve fibers. The cell bodies of these sensory neurons are located in the *vestibular ganglion*.

Auditory Pathways

Sensory Pathways Sensory auditory pathways begin in the spiral organ. The neurons that innervate the hair cells have their cell bodies in the spiral ganglia and their axon terminals in the dorsal and ventral cochlear nuclei of the medulla oblongata.

From the cochlear nuclei auditory information is transmitted by nerve pathways to the inferior colliculi (centers for auditory reflexes), the medial geniculate nuclei in the thalamus, and the auditory cortex. The primary auditory cortex (Brodmann's area 41) is located in the temporal lobe in the floor of the lateral sulcus. From the primary auditory cortex signals are carried to adjacent auditory association areas.

Motor Pathways Motor pathways begin in the brain stem. The olivocochlear bundle is a bundle of nerve fibers that starts in the superior olives of the midbrain and ends around the bases of hair cells in the spiral organ. Its function is uncertain.

Vestibular Pathways

The vestibular pathways begin in the hair cells of the maculae and cristae; the maculae are located in the utricle and saccule, and the cristae are located in the membranous ampullae of the the semicircular ducts. The neurons that innervate these hair cells have their cell bodies in the vestibular ganglia and their axon terminals in the vestibular nuclei of the medulla and in the flocculonodular lobe of the cerebellum.

Medulla (Vestibular Nuclei)

Most of the vestibular branch fibers end in the medulla oblongata in a region called the vestibular nuclear complex. From the vestibular nuclei impulses are sent in a variety of directions:

(1) Eye Movements Some pathways lead to the cranial nerves that control eye movements: cranial nerves III, IV, & VI. They coordinate head movements with eye movements.

(2) Head & Neck Movements A nerve pathway leads from the vestibular nuclei to the nucleus of the accessory nerve (XI) that helps to control movements of the head and neck.

(3) Postural Muscles Impulses sent to motor neurons that lead to skeletal muscles help control posture and balance in response to head movements.

(4) Cerebral Cortex Poorly defined pathways lead to the cerebral cortex.

Cerebellum (Flocculonodular Lobe)

The cerebellum receives continuous input from the utricle and saccule. Based on the information received, it sends impulses to the motor areas of the cerebral cortex. In response the motor cortex sends impulses to skeletal muscles to help maintain posture and balance.

VESTIBULO-COCHLEAR NERVE
(8th Cranial Nerve)

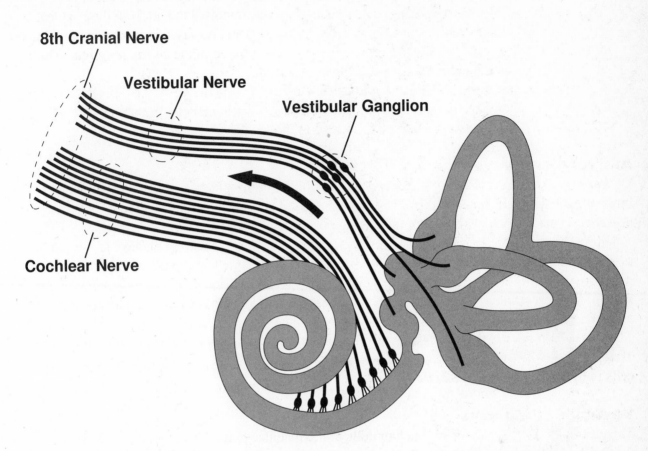

8th Cranial Nerve

Vestibular Nerve

Vestibular Ganglion

Cochlear Nerve

Membranous Labyrinth

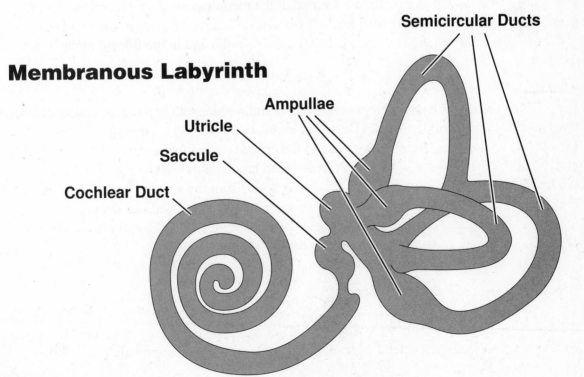

Semicircular Ducts

Ampullae

Utricle

Saccule

Cochlear Duct

Part II : Self-Testing Exercises

Unlabeled illustrations from Part I

NERVOUS SYSTEM ORGANIZATION

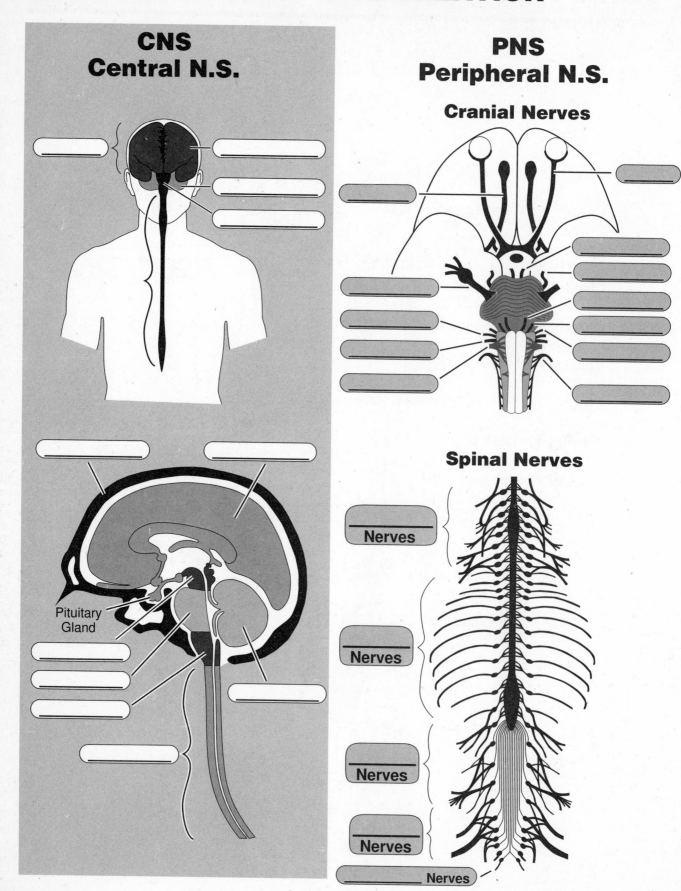

CNS
Central N.S.

PNS
Peripheral N.S.

Cranial Nerves

Spinal Nerves

Nerves

Nerves

Nerves

Nerves

Nerves

Pituitary
Gland

NEURON (nerve cell)

Neurons carry impulses to other neurons, _____ cells, & _____ cells.

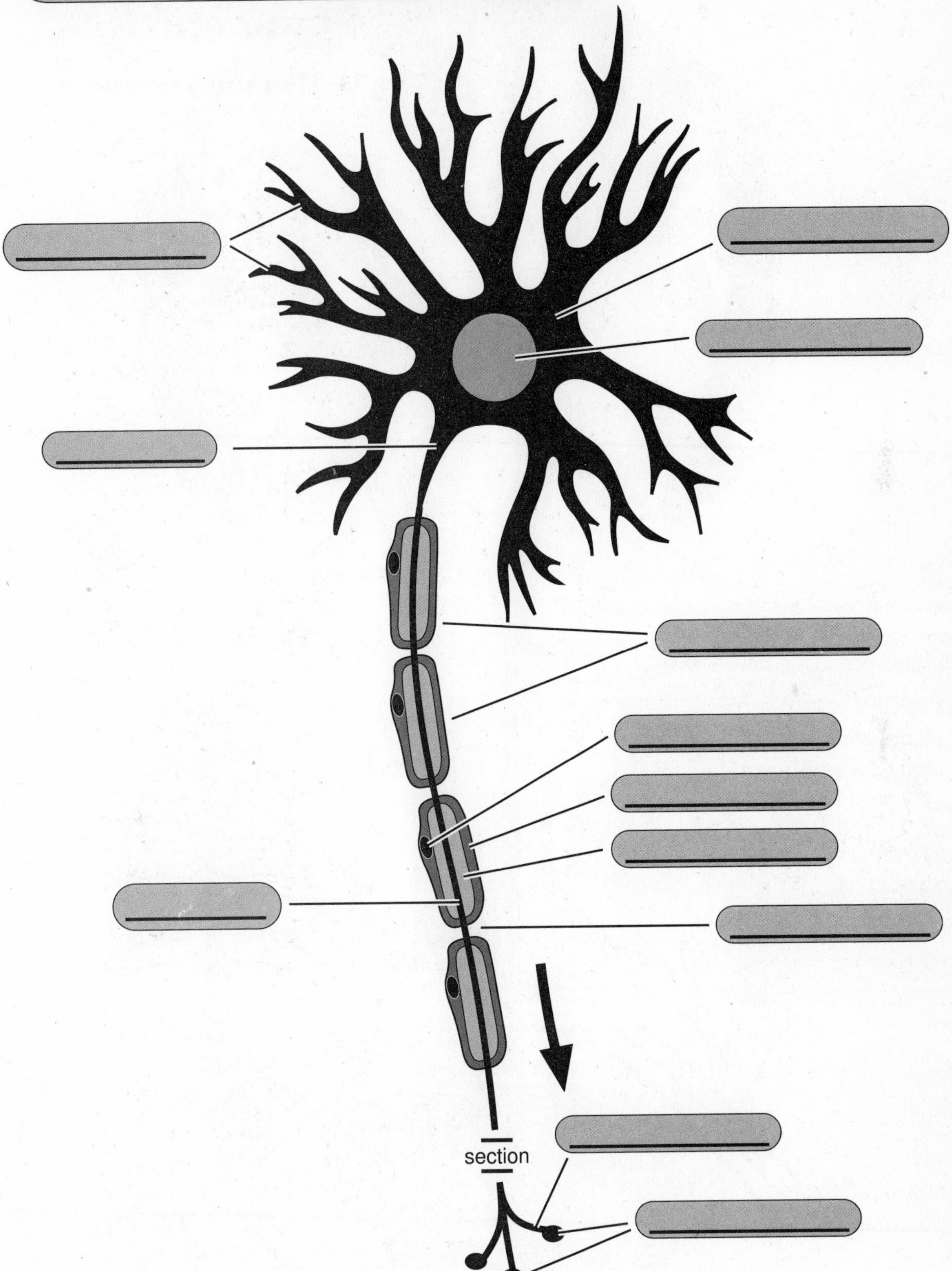

section

199

NEURON CLASSIFICATION

Brain

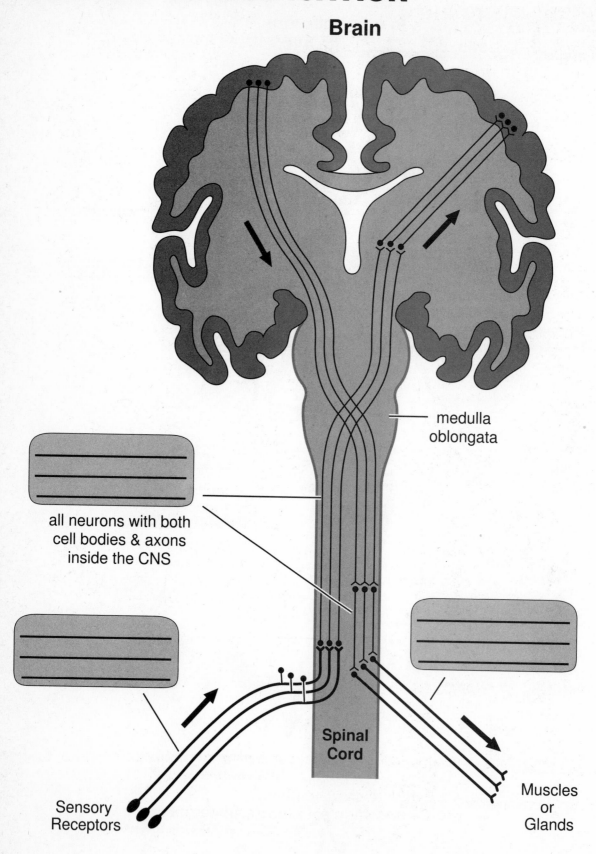

medulla
oblongata

all neurons with both
cell bodies & axons
inside the CNS

Spinal
Cord

Sensory
Receptors

Muscles
or
Glands

TYPES OF NEURONS
based on structure

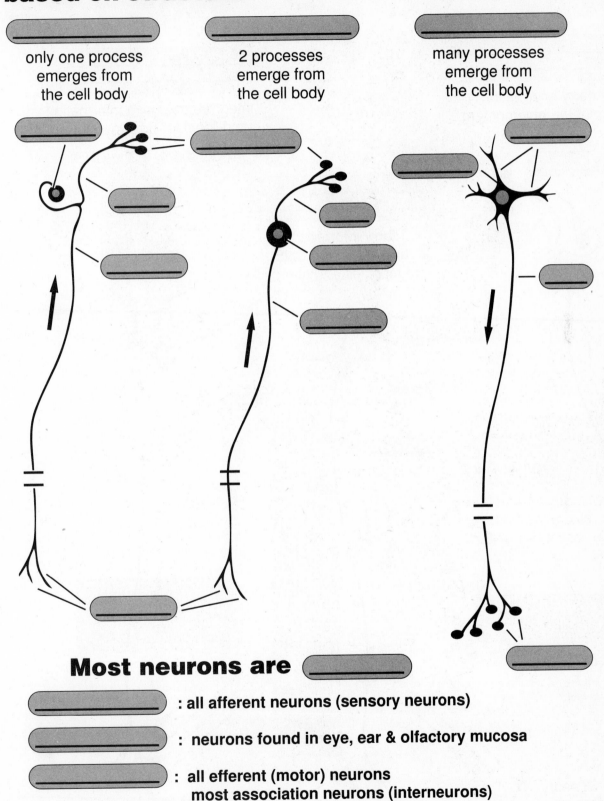

only one process emerges from the cell body

2 processes emerge from the cell body

many processes emerge from the cell body

Most neurons are

_____ : all afferent neurons (sensory neurons)

_____ : neurons found in eye, ear & olfactory mucosa

_____ : all efferent (motor) neurons
most association neurons (interneurons)

TYPES OF NEURONS
based on function

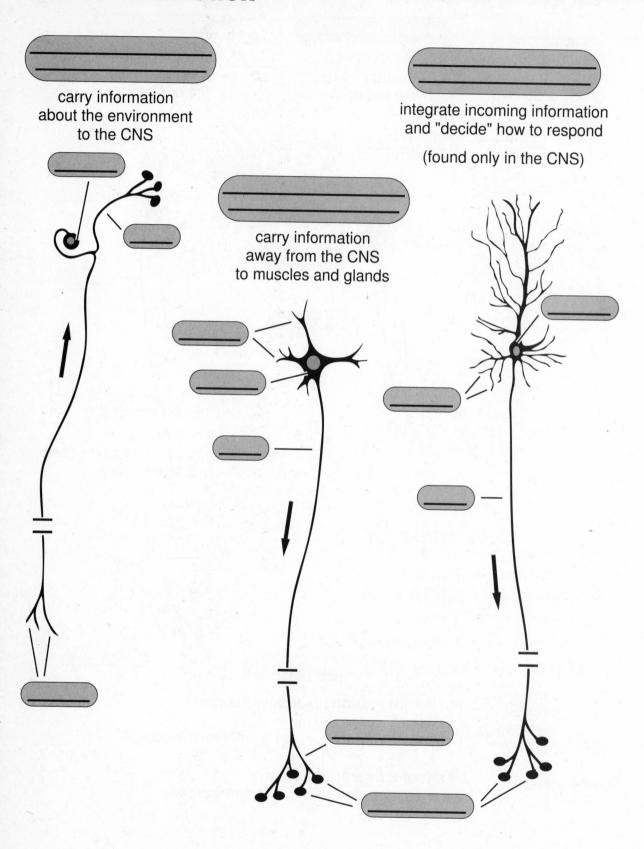

carry information
about the environment
to the CNS

integrate incoming information
and "decide" how to respond

(found only in the CNS)

carry information
away from the CNS
to muscles and glands

202

NEUROGLIAL CELLS
neuroglia of the CNS

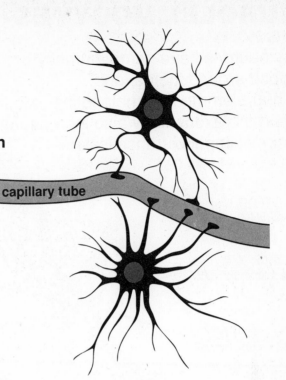

capillary tube

_____

functions :
regulate interstitial fluid composition
maintain blood-brain barrier
provide structural framework
repair damaged neural tissue

_____

functions :
myelinate axons
provide structural framework

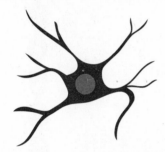

_____

function :
phagocytize pathogens
& cellular debris

_____

epithelial cells that line brain ventricles
& central canal of spinal cord

function :
assist in secretion & circulation of CSF

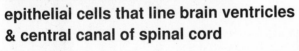

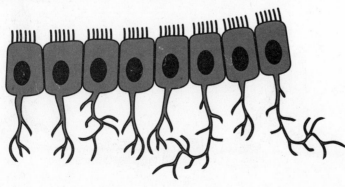

NEUROLEMMOCYTES

Many neurons have neurolemmocytes (Schwann cells) wrapped around their axons.
The neurolemmocytes help to insulate, nourish, and support the axons; they also increase the velocity of impulse transmission.

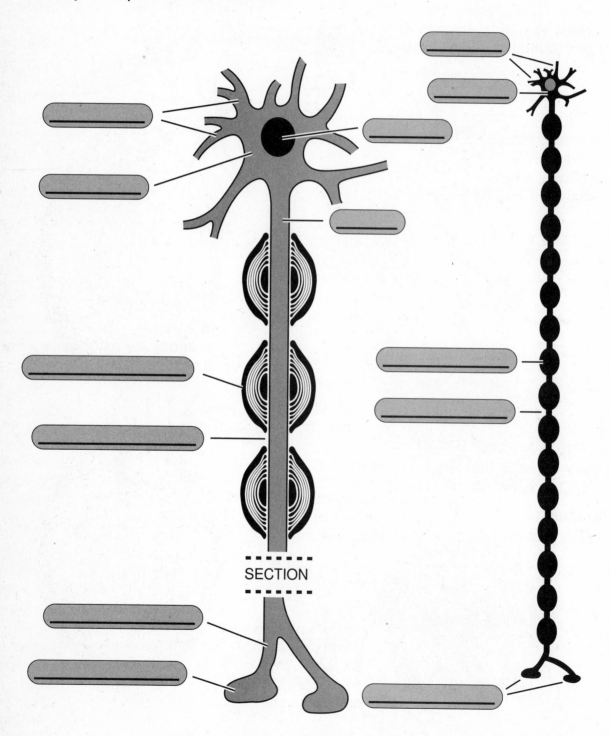

SECTION

MYELIN SHEATH : myelination

A neurolemmocyte (Schwann cell)
wrapping around an axon, forming a myelin sheath

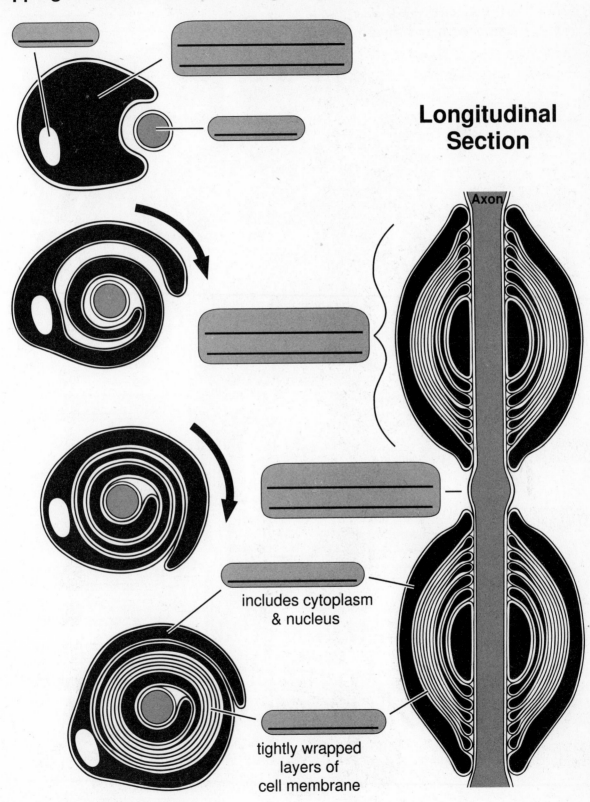

Longitudinal Section

Axon

includes cytoplasm
& nucleus

tightly wrapped
layers of
cell membrane

PATHWAYS
Sensory & Direct Motor Pathways

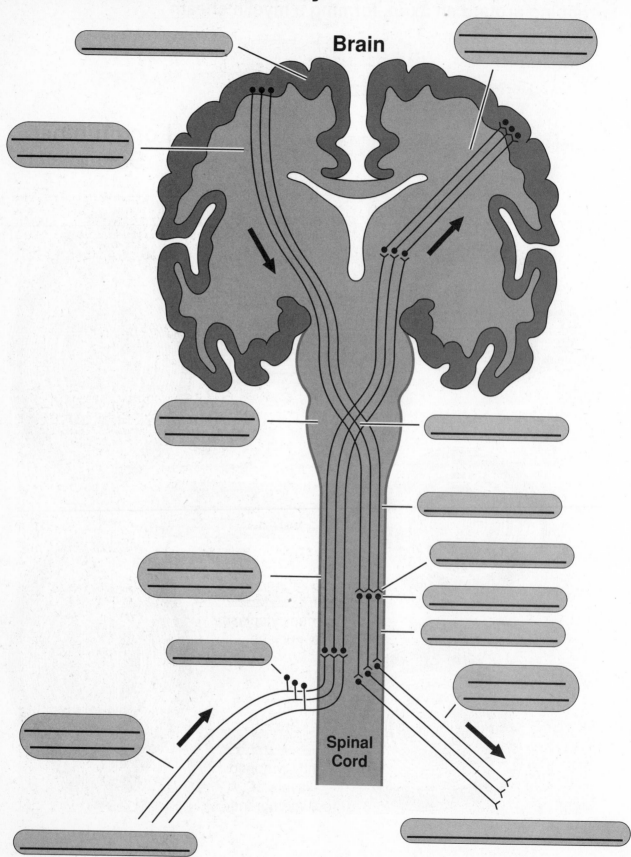

Brain

Spinal
Cord

GANGLIA & NUCLEI
(clusters of neuron cell bodies)

A cluster of neuron cell bodies in the PNS
(outside the brain or spinal cord)
is called a (_____) .

A cluster of neuron cell bodies in the CNS
(inside the brain or spinal cord)
is called a (_____) .

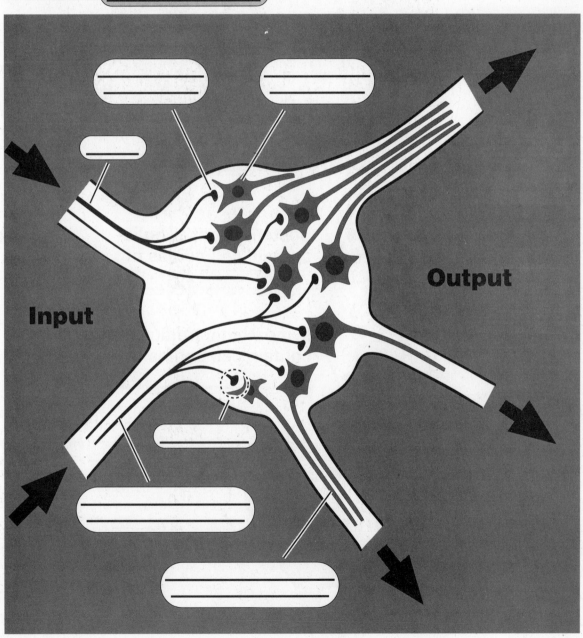

Input

Output

GANGLIA
Ganglia are clusters of neuron cell bodies in the PNS.

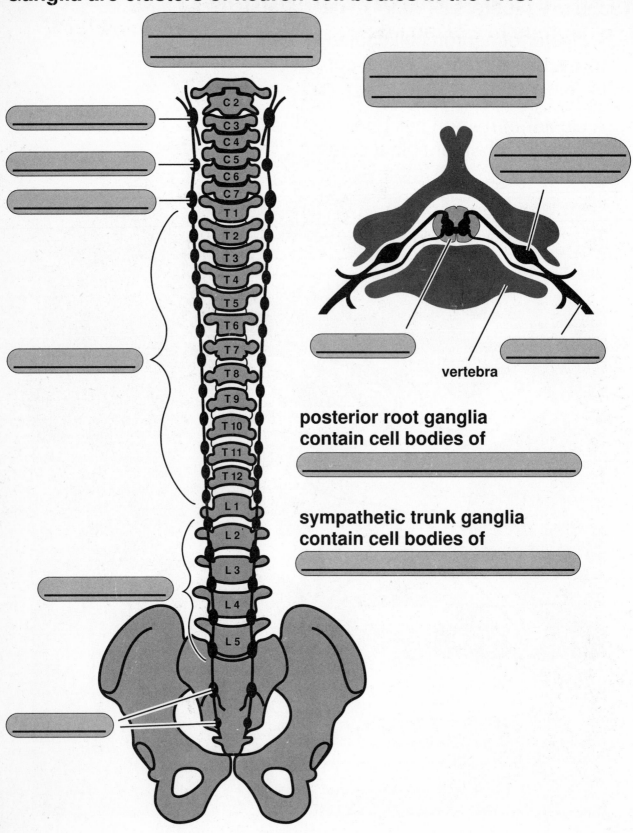

vertebra

**posterior root ganglia
contain cell bodies of**

**sympathetic trunk ganglia
contain cell bodies of**

NUCLEI (in the brain)

Nuclei are clusters of neuron cell bodies in the CNS.
The neurons in a given nucleus perform a specific function.

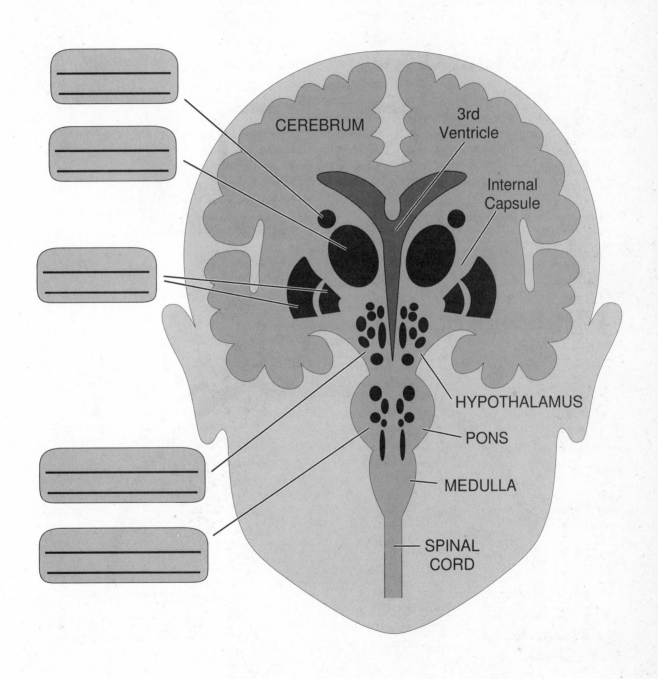

CEREBRUM

3rd Ventricle

Internal Capsule

HYPOTHALAMUS

PONS

MEDULLA

SPINAL CORD

THE REFLEX ARC

The reflex arc is the basic structural and functional unit of the nervous system.

It summarizes the main steps involved in a nervous system response to a stimulus.

Thermostat

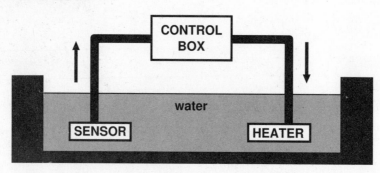

Reflex Arc

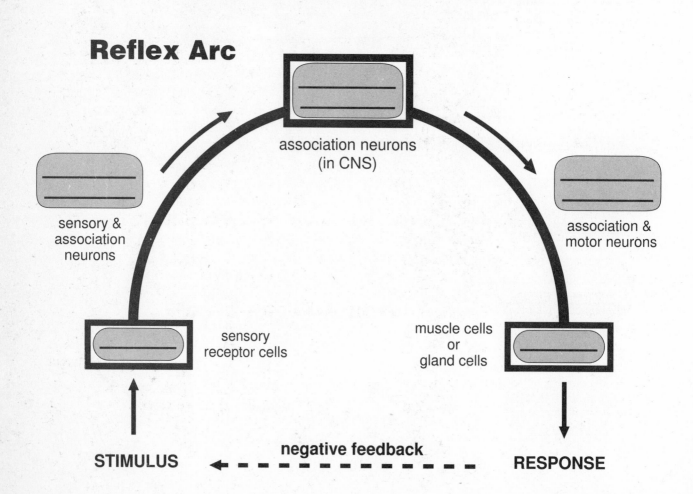

association neurons
(in CNS)

sensory &
association
neurons

association &
motor neurons

sensory
receptor cells

muscle cells
or
gland cells

negative feedback

STIMULUS

RESPONSE

CHARGED PARTICLES

Electrons

Name the elements :

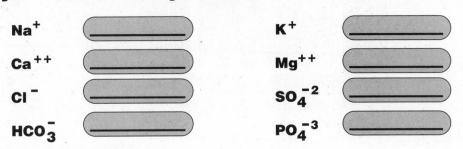

Major Ions in Body Fluids :

Na^+ _____ K^+ _____

Ca^{++} _____ Mg^{++} _____

Cl^- _____ SO_4^{-2} _____

HCO_3^- _____ PO_4^{-3} _____

Molecules with Ionized Groups

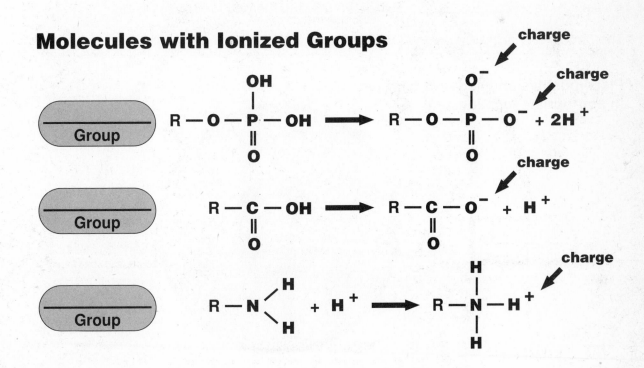

VOLTAGE electric potential energy

BATTERY

Batteries contain opposite charges separated by an insulating material.

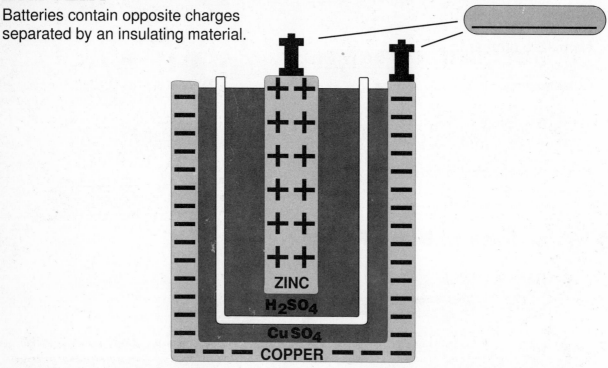

ZINC

H_2SO_4

$CuSO_4$

COPPER

HUMAN CELL

All cells have a _____ charge on the outside relative to the inside.

The opposite charges are insulated by the high fat content of the _____

Place positive and negative charges in appropriate locations.

Nucleus

Plasma Membrane

EQUILIBRIUM POTENTIALS

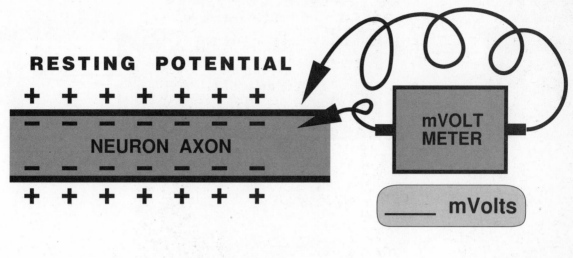

RESTING POTENTIAL

+ + + + + + +

− − − − − −

NEURON AXON

− − − − − −

+ + + + + + +

mVOLT METER

_____ mVolts

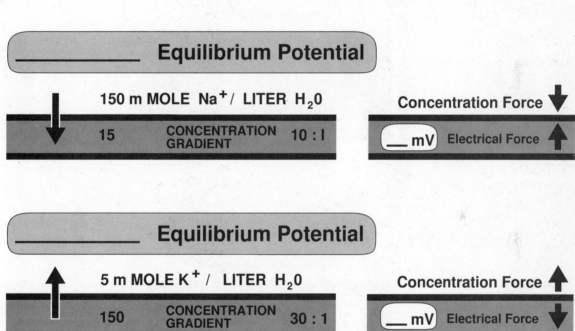

_____ **Equilibrium Potential**

150 m MOLE Na^+ / LITER H_2O

| 15 | CONCENTRATION GRADIENT | 10 : 1 |

Concentration Force ↓

___ mV   Electrical Force ↑

_____ **Equilibrium Potential**

5 m MOLE K^+ / LITER H_2O

| 150 | CONCENTRATION GRADIENT | 30 : 1 |

Concentration Force ↑

___ mV   Electrical Force ↓

RESTING POTENTIAL

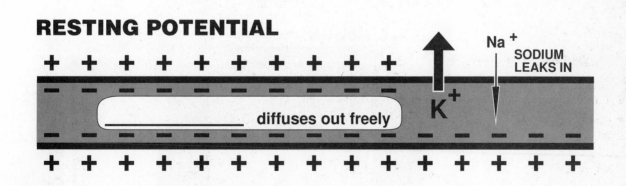

+ + + + + + + + + + + + + +

− − − − − − − − − − − − − −

_____ diffuses out freely

− − − − − − − − − − − − − −

+ + + + + + + + + + + + + + +

K^+

Na^+ SODIUM LEAKS IN

VOLTAGE – GATED ION CHANNELS
Changes in voltage-gated channels during an action potential

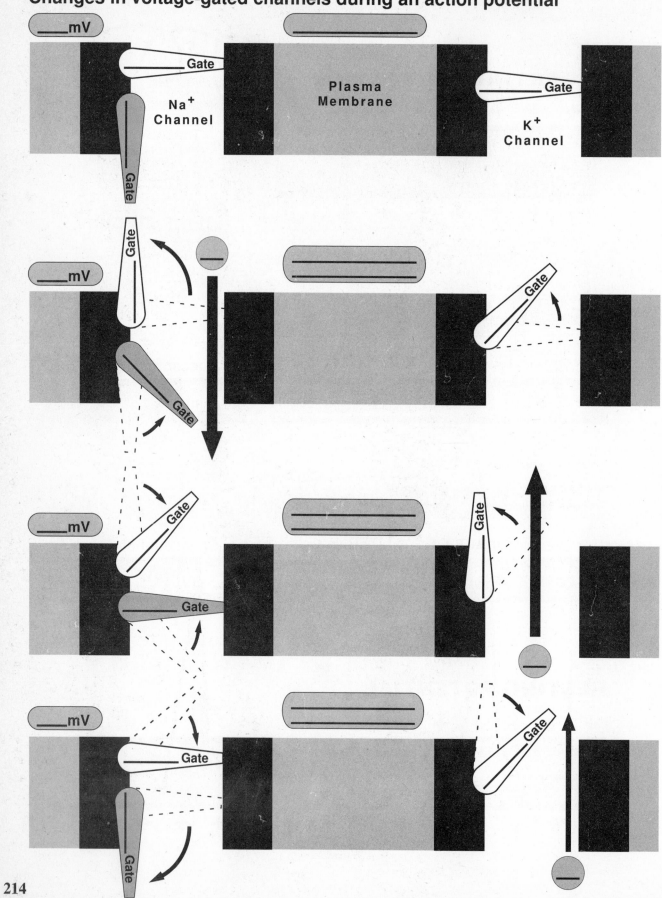

A NERVE IMPULSE
PROPAGATED ACTION POTENTIALS

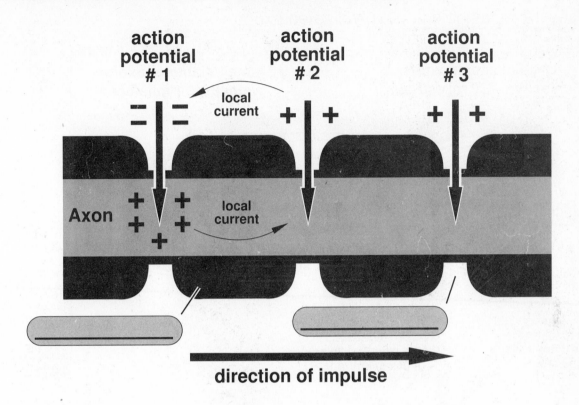

action
potential
1

action
potential
2

action
potential
3

local
current

$-$ $-$ $+$ $+$ $+$ $+$

Axon

$+$ $+$
$+$ $+$
$+$

local
current

direction of impulse

ACTION POTENTIALS
oscilloscope trace

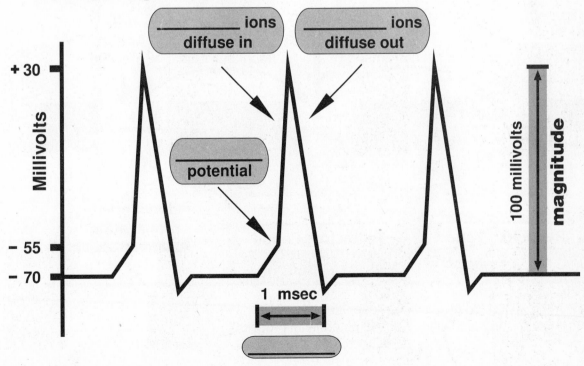

_____ ions
diffuse in

_____ ions
diffuse out

_____
potential

Millivolts

+ 30

$-$ 55

$-$ 70

1 msec

100 millivolts

magnitude

NERVE IMPULSE : Velocity & Frequency

Velocity of Impulses

Impulses travel faster in large, myelinated axons.

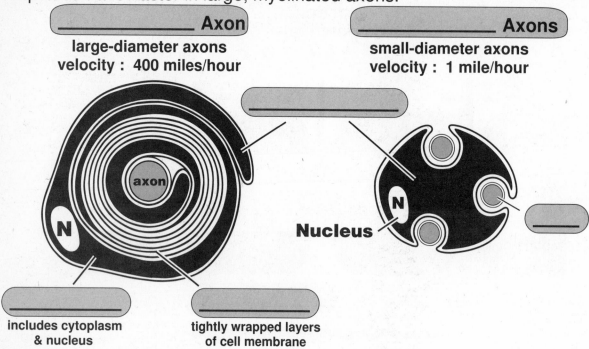

_____ Axon

large-diameter axons
velocity : 400 miles/hour

_____ Axons

small-diameter axons
velocity : 1 mile/hour

axon

N

N

Nucleus

_____

**includes cytoplasm
& nucleus**

**tightly wrapped layers
of cell membrane**

Frequency of Impulses

The frequency of nerve impulses is limited by the refractory period.
During refractory periods new action potentials cannot be generated.

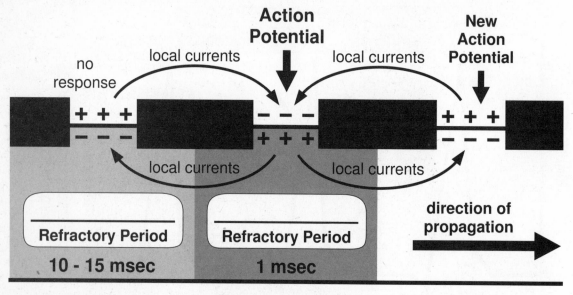

**Action
Potential**

**New
Action
Potential**

no
response

local currents

local currents

+ + +

− − −

+ + +

− − −

+ + +

− − −

local currents

local currents

**direction of
propagation**

Refractory Period

10 - 15 msec

Refractory Period

1 msec

repolarized region
(recent action potential)

depolarized region
(action potential in process)

216

SYNAPSE : contact point between neurons
Presynaptic & Postsynaptic Neurons

_____ Neurons : conduct impulses toward a synapse

_____ Neurons : conduct impulses away from a synapse

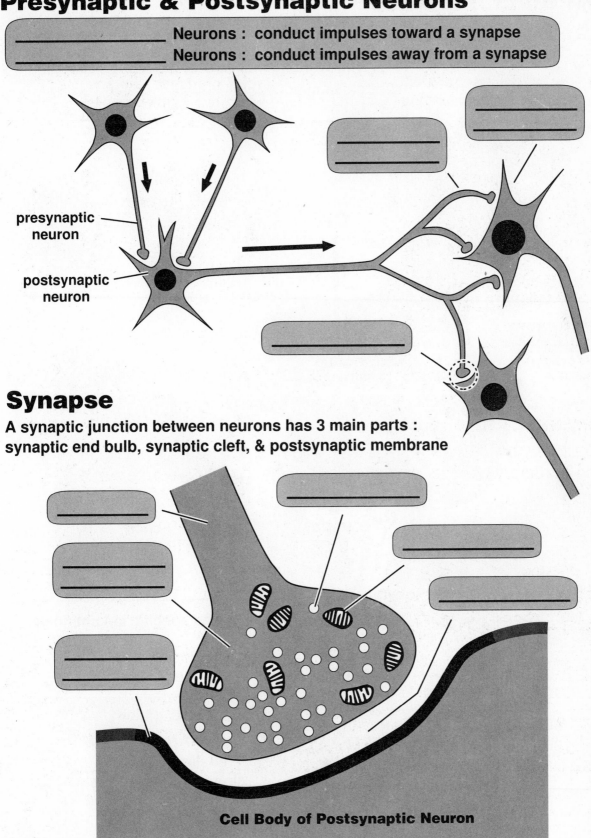

presynaptic
neuron

postsynaptic
neuron

Synapse

A synaptic junction between neurons has 3 main parts :
synaptic end bulb, synaptic cleft, & postsynaptic membrane

Cell Body of Postsynaptic Neuron

SYNAPTIC TRANSMISSION
Sequence of Events

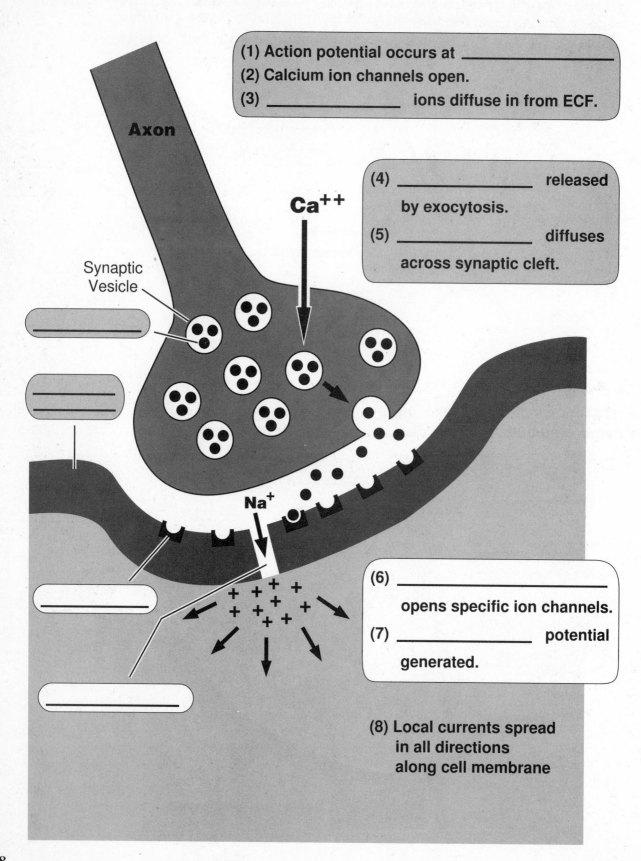

(1) Action potential occurs at _____

(2) Calcium ion channels open.

(3) _____ ions diffuse in from ECF.

(4) _____ released by exocytosis.

(5) _____ diffuses across synaptic cleft.

(6) _____ opens specific ion channels.

(7) _____ potential generated.

(8) Local currents spread in all directions along cell membrane

Axon

Ca^{++}

Synaptic Vesicle

Na^+

SUMMATION

One synaptic event will not cause a postsynaptic neuron to fire.
A postsynaptic neuron fires when many excitatory & inhibitory inputs
are added together (summated).

A motor neuron cell body may have
15,000 synaptic junctions.

(only 10 are shown)

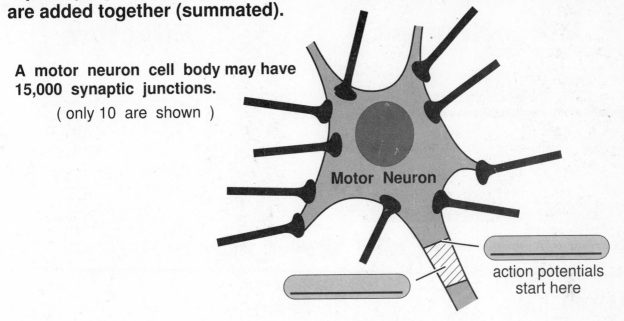

Motor Neuron

action potentials
start here

Excitatory Synapse

At excitatory synapses the binding of
neurotransmitter with receptor causes
_____ channels to open.
_____ diffuse into the
cell body, generating an EPSP.

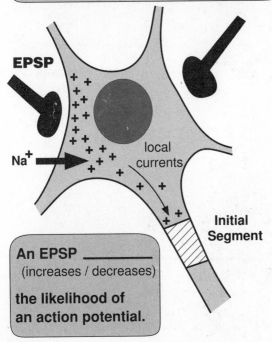

EPSP

Na⁺

local
currents

Initial
Segment

An EPSP _____
(increases / decreases)

the likelihood of
an action potential.

Inhibitatory Synapse

At inhibitory synapses the binding of
neurotransmitter with receptor causes
_____ channels to open.
_____ diffuse into the
cell body, generating an IPSP.

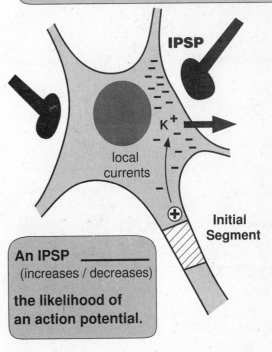

IPSP

K^+

local
currents

Initial
Segment

An IPSP _____
(increases / decreases)

the likelihood of
an action potential.

NEUROTRANSMITTERS
Neurotransmitters released by Motor Neurons

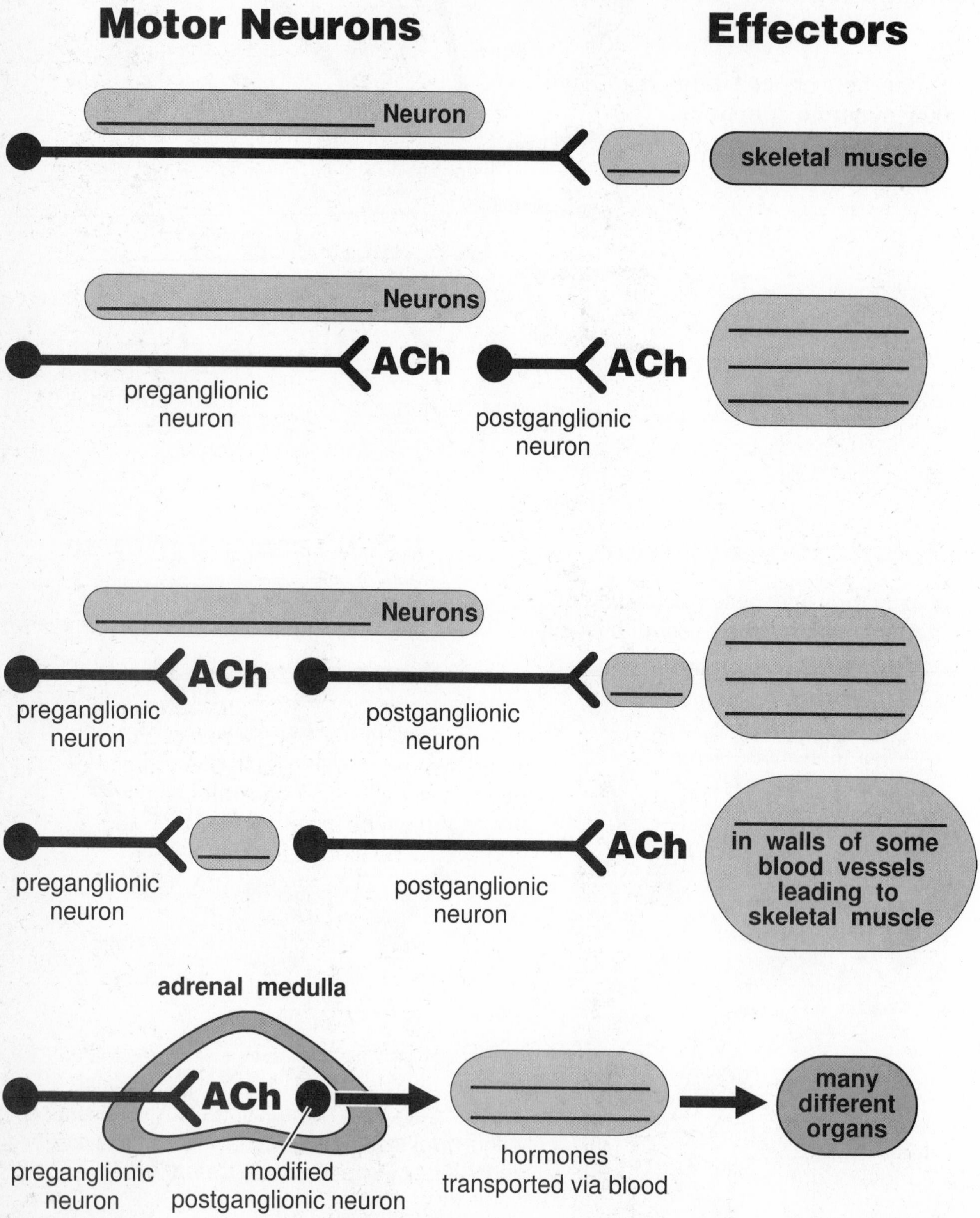

Motor Neurons   **Effectors**

_____ Neuron

_____ skeletal muscle

_____ Neurons

preganglionic
neuron   〈ACh   postganglionic
                    neuron 〈ACh

_____ Neurons

preganglionic   〈ACh   postganglionic
neuron   neuron _____

preganglionic   _____   postganglionic
neuron   neuron 〈ACh

in walls of some
blood vessels
leading to
skeletal muscle

adrenal medulla

preganglionic
neuron   〈ACh   modified
                    postganglionic neuron

hormones
transported via blood

many
different
organs

MORPHINE ADDICTION (hypothesis)

Normal Release

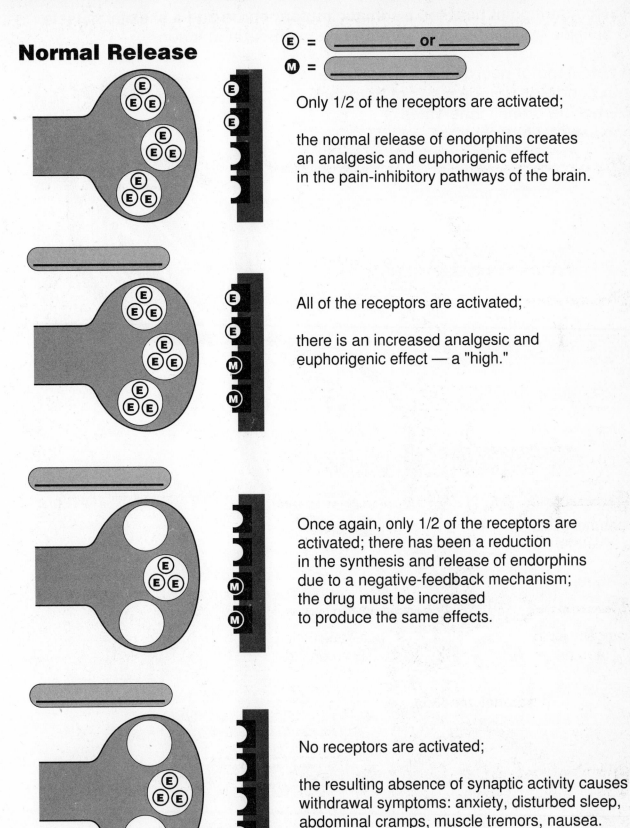

E = _____ or _____
M = _____

Only 1/2 of the receptors are activated;

the normal release of endorphins creates
an analgesic and euphorigenic effect
in the pain-inhibitory pathways of the brain.

All of the receptors are activated;

there is an increased analgesic and
euphorigenic effect — a "high."

Once again, only 1/2 of the receptors are
activated; there has been a reduction
in the synthesis and release of endorphins
due to a negative-feedback mechanism;
the drug must be increased
to produce the same effects.

No receptors are activated;

the resulting absence of synaptic activity causes
withdrawal symptoms: anxiety, disturbed sleep,
abdominal cramps, muscle tremors, nausea.

NEUROMUSCULAR JUNCTION

The contact point between a somatic motor neuron and a skeletal muscle is called a neuromuscular junction or a myoneural junction.

A single motor neuron axon may divide into hundreds or thousands of branches. Each axon branch innervates one skeletal muscle fiber.

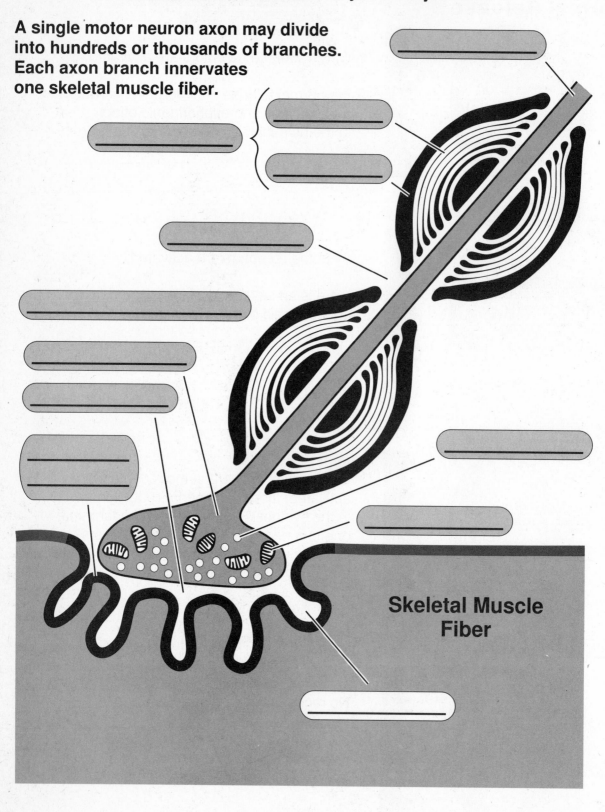

Skeletal Muscle Fiber

NEURONAL CIRCUITS

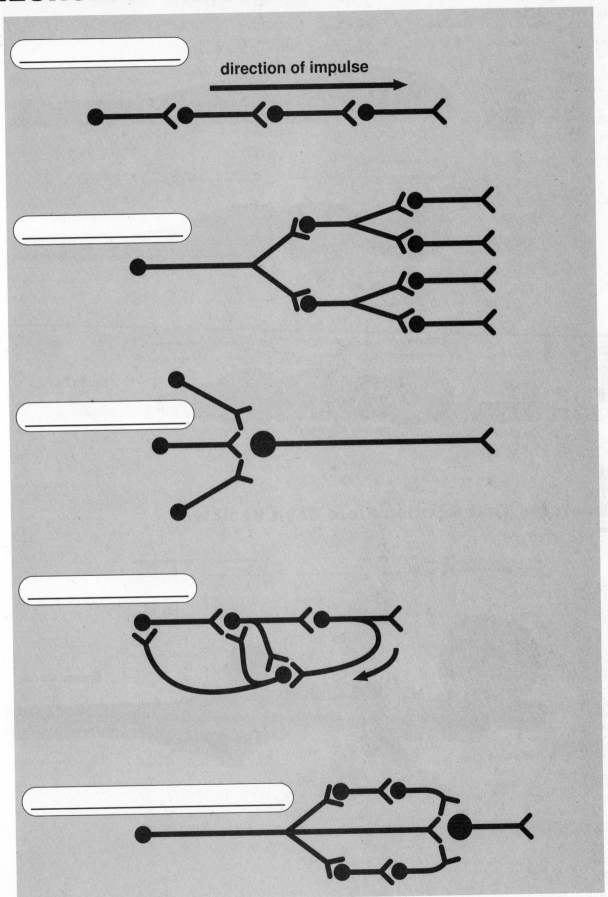

direction of impulse

223

BRAIN : Neural Tube Development

Lateral Views

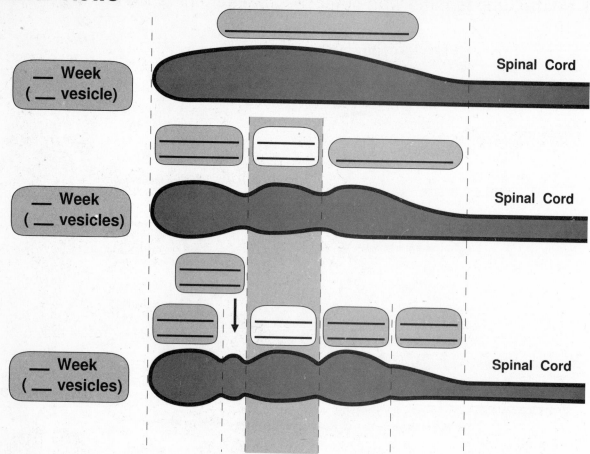

_____ Week
(_____ vesicle)

Spinal Cord

_____ Week
(_____ vesicles)

Spinal Cord

_____ Week
(_____ vesicles)

Spinal Cord

Structures That Develop From Each Vesicle

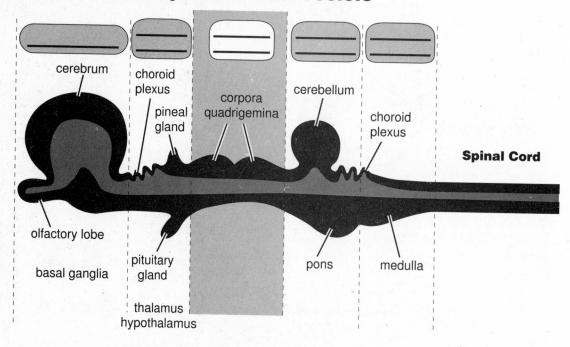

cerebrum

choroid
plexus

pineal
gland

corpora
quadrigemina

cerebellum

choroid
plexus

Spinal Cord

olfactory lobe

pituitary
gland

pons

medulla

basal ganglia

thalamus
hypothalamus

BRAIN : Embryonic Development

The neural tube is filled with cerebrospinal fluid (shaded areas).

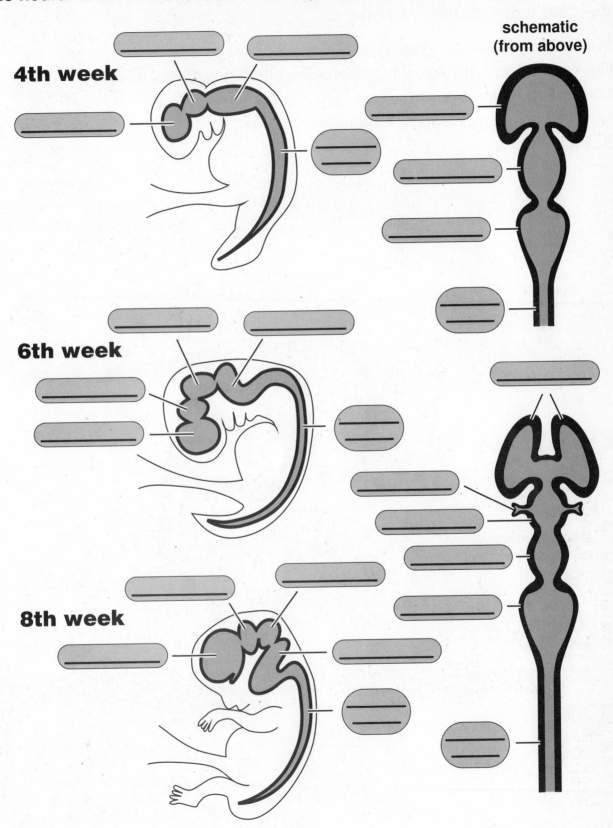

schematic
(from above)

4th week

6th week

8th week

225

BRAIN : 8th Week

By the end of the 8th week of embryonic development
the CNS has 5 distinct regions :

Forebrain : develops into the cerebrum
Diencephalon : thalamus, hypothalamus, pituitary & pineal glands
Midbrain : corpora quadrigemina (superior & inferior colliculi)
Hindbrain : pons, medulla, & cerebellum
Spinal Cord

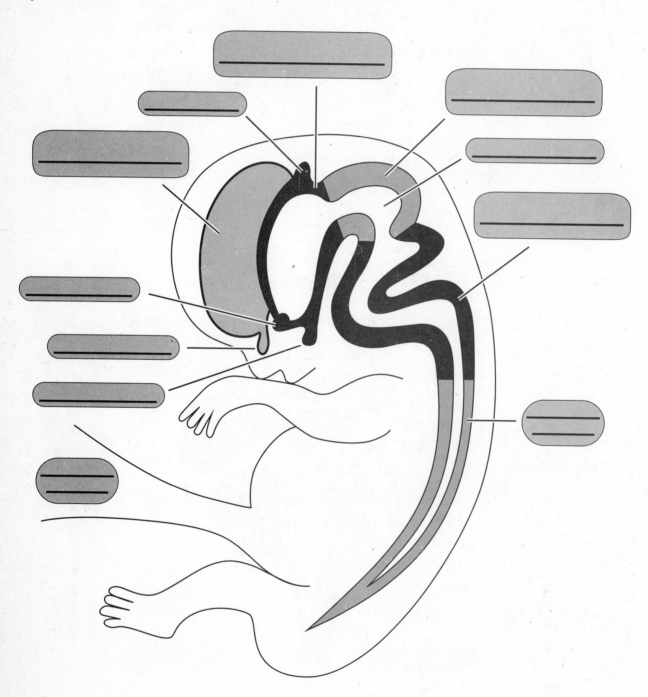

BRAIN : Fetal Development

2nd MONTH

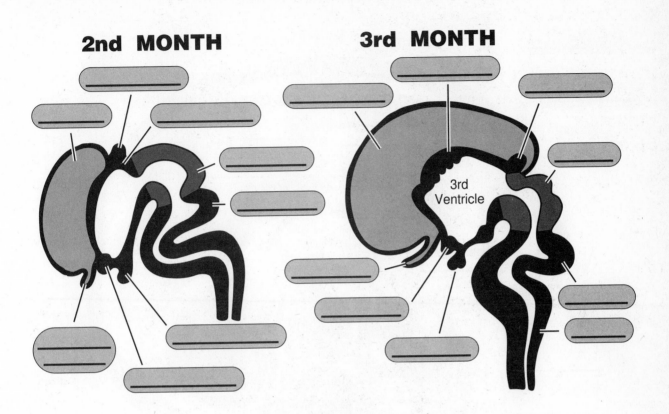

3rd MONTH

3rd
Ventricle

7th MONTH

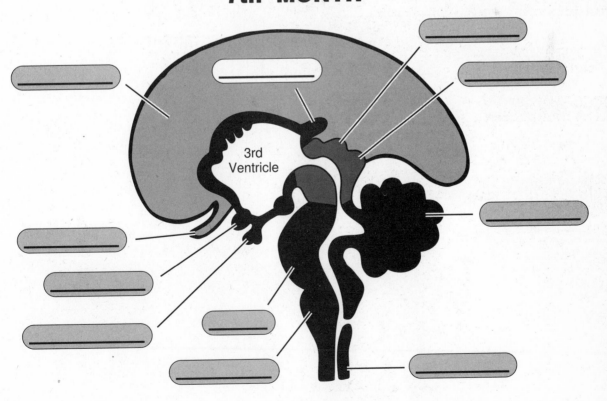

3rd
Ventricle

MATURE BRAIN : the basic parts

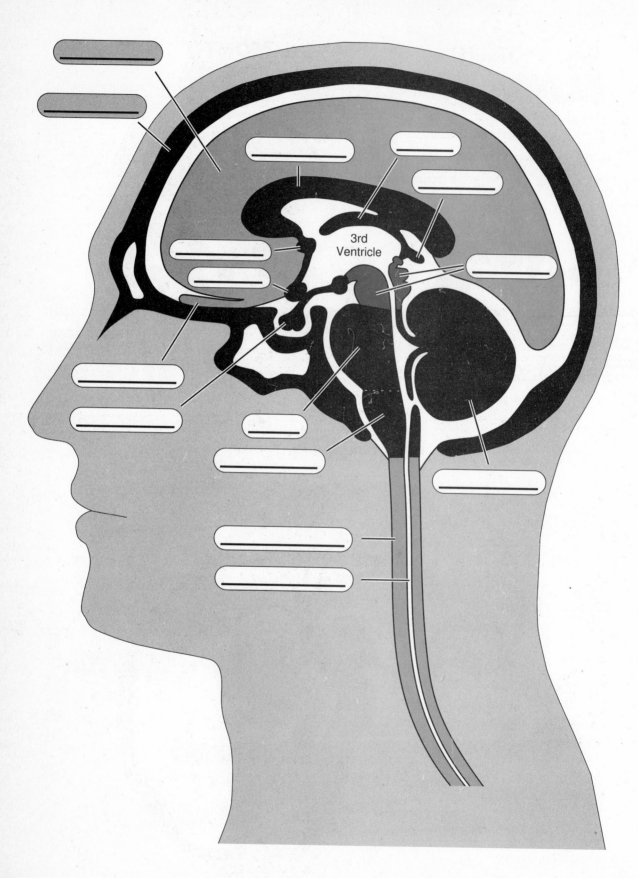

3rd
Ventricle

CRANIUM : bone plates covering the brain

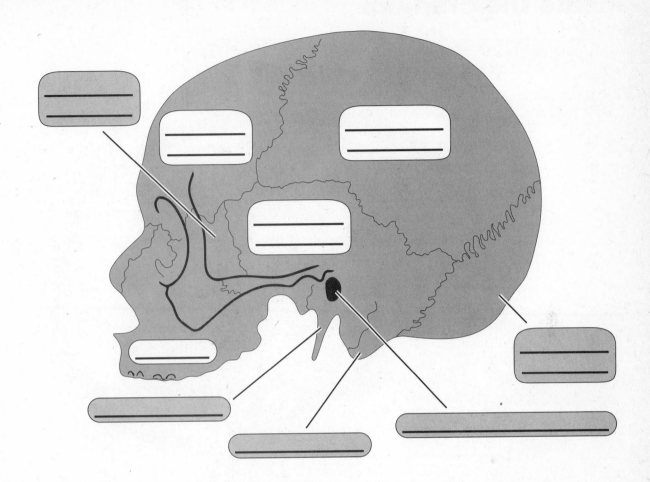

Midsagittal section

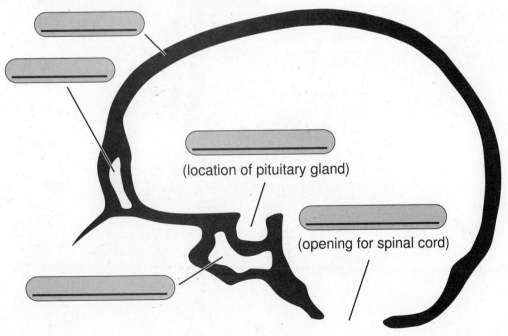

(location of pituitary gland)

(opening for spinal cord)

BRAIN LOCATION
inside the cranium

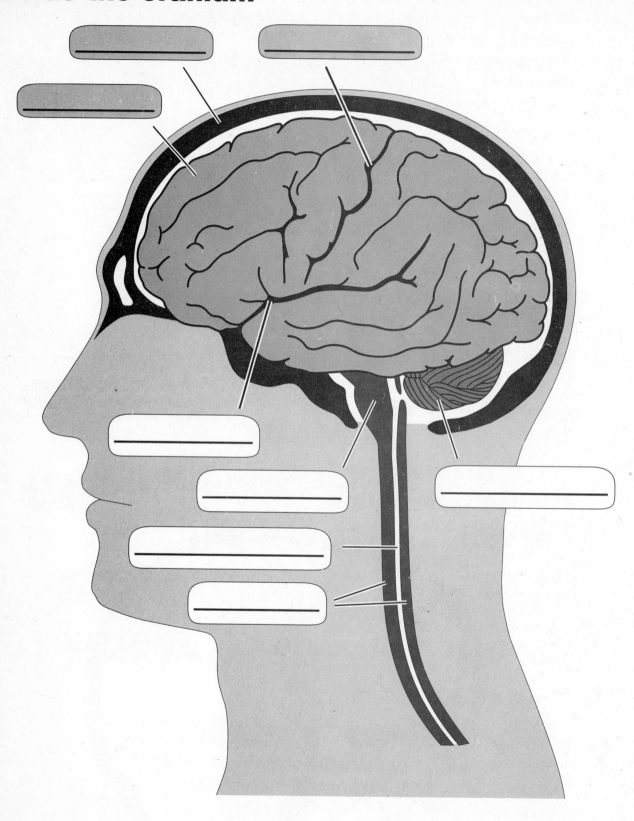

VENTRICLES IN THE BRAIN

There are 4 ventricles in the brain:
a lateral ventricle in each cerebral hemisphere (left & right lateral ventricles),
the 3rd ventricle in the diencephalon,
and the 4th ventricle between the pons & cerebellum.

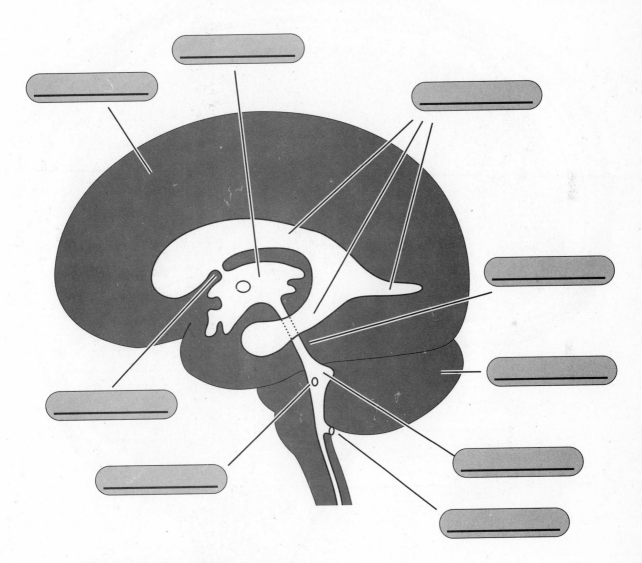

Choroid Plexuses

Networks of specialized capillaries are located
on the roof of each ventricle.
They produce cerebrospinal fluid (CSF)
and filter harmful materials (blood-brain barrier).

CEREBROSPINAL FLUID (CSF)
Cerebrospinal fluid is secreted by choroid plexuses.
It circulates through the brain and enters the superior sagittal sinus.

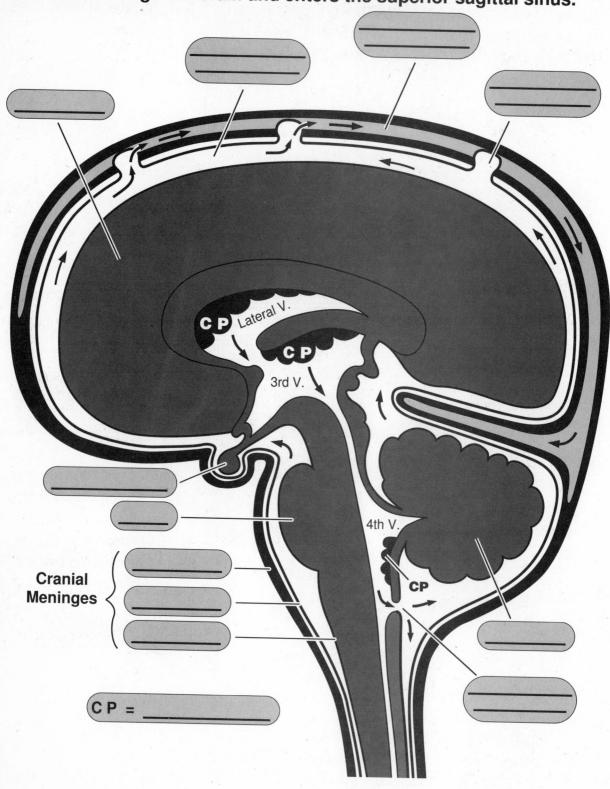

C P Lateral V.

C P

3rd V.

4th V.

CP

Cranial
Meninges

C P = _____

MENINGES :
Dura Mater, Arachnoid, & Pia Mater

Frontal Section
through the brain

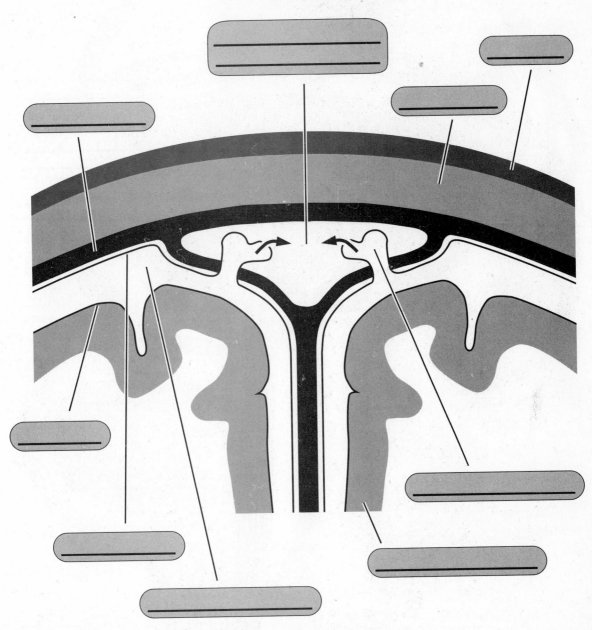

BRAIN STEM : Midbrain, Pons & Medulla

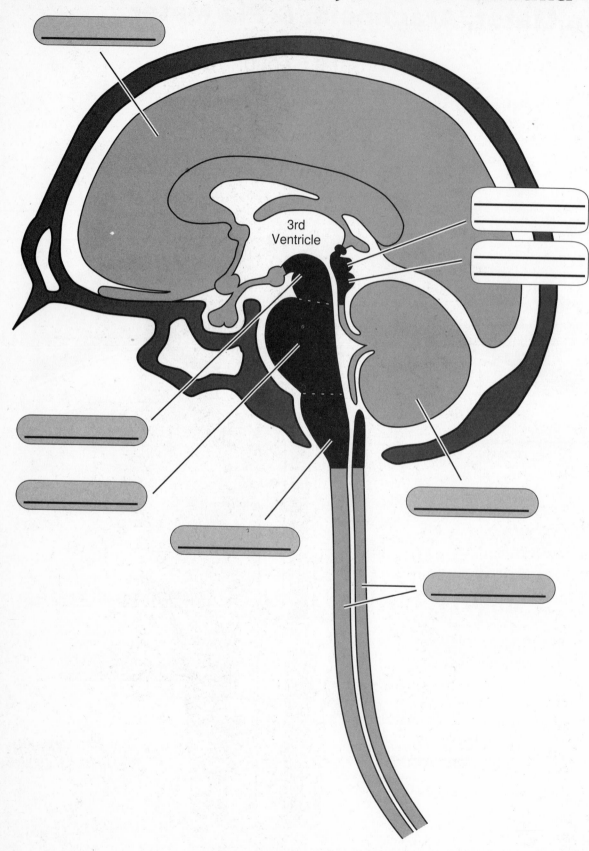

3rd
Ventricle

BRAIN STEM : Midbrain, Pons & Medulla

(cranial nerves are numbered)

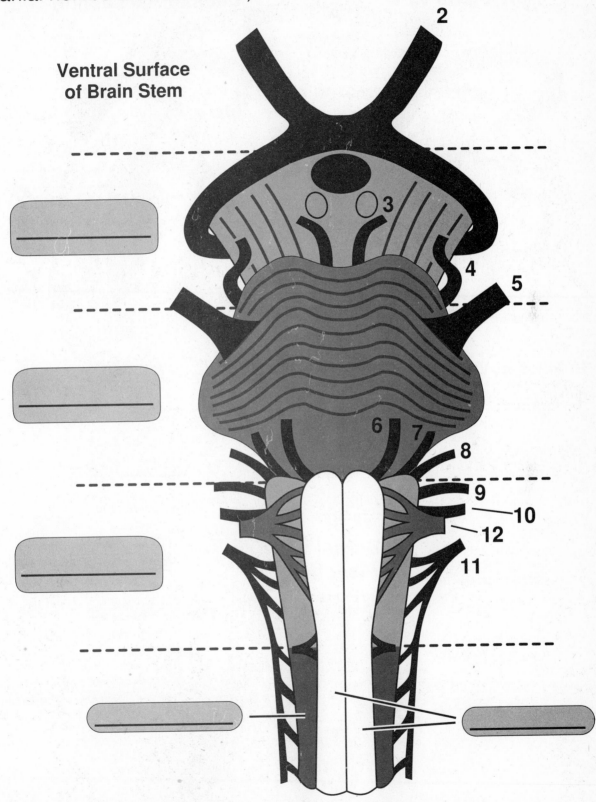

**Ventral Surface
of Brain Stem**

note : the 1st cranial nerves (olfactory nerves) are not visible in this illustration;
they emerge from olfactory bulbs that are located under the frontal lobes of the cerebrum.

CEREBELLUM

left lateral view

midsagittal section

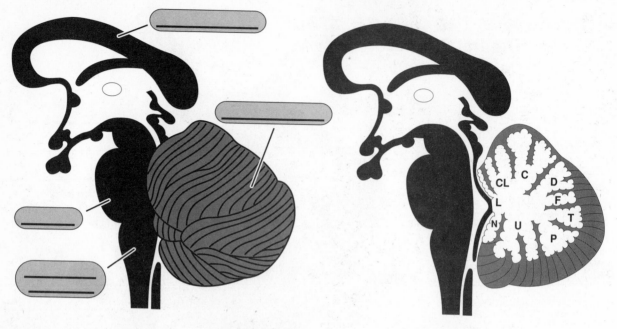

Lobules of Vermis :

L = _____

CL = _____

C = _____

D = _____

F = _____

T = _____

P = _____

U = _____

N = _____

Dorsal View (section)

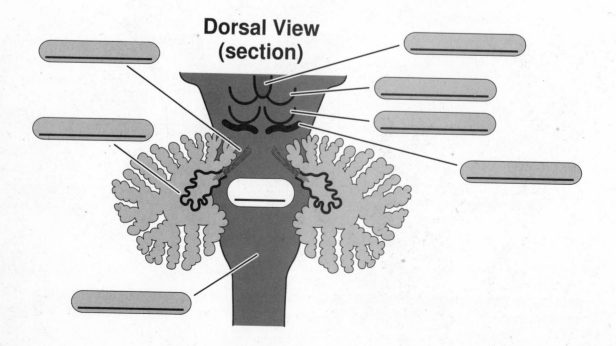

DIENCEPHALON

Thalamus : develops from the side walls of the 3rd ventricle
Hypothalamus : develops from the floor of the 3rd ventricle

Location in the Mature Brain

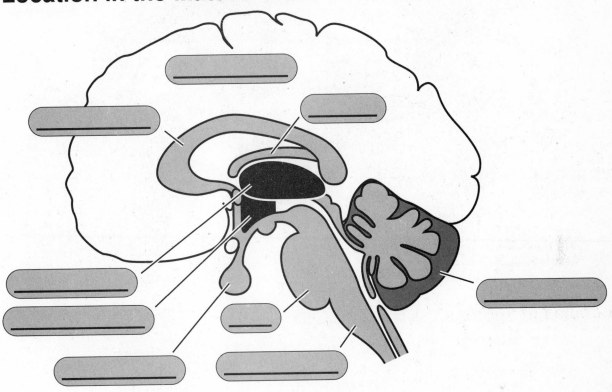

Location in the Embryonic Brain

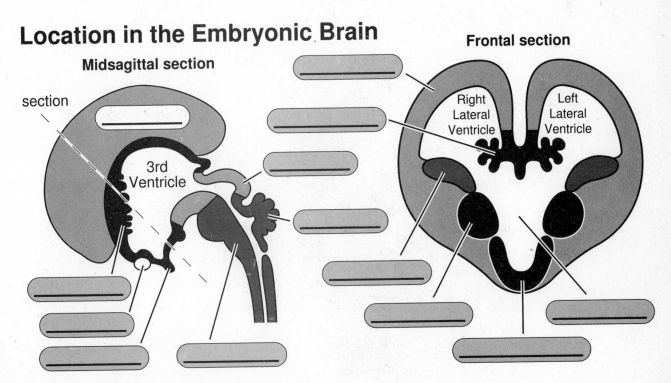

Frontal section

Midsagittal section

section

3rd
Ventricle

Right
Lateral
Ventricle

Left
Lateral
Ventricle

HYPOTHALAMUS : Principal Nuclei

Lateral View

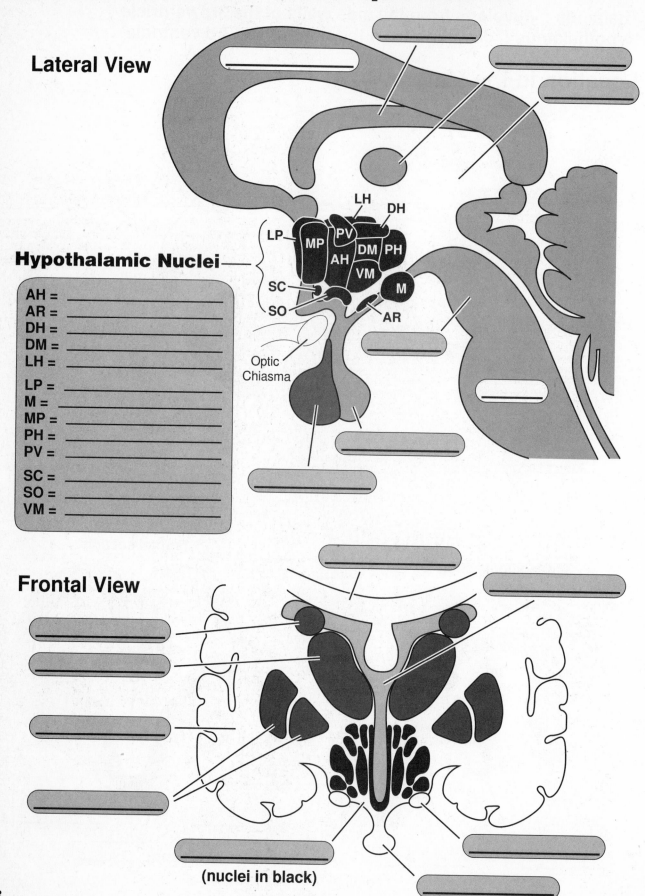

Hypothalamic Nuclei

AH = _____
AR = _____
DH = _____
DM = _____
LH = _____

LP = _____
M = _____
MP = _____
PH = _____
PV = _____

SC = _____
SO = _____
VM = _____

Optic Chiasma

LH   DH

LP   MP   PV   DM   PH
     AH   VM
SC
SO   M
          AR

Frontal View

(nuclei in black)

238

CEREBRUM
midsagittal section

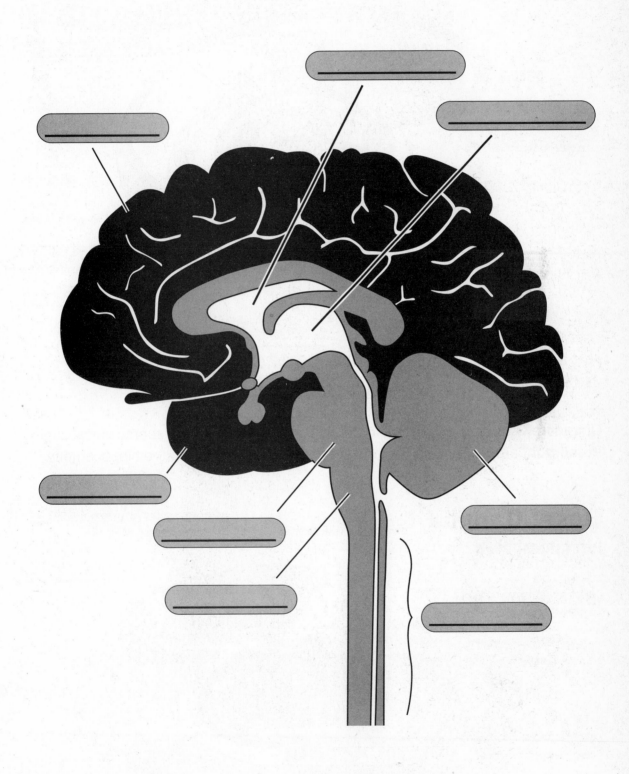

LIMBIC SYSTEM & BASAL GANGLIA

Limbic System
left lateral view

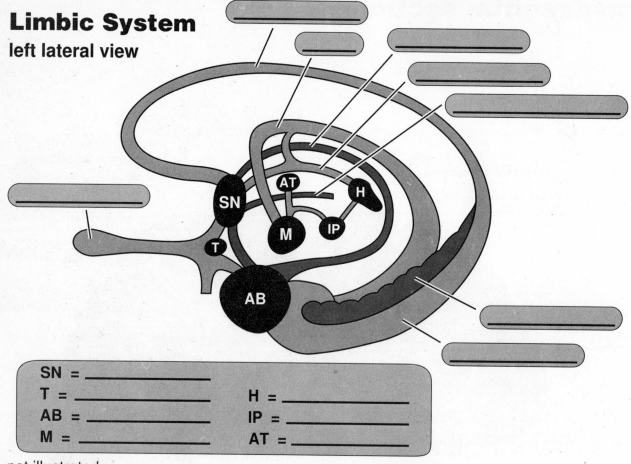

SN = _____

T = _____

AB = _____   H = _____

M = _____   IP = _____

                                     AT = _____

not illustrated :

Cingulate Gyrus : region of the cerebral cortex superior to the supracallosal striae

Parahippocampal Gyrus : region of cerebral cortex inferior to the hippocampus

Basal Ganglia
left lateral view

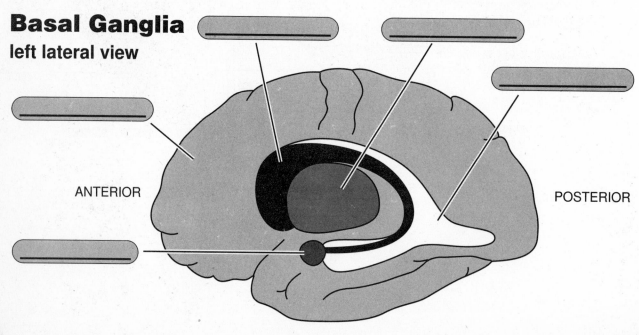

ANTERIOR   POSTERIOR

BRAIN : Horizontal Section

ANTERIOR

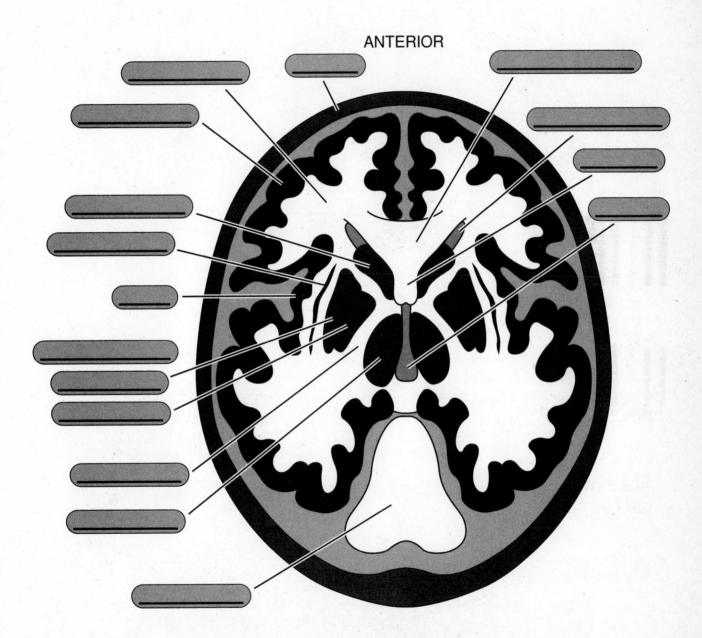

POSTERIOR

FISSURES AND GYRI (grooves & ridges)

Fissures (or Sulci)

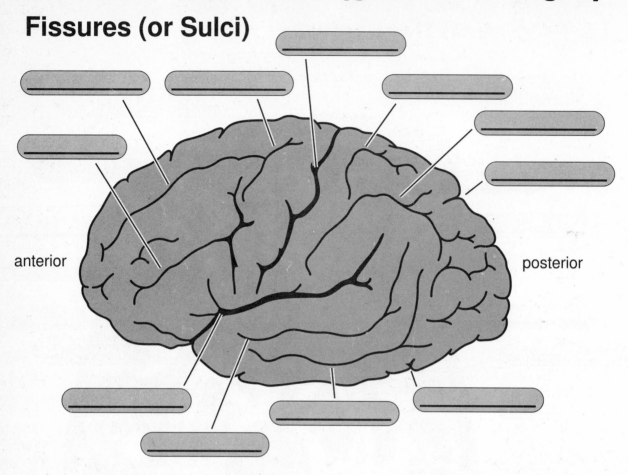

anterior

posterior

Gyri (or Convolutions)

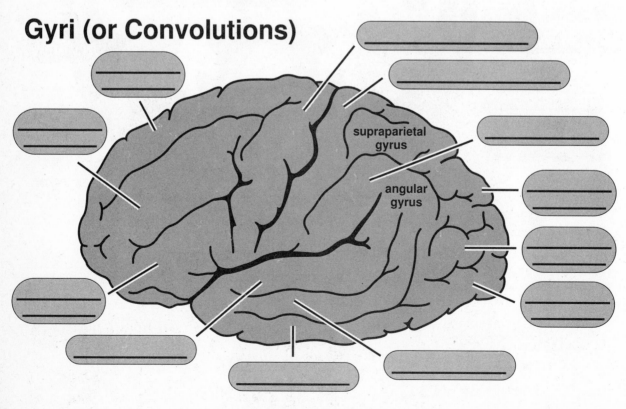

supraparietal
gyrus

angular
gyrus

242

CEREBRUM : 4 Lobes

Left Cerebral Hemisphere

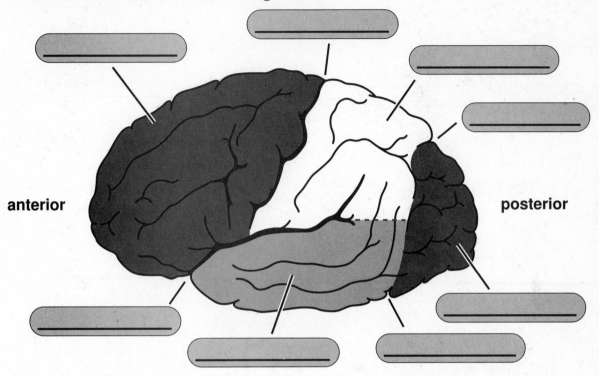

anterior

posterior

View From Above

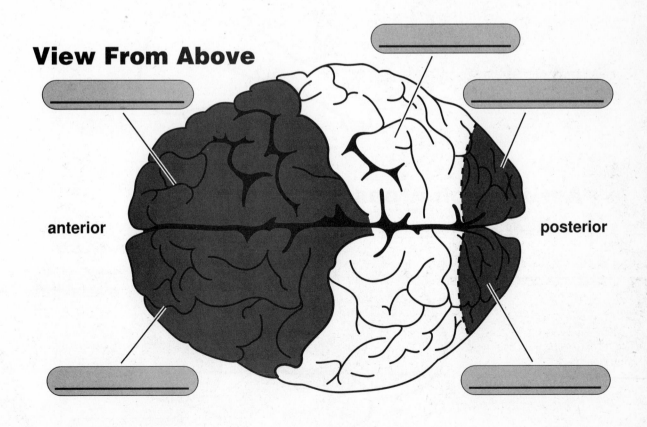

anterior

posterior

CEREBRAL CORTEX
Sensory, Motor, & Association Areas

Sensory Areas

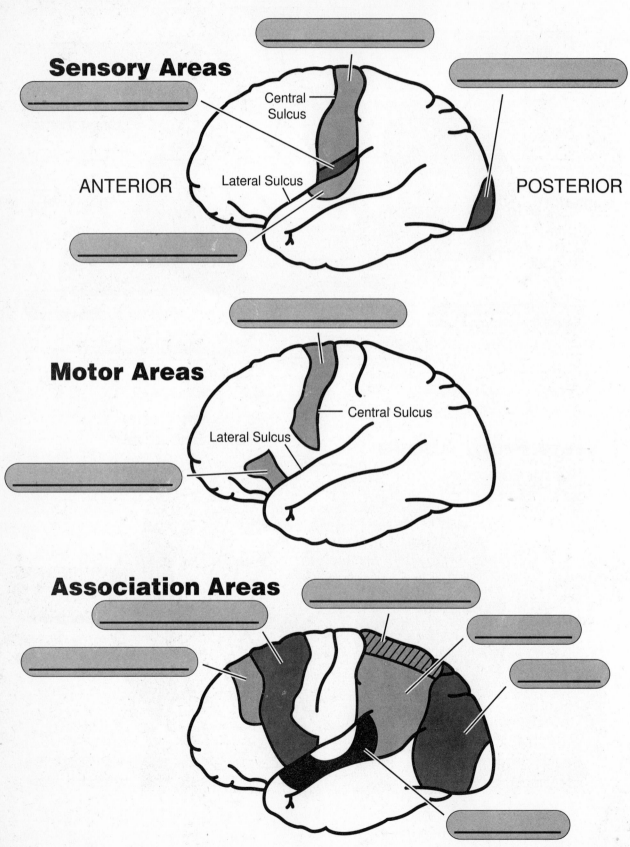

Central Sulcus

ANTERIOR

Lateral Sulcus

POSTERIOR

Motor Areas

Central Sulcus

Lateral Sulcus

Association Areas

SENSORY CORTEX

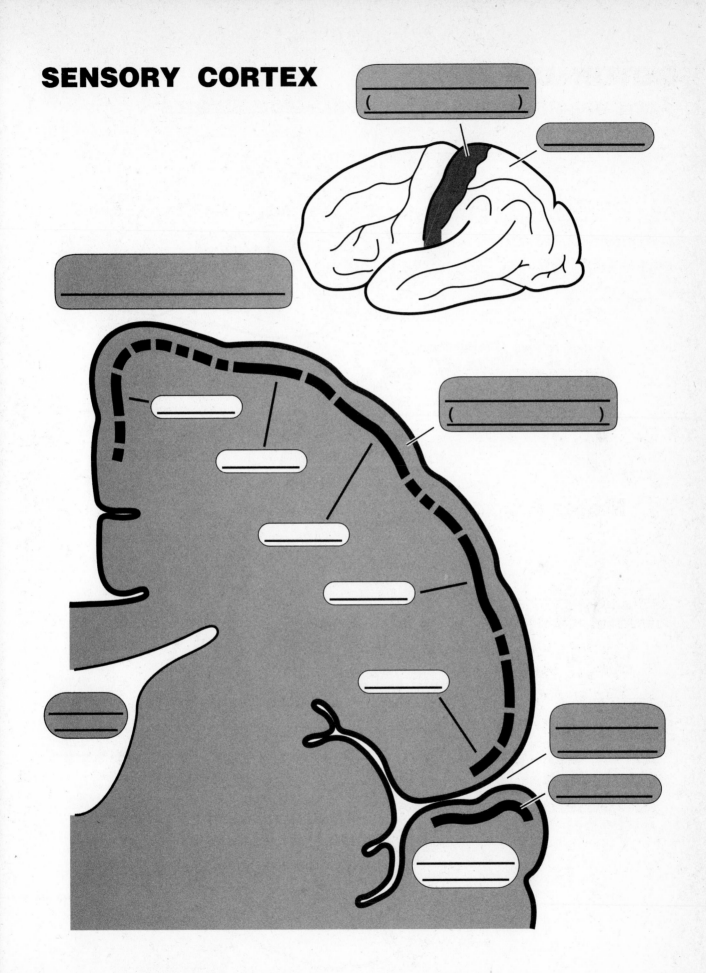

MOTOR CORTEX

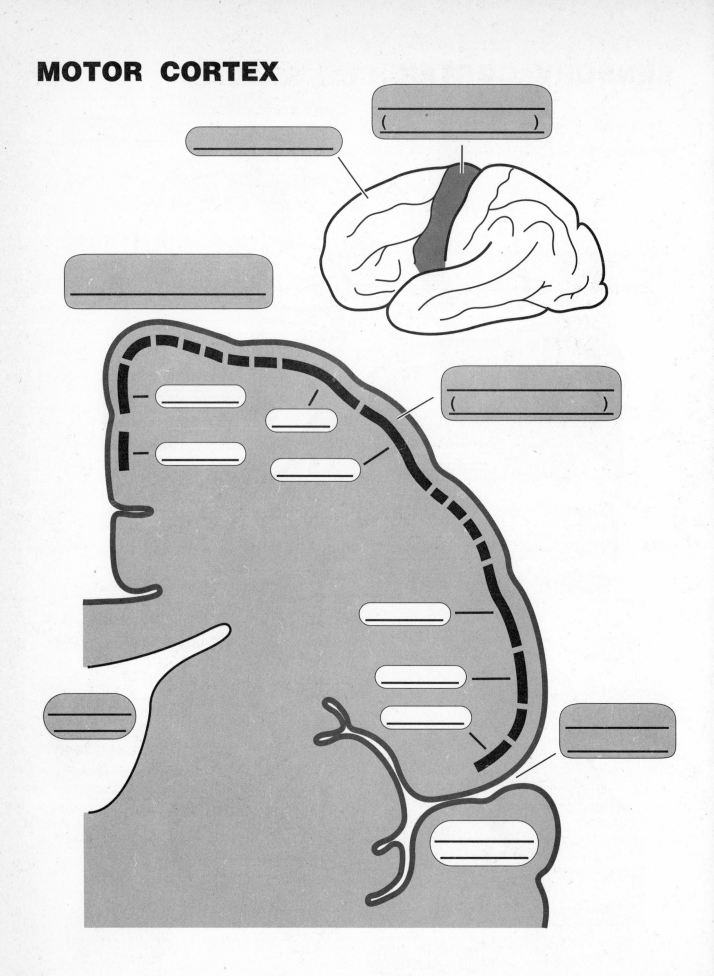

MENINGES & EPIDURAL SPACE

Spinal Cord
cross section inside a vertebra

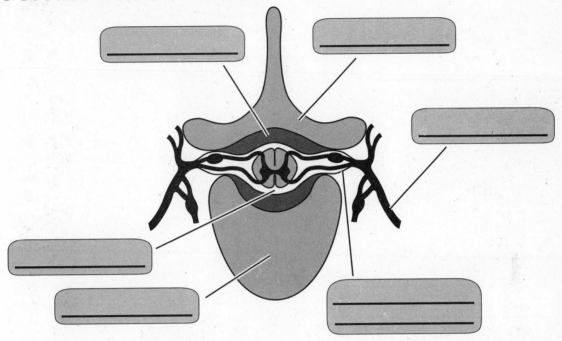

Spinal Cord
cross section showing meninges

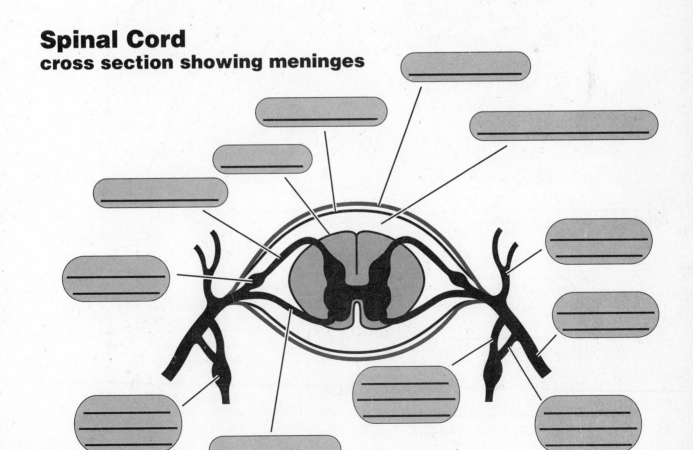

VERTEBRAL COLUMN
33 vertebrae (26 separate bones)

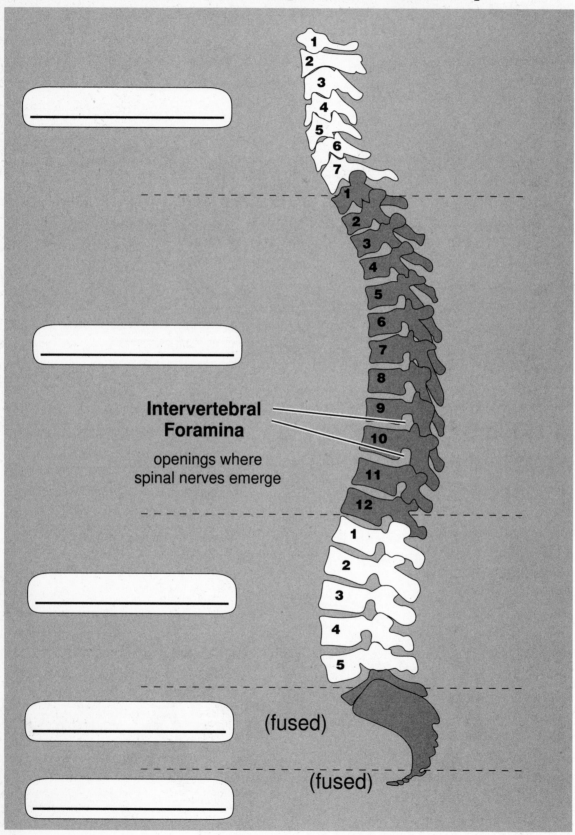

**Intervertebral
Foramina**

openings where
spinal nerves emerge

(fused)

(fused)

SPINAL CORD DIVISIONS

There are ____ pairs of spinal nerves.
They are named and numbered according to where they emerge from the _____ .

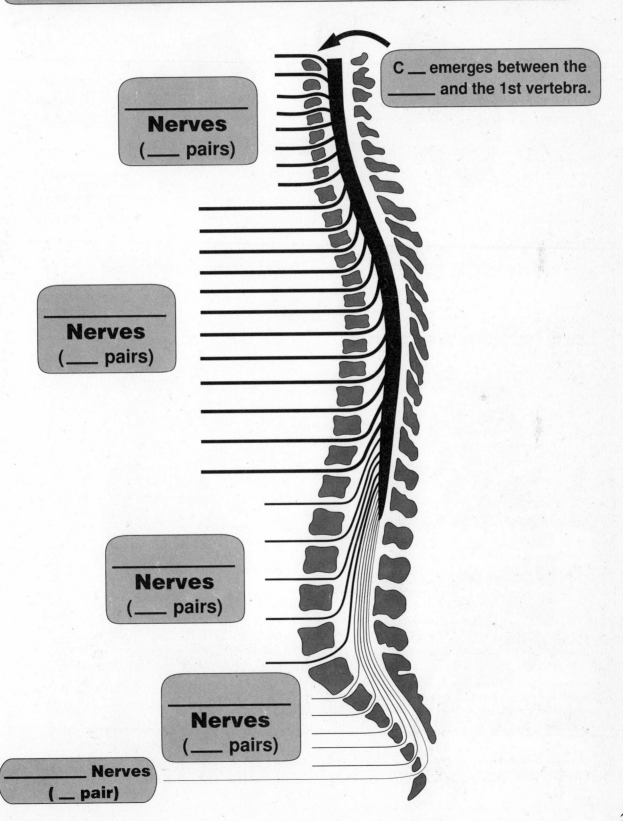

C ___ emerges between the _____ and the 1st vertebra.

_____
Nerves
(____ pairs)

_____
Nerves
(____ pairs)

_____
Nerves
(____ pairs)

_____
Nerves
(____ pairs)

_____ **Nerves**
(__ pair)

SPINAL CORD ANATOMY

Cross Section

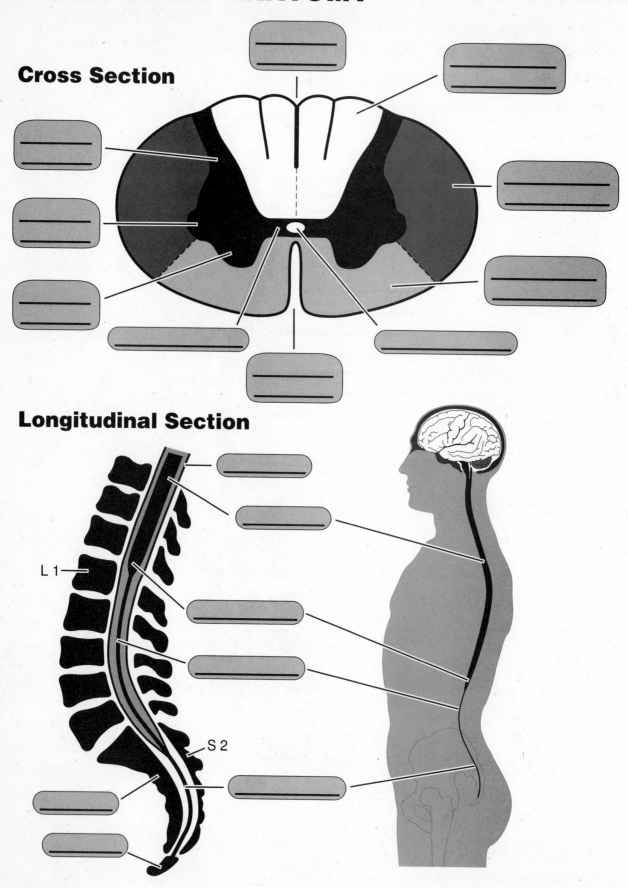

Longitudinal Section

L 1

S 2

SPINAL CORD TRACTS

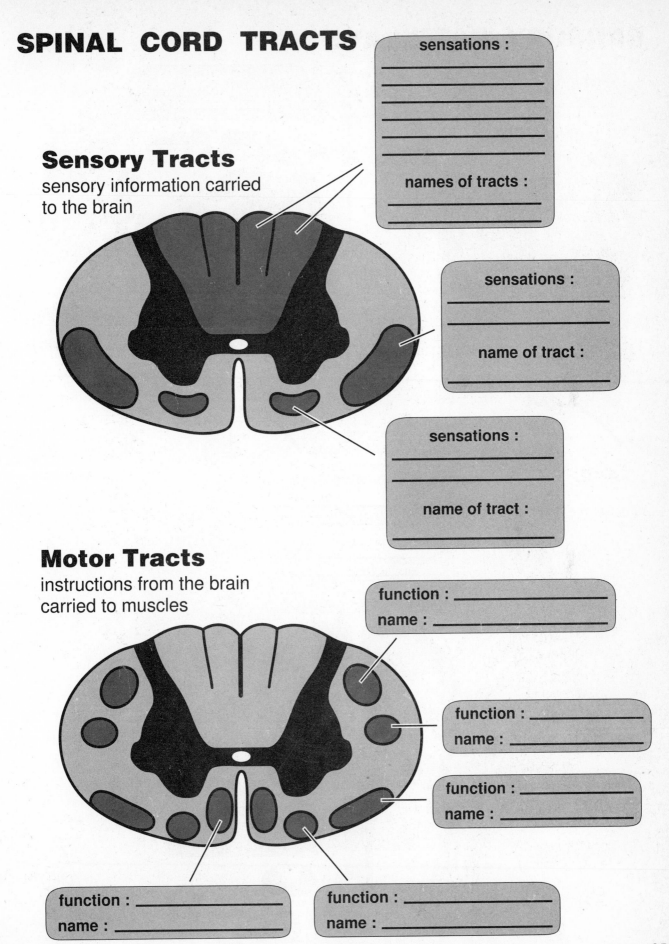

Sensory Tracts
sensory information carried
to the brain

sensations :
_____
_____
_____
_____
_____

names of tracts :
_____
_____

sensations :
_____
_____

name of tract :
_____

sensations :
_____
_____

name of tract :
_____

Motor Tracts
instructions from the brain
carried to muscles

function : _____
name : _____

function : _____
name : _____

function : _____
name : _____

function : _____
name : _____

function : _____
name : _____

SENSORY PATHWAYS

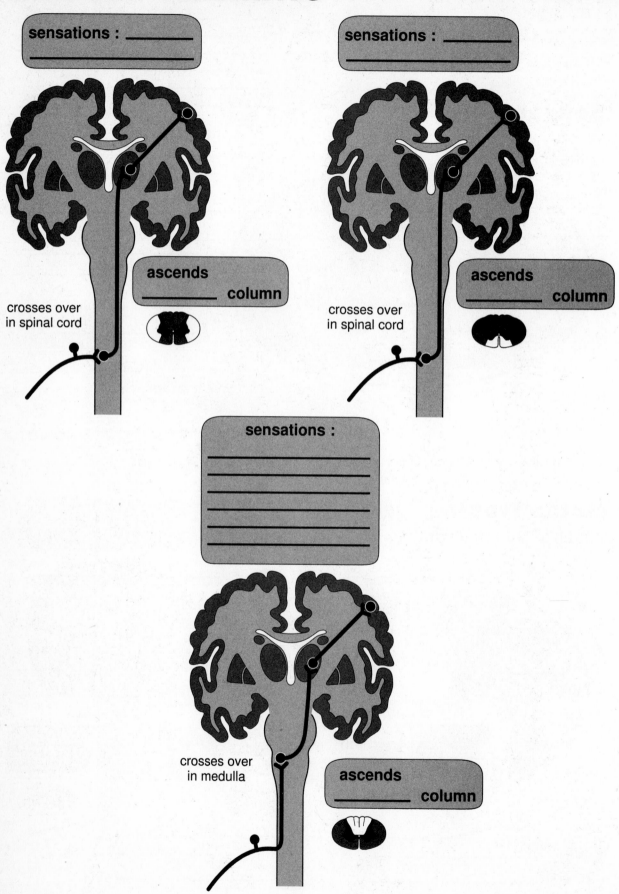

sensations : _____
_____

ascends
_____ column

crosses over
in spinal cord

sensations : _____
_____

ascends
_____ column

crosses over
in spinal cord

sensations :
_____
_____
_____
_____
_____
_____

crosses over
in medulla

ascends
_____ column

MOTOR PATHWAYS

Direct (Pyramidal) Pathways :
Voluntary Control of Skeletal Muscles

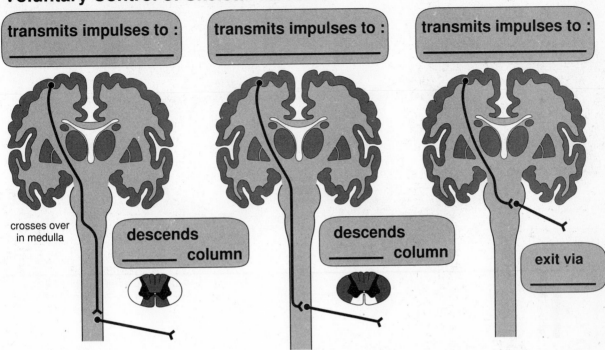

transmits impulses to :
_____

transmits impulses to :
_____

transmits impulses to :
_____

crosses over
in medulla

descends
_____ column

descends
_____ column

exit via
_____

Indirect (Extrapyramidal) Pathways :
Subconscious Control of Skeletal Muscles

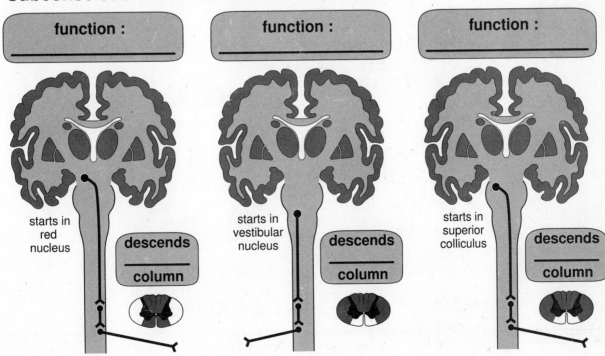

function :
_____

function :
_____

function :
_____

starts in
red
nucleus

descends
_____
column

starts in
vestibular
nucleus

descends
_____
column

starts in
superior
colliculus

descends
_____
column

SPINAL REFLEX

Spinal Cord Cross Section

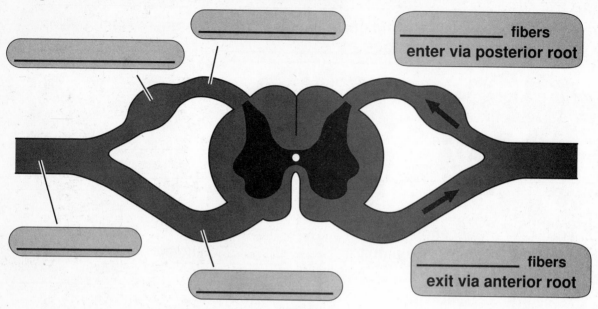

_____

_____

_____ fibers
enter via posterior root

_____

_____

_____ fibers
exit via anterior root

Generalized Reflex Arc

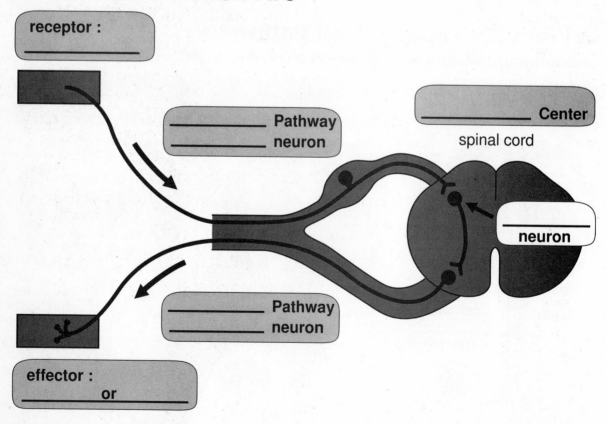

receptor :
_____

_____ Pathway
_____ neuron

_____ Center
spinal cord

_____ neuron

_____ Pathway
_____ neuron

effector :
_____ or

254

STRETCH REFLEX

The knee jerk reflex is an example of a stretch reflex.

When the muscle is stretched, muscle spindles are stimulated. The stretch reflex causes contraction of the same muscle that has been stretched.

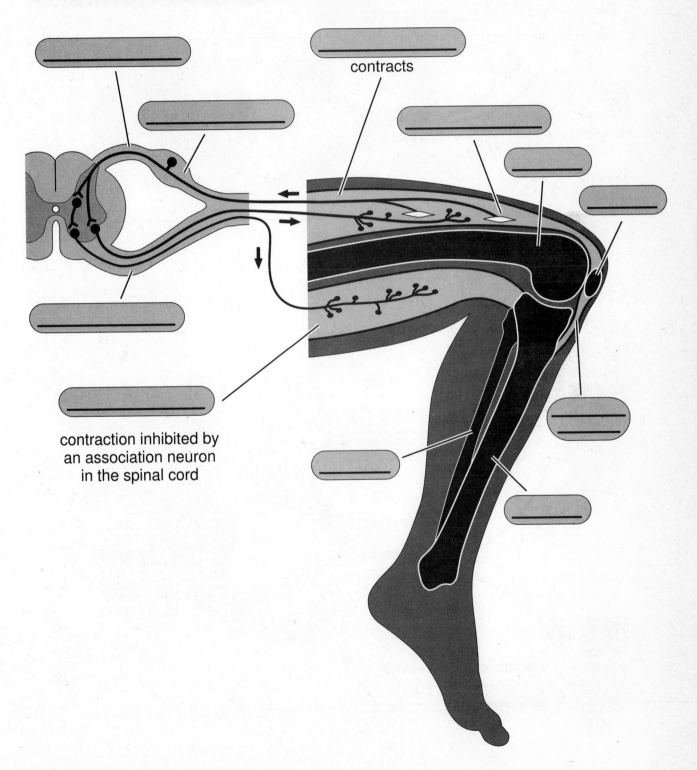

contracts

contraction inhibited by
an association neuron
in the spinal cord

SPINAL REFLEX : Examples

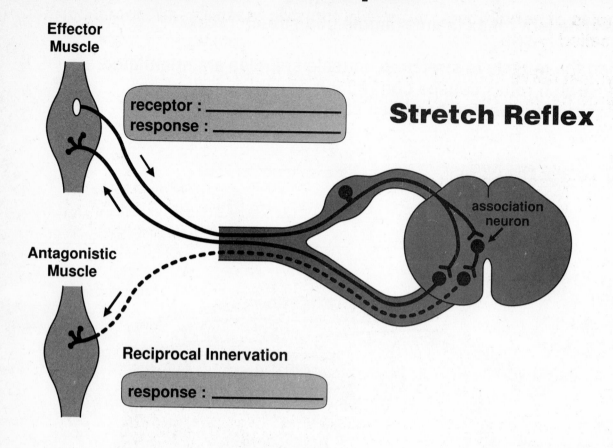

Effector Muscle

receptor : _____
response : _____

Stretch Reflex

association neuron

Antagonistic Muscle

Reciprocal Innervation

response : _____

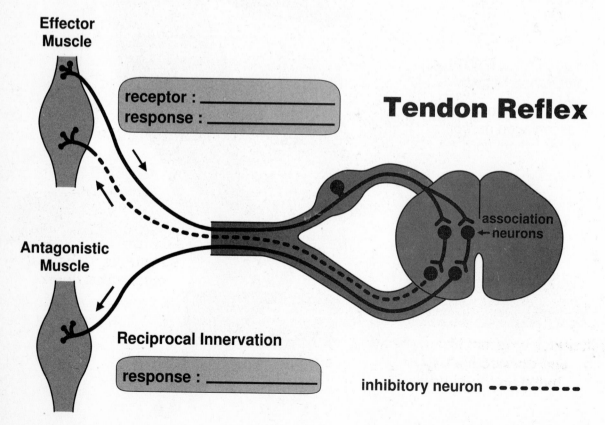

Effector Muscle

receptor : _____
response : _____

Tendon Reflex

association neurons

Antagonistic Muscle

Reciprocal Innervation

response : _____

inhibitory neuron ----------

NERVE (cross section)

Bundles of nerve fibers in the PNS (outside the brain and spinal cord) are called nerves.

A typical nerve contains several bundles of nerve fibers.
A large nerve contains thousands of nerve fibers.

(bundles of nerve fibers)

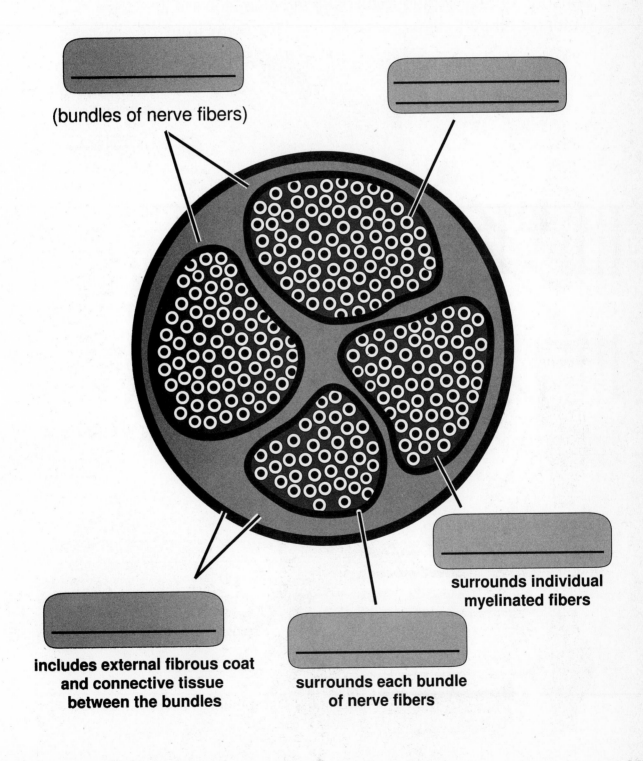

surrounds individual
myelinated fibers

includes external fibrous coat
and connective tissue
between the bundles

surrounds each bundle
of nerve fibers

PNS ORGANIZATION

Nerves :

(1) Cranial nerves emerge from the brain.
(2) Spinal nerves emerge from the spinal cord.

Neurons :

(1) Sensory (or afferent) neurons carry impulses toward the CNS.
(2) Motor (or efferent) neurons carry impulses away from the CNS.

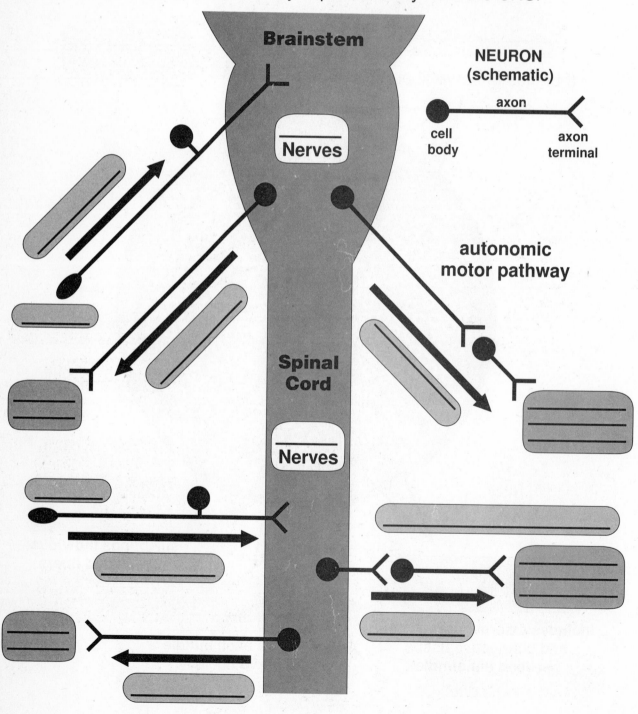

SPINAL NERVES   31 pairs of spinal nerves

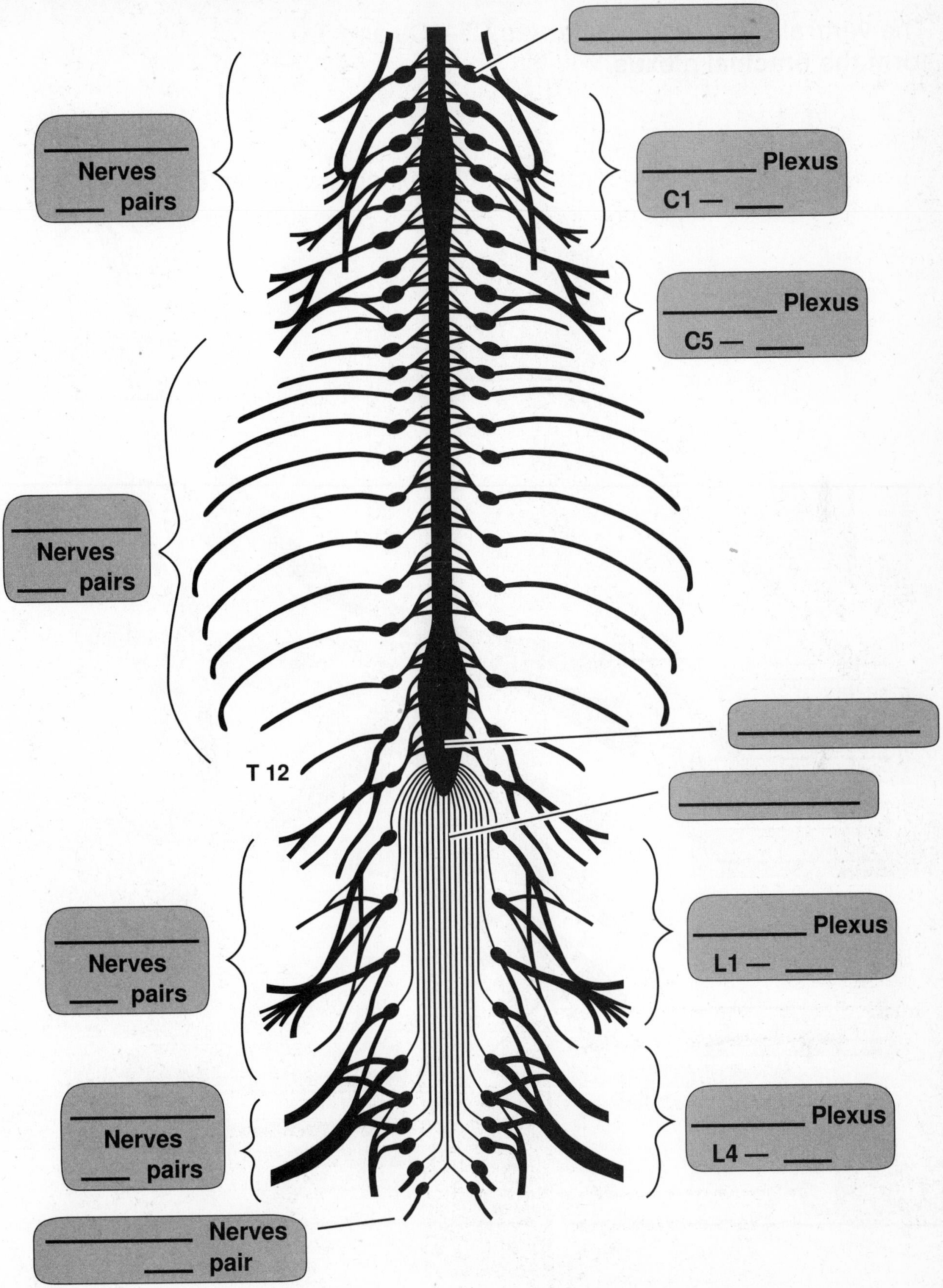

_____

_____ Nerves
_____ pairs

_____ Plexus

C1 — _____

_____ Plexus

C5 — _____

_____ Nerves
_____ pairs

T 12

_____

_____

_____ Nerves
_____ pairs

_____ Plexus

L1 — _____

_____ Nerves
_____ pairs

_____ Plexus

L4 — _____

_____ Nerves
_____ pair

SPINAL NERVES : Brachial Plexus

The ventral rami of spinal nerves C5—C8 and T1
form the brachial plexus.

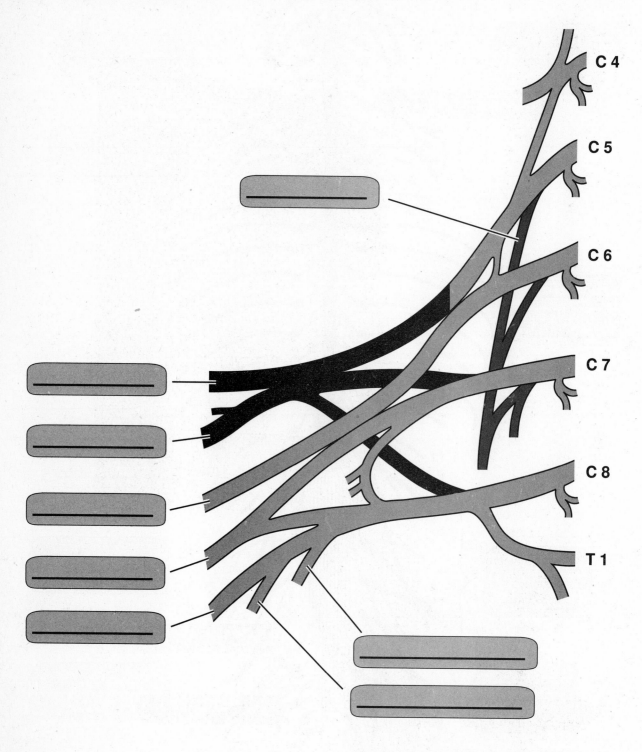

SPINAL NERVES
5 Major Nerves to the Arm

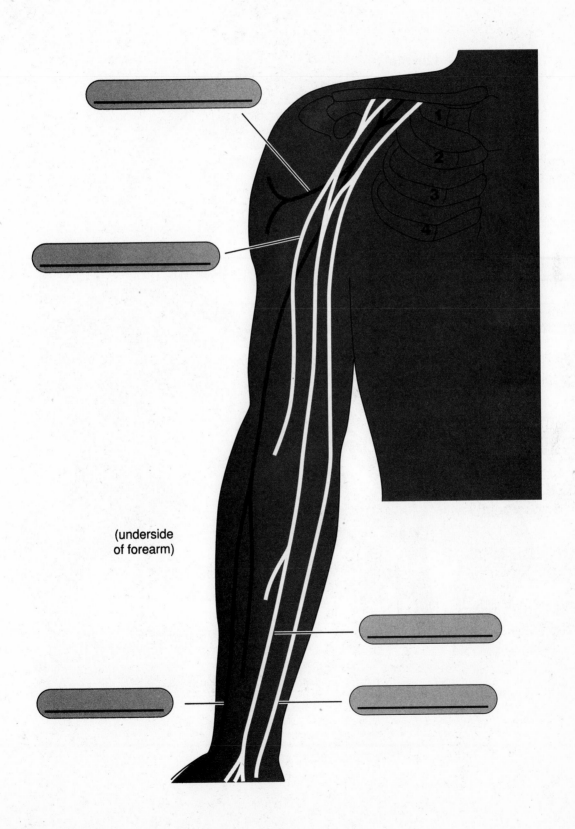

(underside
of forearm)

SPINAL NERVES : Lumbo-Sacral Plexus

The roots of the lumbosacral plexus are formed by
the ventral rami of spinal nerves L1 — S4.

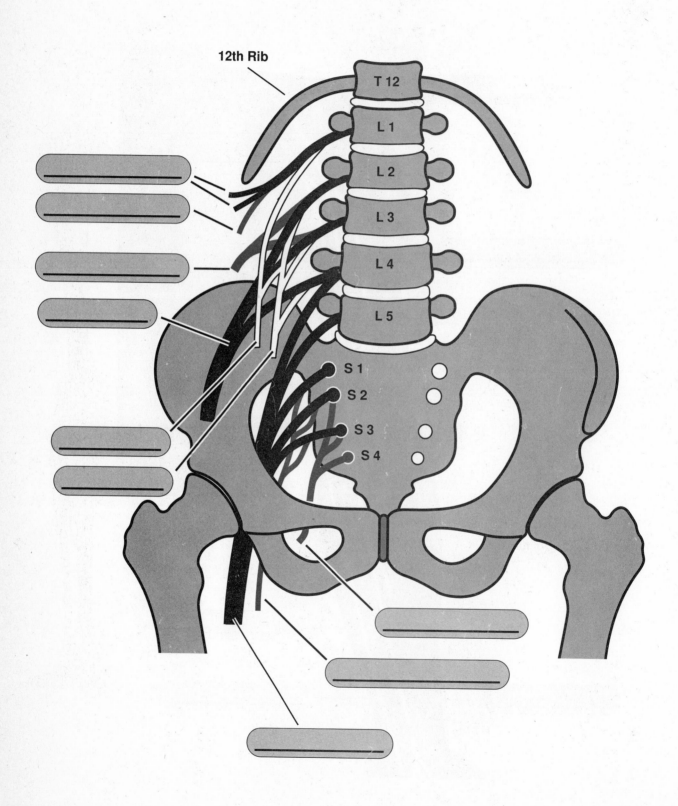

12th Rib

T 12

L 1

L 2

L 3

L 4

L 5

S 1

S 2

S 3

S 4

SPINAL NERVES
Sciatic Nerve

Anterior View

Posterior View

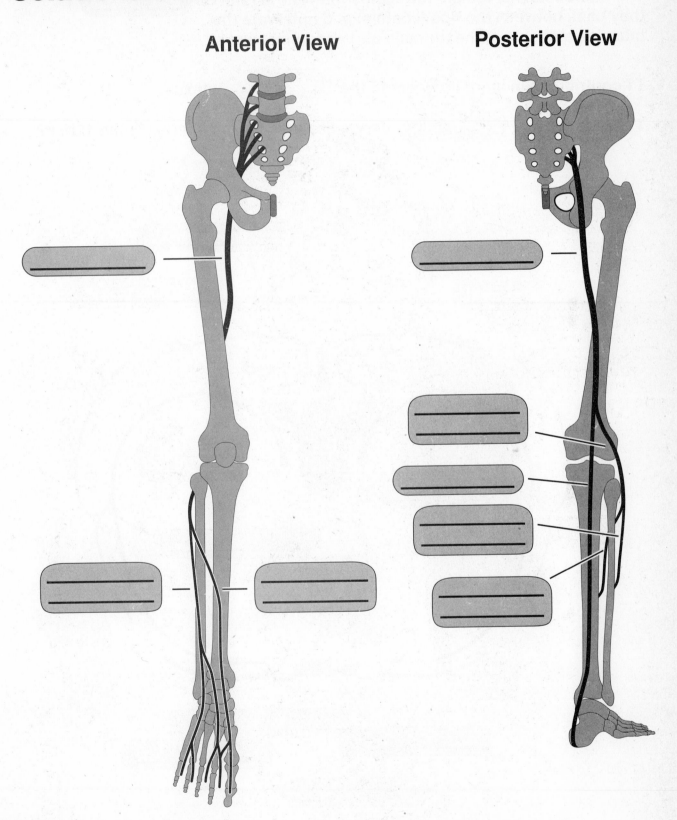

SPINAL NERVES : Intercostal Nerves

The intercostal nerves are formed by the ventral rami of 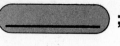 ;
they pass between the ribs (costals) and innervate the
muscles and skin of the thoracic and abdominal walls.

T1 contributes most of its fibers to the _____ plexus.

T12 is called the _____ nerve, because it runs inferior to the 12th rib.

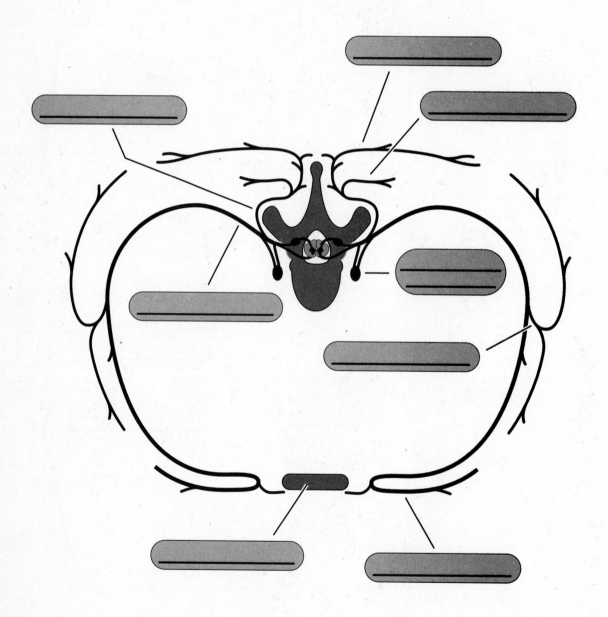

DERMATOMES
Segments of Skin Supplied by Spinal Nerves

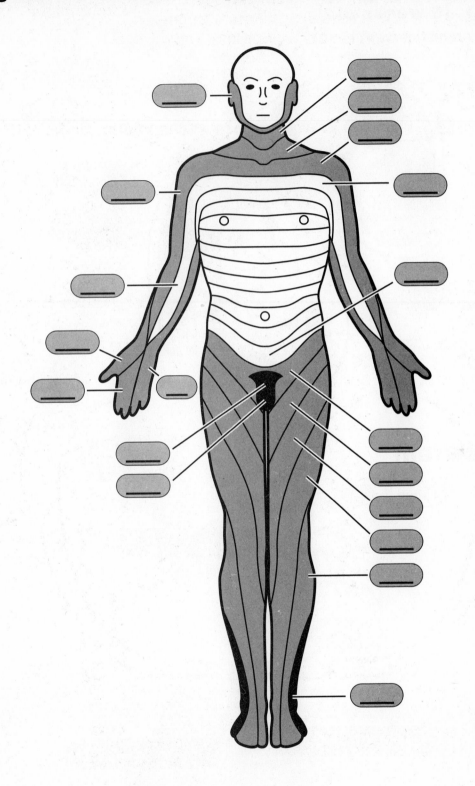

CRANIAL NERVES

Embryo (6 weeks old)
Number the cranial nerves (1 - 12).

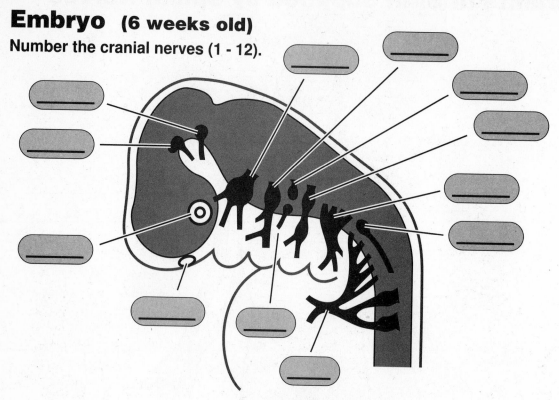

Mature Brain

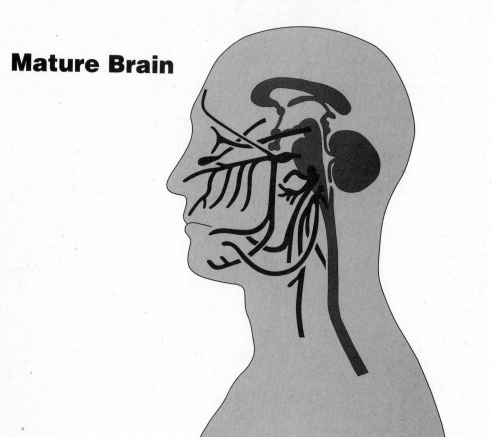

CRANIAL NERVES
ventral view

Number the cranial nerves.

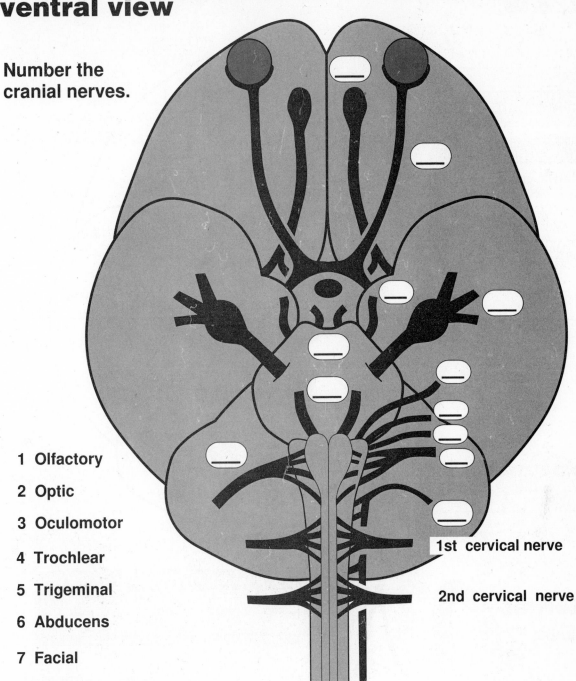

1st cervical nerve

2nd cervical nerve

1 Olfactory

2 Optic

3 Oculomotor

4 Trochlear

5 Trigeminal

6 Abducens

7 Facial

8 Vestibulocochlear

9 Glossopharyngeal

10 Vagus

11 Spinal Accessory

12 Hypoglossal

Note :
There are 12 pairs of cranial nerves.
For clarity only one nerve is shown
for cranial nerves 7 - 12.

PURELY SENSORY CRANIAL NERVES 1, 2, & 8

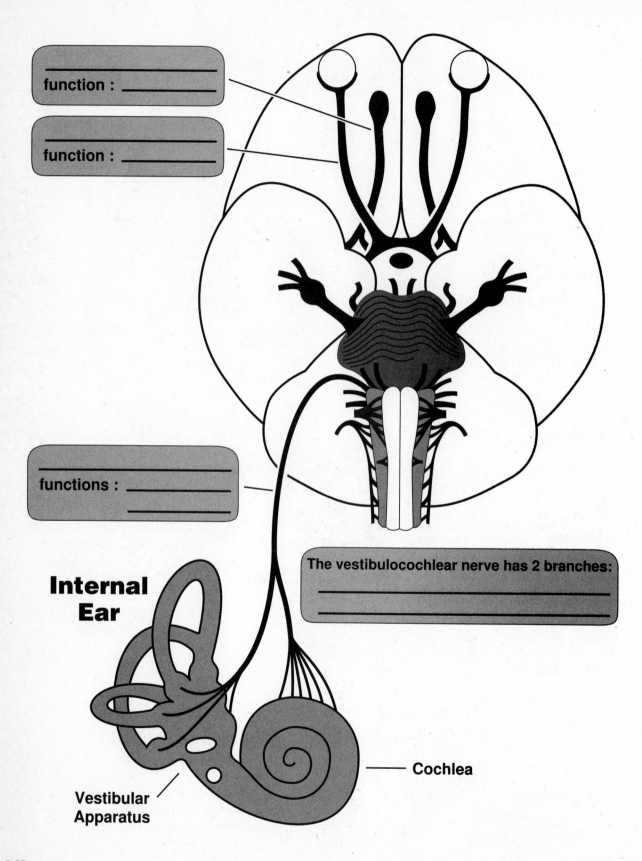

function : _____

function : _____

functions : _____

The vestibulocochlear nerve has 2 branches:
_____
_____

Internal Ear

Cochlea

Vestibular Apparatus

PRIMARILY MOTOR CRANIAL NERVES
3rd Cranial Nerve
also called : _____

4 eyeball muscles :
_____
_____
_____

eyelid muscle :
_____

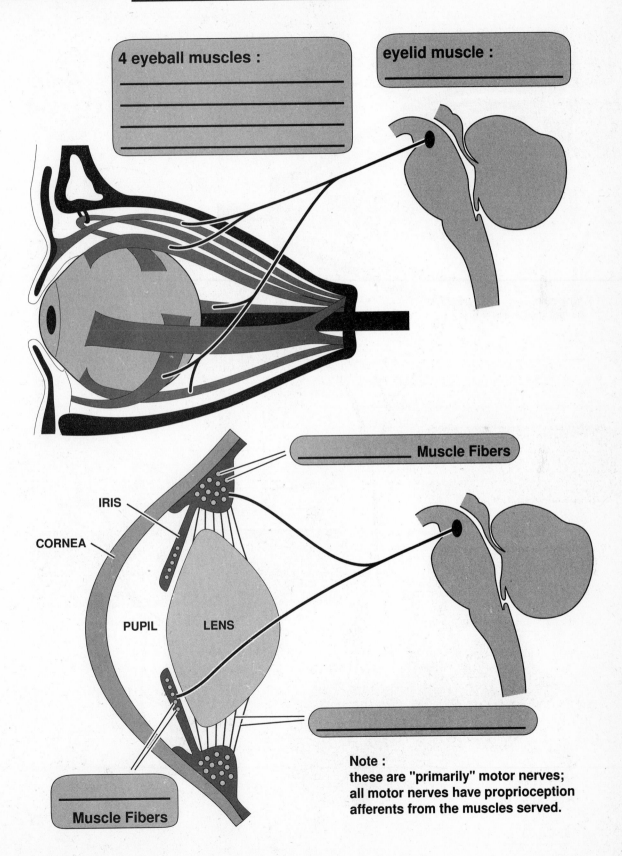

_____ Muscle Fibers

IRIS

CORNEA

PUPIL   LENS

Muscle Fibers

Note :
these are "primarily" motor nerves;
all motor nerves have proprioception
afferents from the muscles served.

PRIMARILY MOTOR CRANIAL NERVES
4, 6, 11, & 12

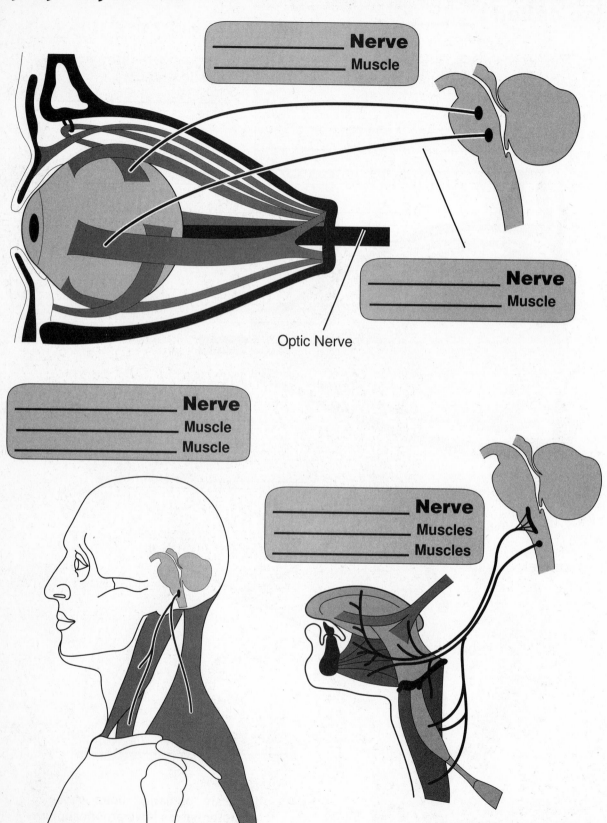

_____ Nerve
_____ Muscle

_____ Nerve
_____ Muscle

Optic Nerve

_____ Nerve
_____ Muscle
_____ Muscle

_____ Nerve
_____ Muscles
_____ Muscles

MIXED CRANIAL NERVES : 5, 7, 9, & 10
Sensory Components

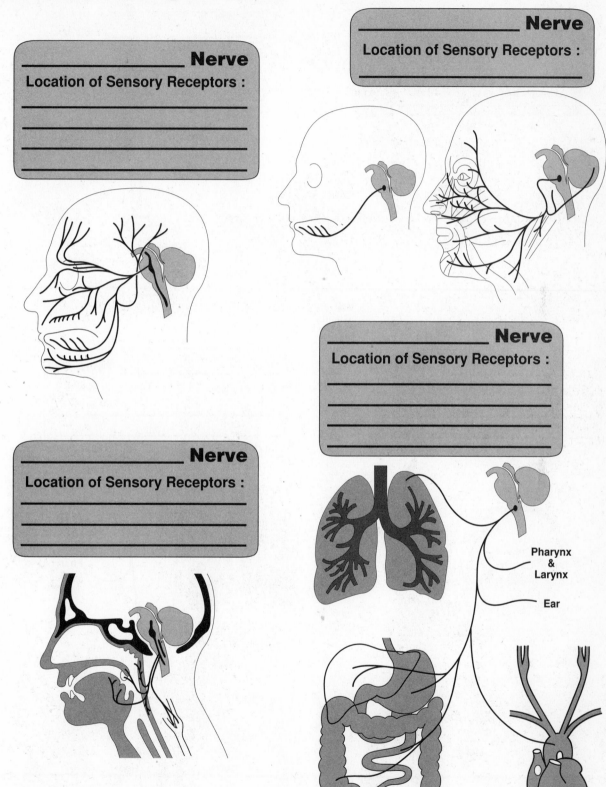

_____ Nerve

Location of Sensory Receptors :

_____

_____

_____

_____

_____ Nerve

Location of Sensory Receptors :

_____

_____ Nerve

Location of Sensory Receptors :

_____

_____

_____

_____ Nerve

Location of Sensory Receptors :

_____

_____

_____

Pharynx
&
Larynx

Ear

MIXED CRANIAL NERVES : 5, 7, 9, & 10
Motor Components

_____ Nerve

Effectors :
_____

_____ Nerve

Effectors :
_____
_____

_____ Nerve

Effectors :
_____
_____

_____ Nerve

Effectors :
_____
_____

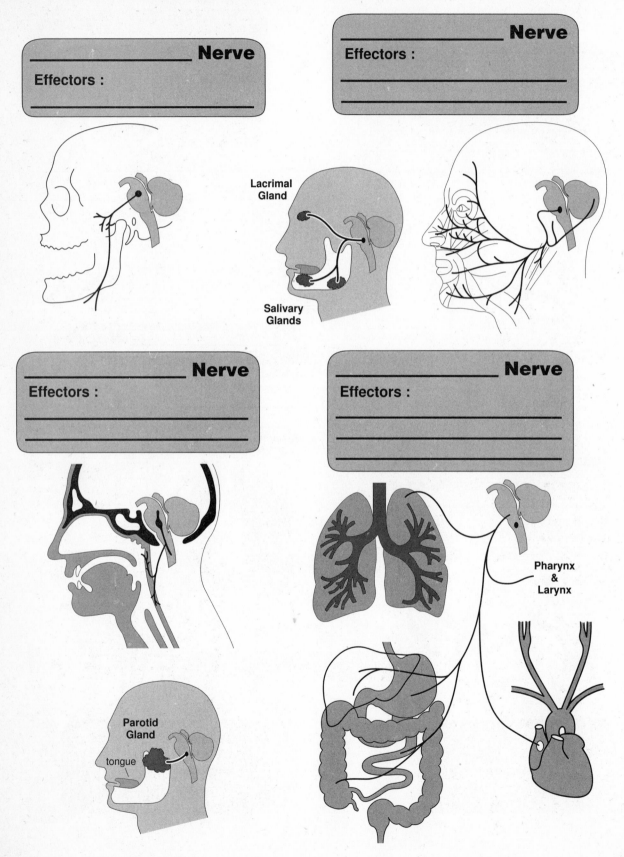

Lacrimal Gland

Salivary Glands

Parotid Gland

tongue

Pharynx & Larynx

AUTONOMIC NERVOUS SYSTEM
origins and outgoing pathways

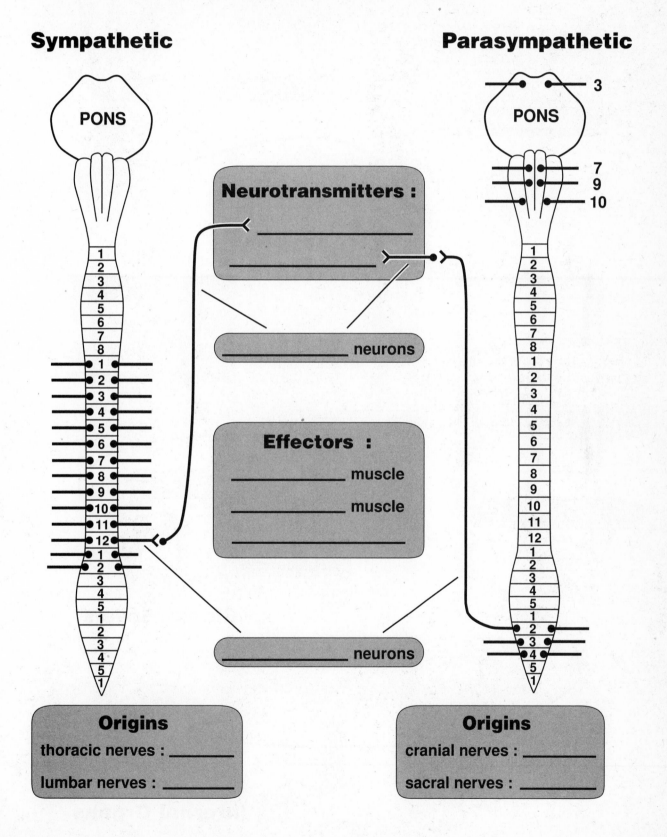

Sympathetic

Parasympathetic

PONS

PONS

Neurotransmitters :

_____

_____

_____ neurons

Effectors :

_____ muscle

_____ muscle

_____

_____ neurons

Origins

thoracic nerves : _____

lumbar nerves : _____

Origins

cranial nerves : _____

sacral nerves : _____

SYMPATHETIC NERVE PATHWAYS

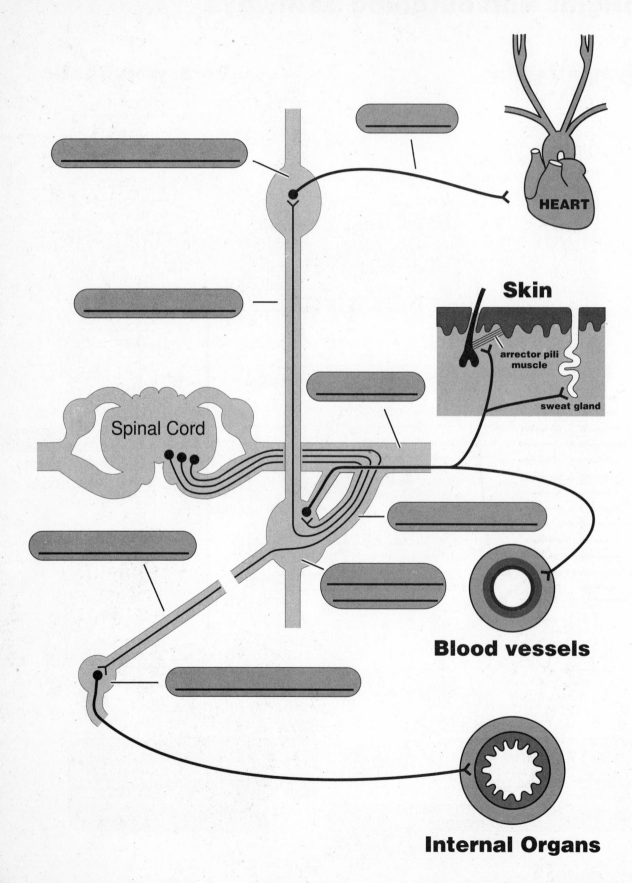

HEART

Skin

arrector pili
muscle

sweat gland

Spinal Cord

Blood vessels

Internal Organs

PARASYMPATHETIC SPINAL NERVES
Sacral Nerves 2, 3, and 4

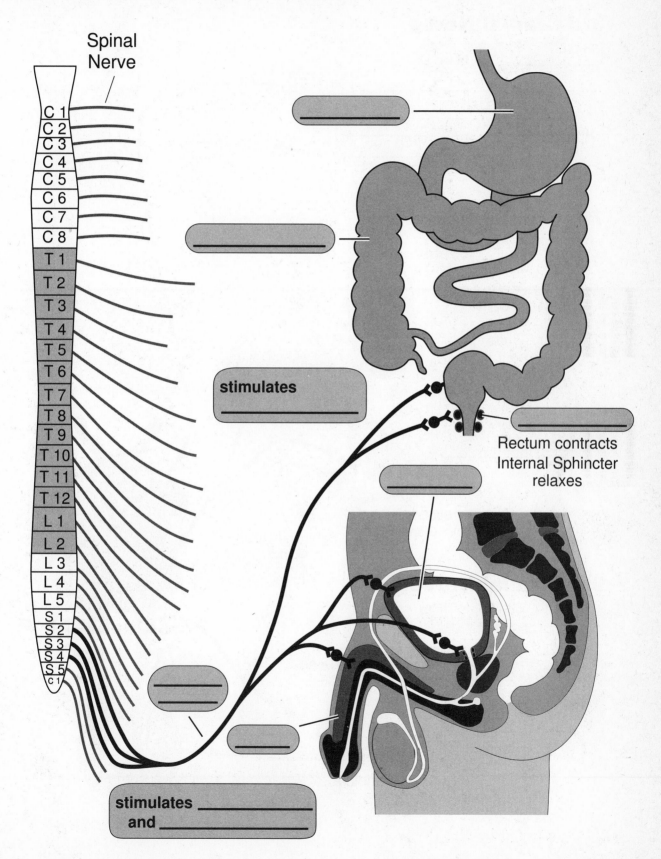

Spinal
Nerve

C 1
C 2
C 3
C 4
C 5
C 6
C 7
C 8
T 1
T 2
T 3
T 4
T 5
T 6
T 7
T 8
T 9
T 10
T 11
T 12
L 1
L 2
L 3
L 4
L 5
S 1
S 2
S 3
S 4
S 5
C 1

stimulates
_____

Rectum contracts
Internal Sphincter
relaxes

stimulates _____
and _____

PARASYMPATHETIC CRANIAL NERVES
Cranial Nerves 3, 7, & 9

3rd Cranial Nerve

_____ Nerve

functions

Lens : _____

Iris : _____

7th Cranial Nerve

_____ Nerve

functions

Lacrimal Glands :

_____

Sublingual Glands :

_____

Submandibular Glands :

_____

9th Cranial Nerve

_____ Nerve

functions

Parotid Glands :

_____

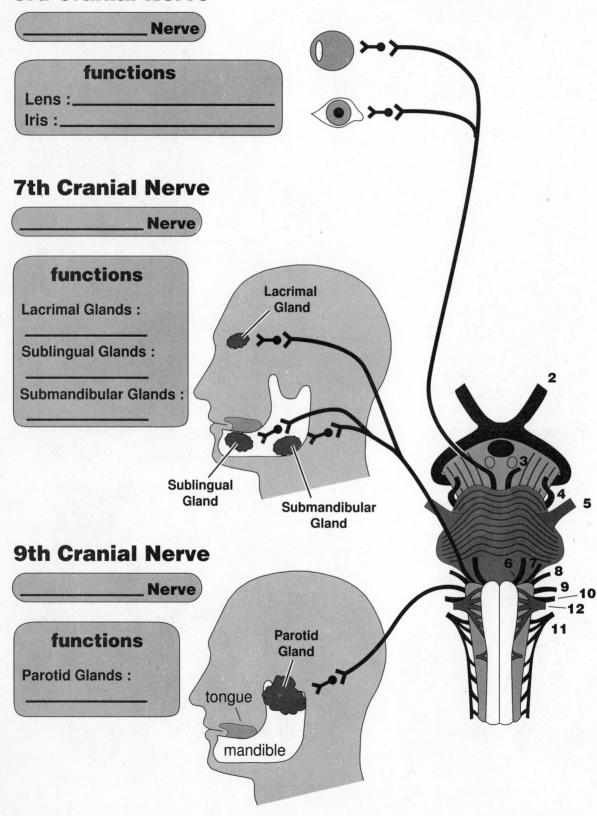

Lacrimal Gland

Sublingual Gland

Submandibular Gland

Parotid Gland

tongue

mandible

2

3

4

5

6   7

8

9   10

12

11

PARASYMPATHETIC CRANIAL NERVES

10th Cranial Nerve

_____ Nerve

functions

Heart : _____

Pacemaker

functions

Lungs : _____

_____

functions

Stomach : _____
Liver : _____
Gall Bladder : _____
Small Intestine : _____
Proximal Colon : _____

Liver

Stomach

Proximal Colon

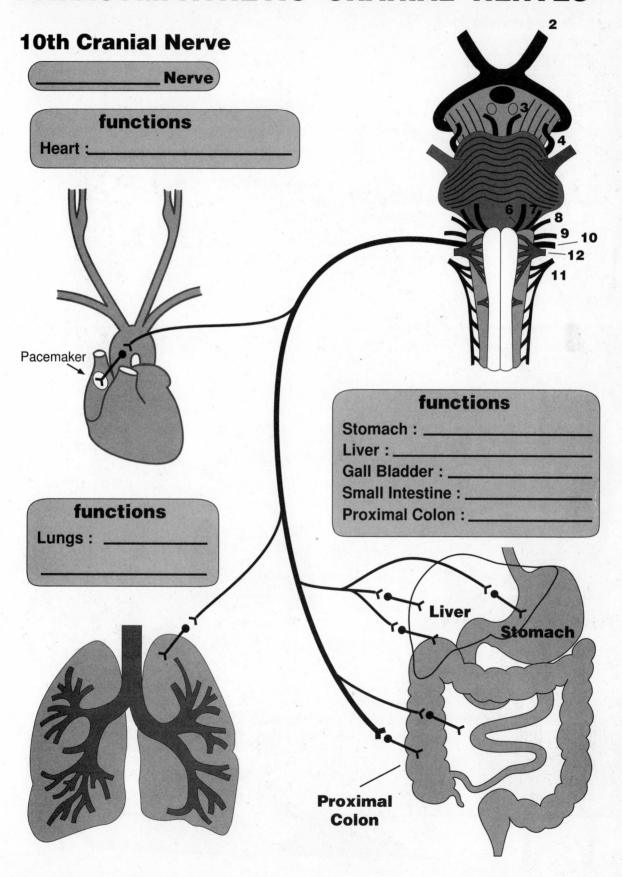

SENSORY RECEPTORS

name : _____
function : _____

name : _____
function : _____

name : _____
function : _____

name : _____
function : _____

name : _____
function : _____

name : _____
function : _____

name : _____
function : _____

name : _____
function : _____

name : _____
function : _____

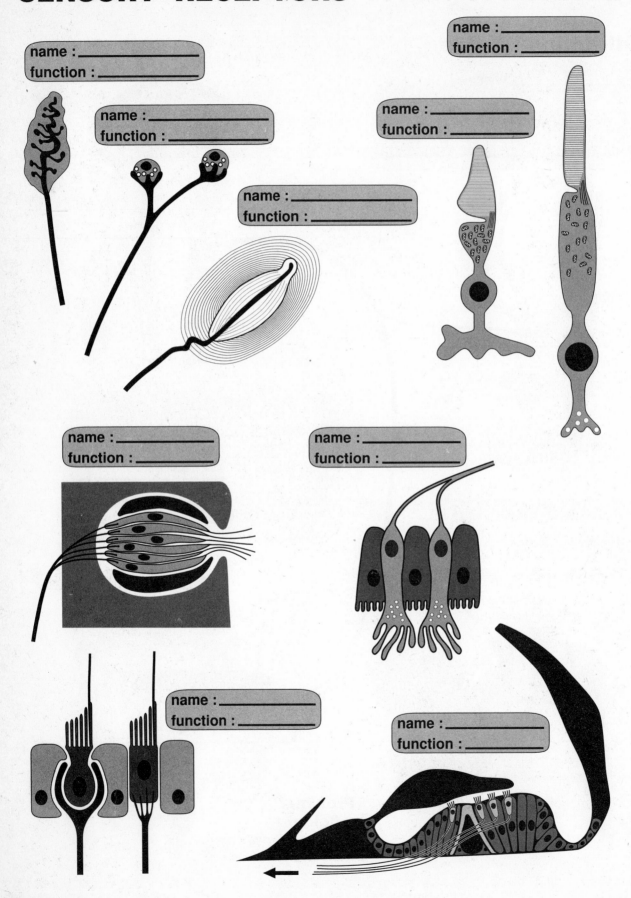

GENERATOR POTENTIAL

The magnitude of the generator potential is controlled by :
the stimulus intensity,
the rate of change of stimulus application,

_____

and _____

Stimulus

The strength of the decremental current depends upon the magnitude of

_____

The first action potential occurs at the first node if the

_____

is strong enough.

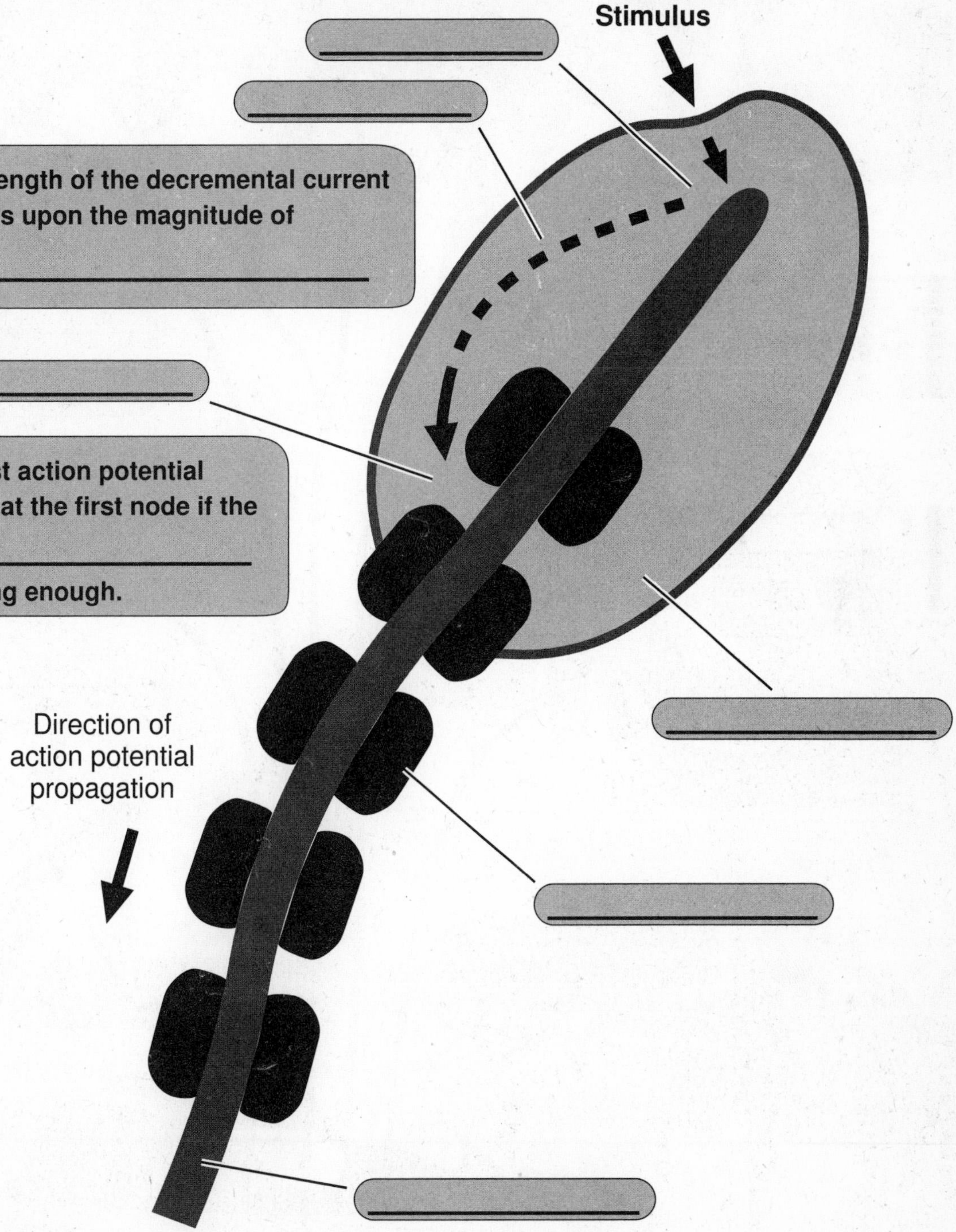

Direction of
action potential
propagation

SKIN RECEPTORS
Touch, Temperature, Pain, & Pressure

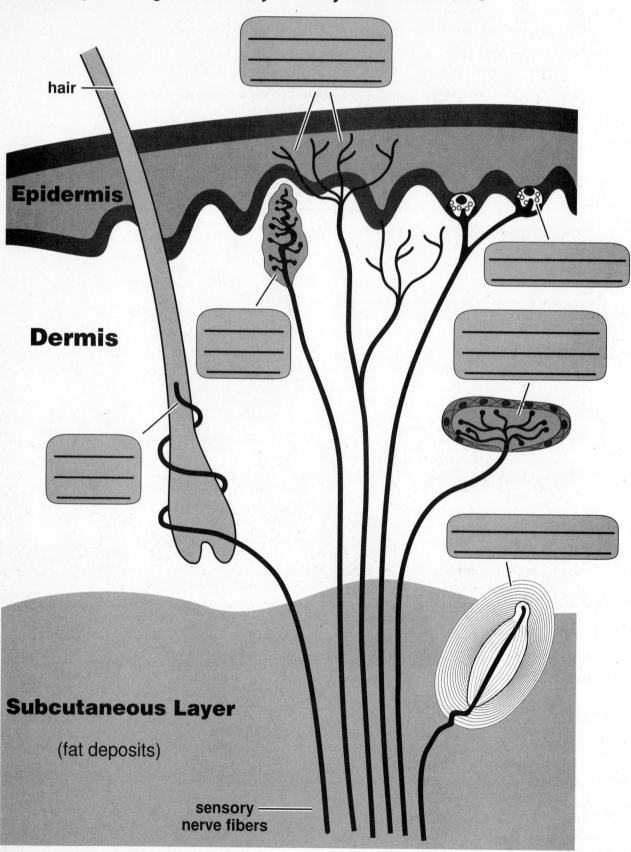

hair

Epidermis

Dermis

Subcutaneous Layer

(fat deposits)

sensory
nerve fibers

OLFACTORY BULB

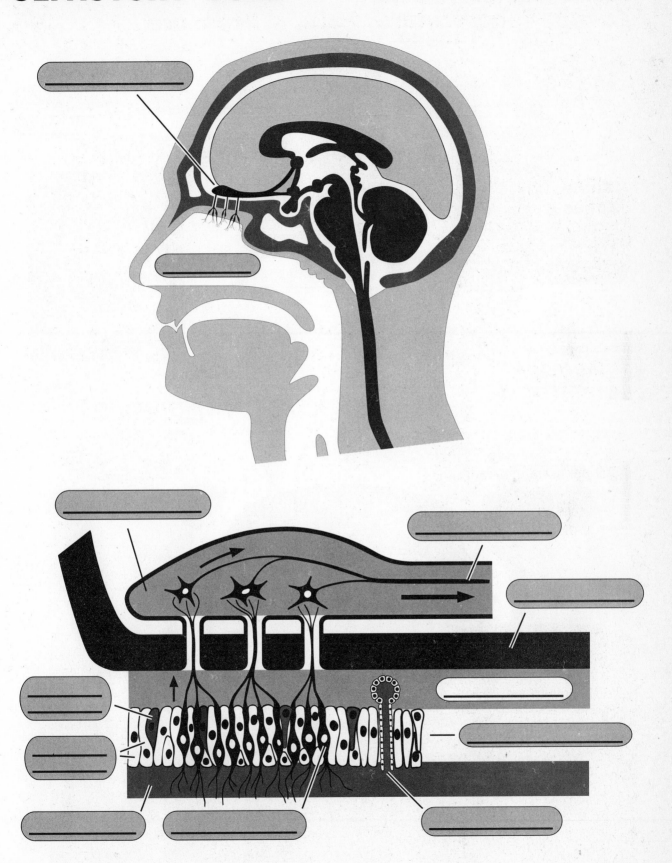

TASTE RECEPTORS

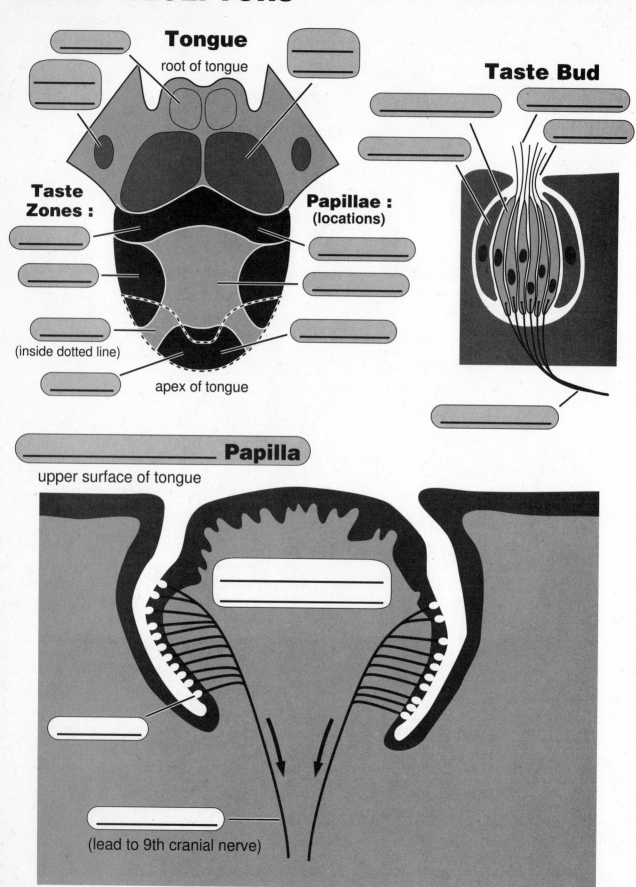

Tongue

root of tongue

Taste Bud

Taste Zones :

(inside dotted line)

apex of tongue

Papillae : (locations)

Papilla

upper surface of tongue

(lead to 9th cranial nerve)

TENDON ORGAN & MUSCLE SPINDLE

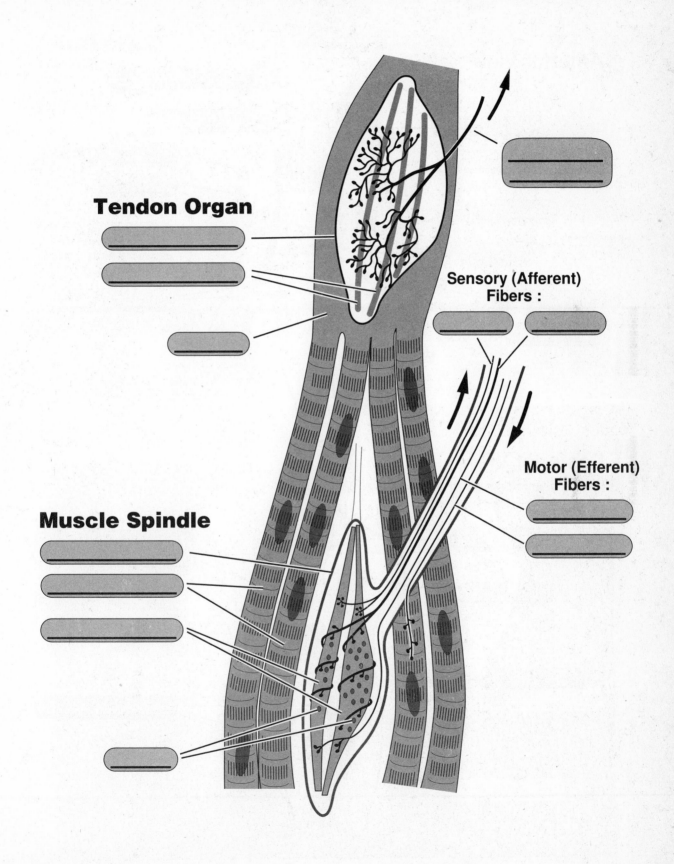

Tendon Organ

Sensory (Afferent) Fibers :

Motor (Efferent) Fibers :

Muscle Spindle

REFERRED PAIN
Areas of the skin to which visceral pain is referred.

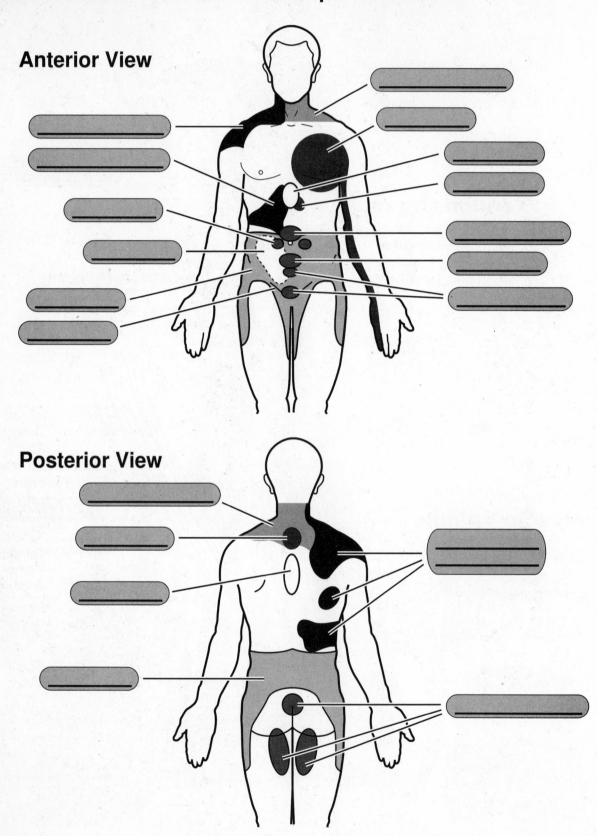

Anterior View

Posterior View

INTERNAL ENVIRONMENT RECEPTORS

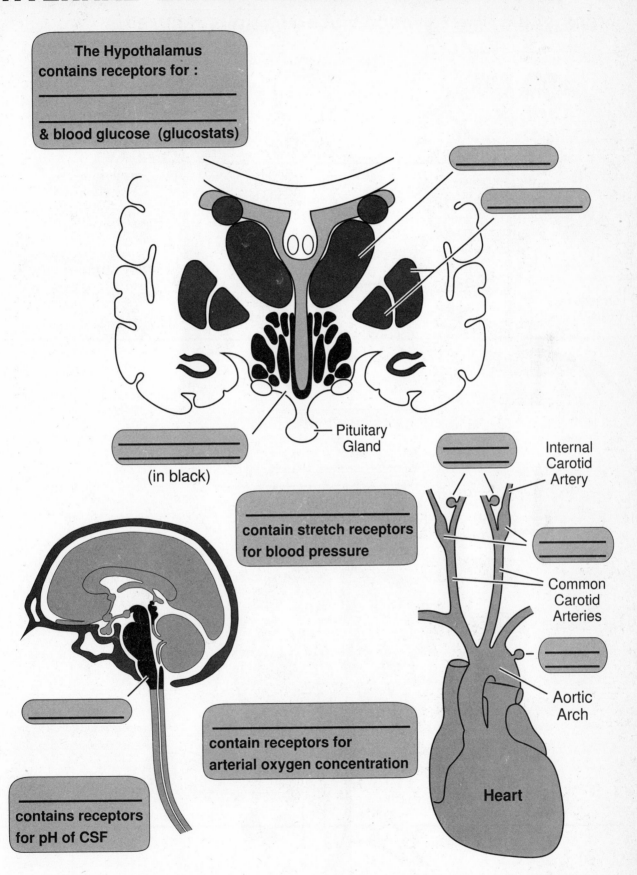

The Hypothalamus contains receptors for :

_____

_____

& blood glucose (glucostats)

Pituitary Gland

(in black)

_____ contain stretch receptors for blood pressure

Internal Carotid Artery

Common Carotid Arteries

Aortic Arch

Heart

_____ contain receptors for arterial oxygen concentration

_____ contains receptors for pH of CSF

SENSORY PATHWAYS

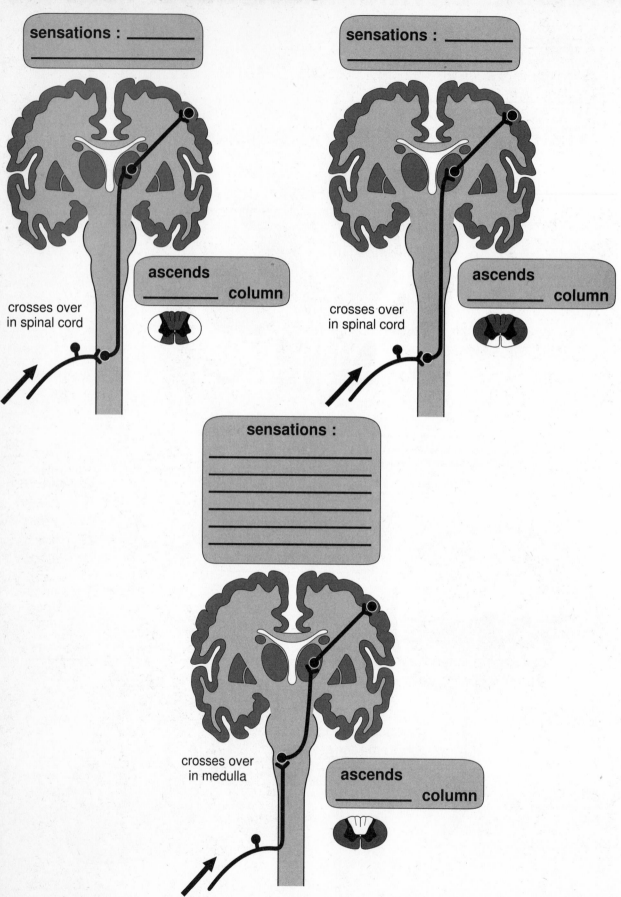

sensations : _____
_____

ascends
_____ column

crosses over
in spinal cord

sensations : _____
_____

ascends
_____ column

crosses over
in spinal cord

sensations :
_____
_____
_____
_____
_____
_____

crosses over
in medulla

ascends
_____ column

OPTICS

light rays bend as they enter obliquely
into a medium of a different density

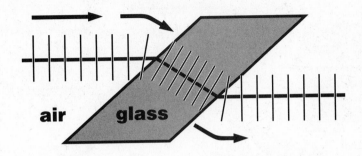

air **glass**

a beam of light passed through a glass prism
breaks up into the colors of the spectrum

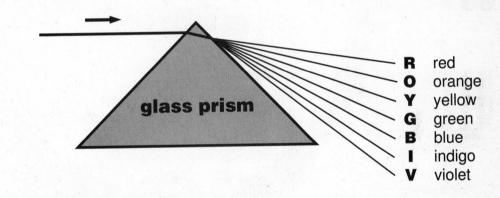

glass prism

R red
O orange
Y yellow
G green
B blue
I indigo
V violet

an image passed through a lens
is turned upside down

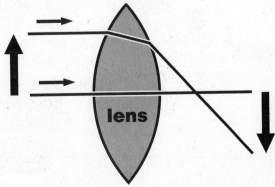

lens

EYEBALL ANATOMY
right eyeball viewed from above

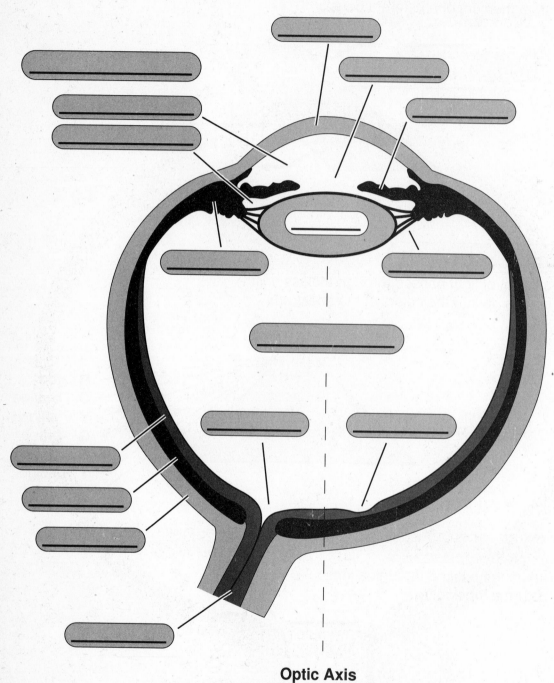

Optic Axis
(anterior - posterior)

RIGHT EYEBALL
viewed from above

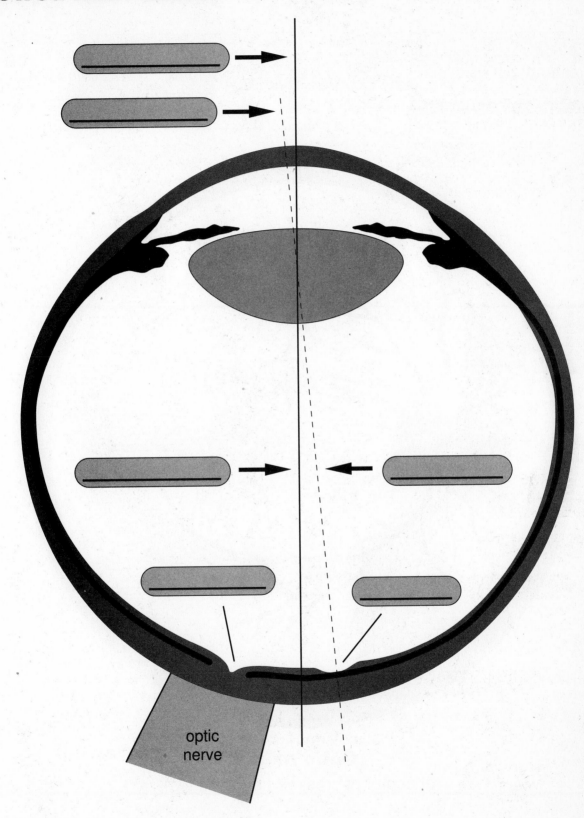

optic
nerve

289

RETINA
left eyeball as seen through an ophthalmoscope

Blood vessels and optic nerve enter & exit via the
_____

A concentration of cones for color & finely detailed vision are located in the _____

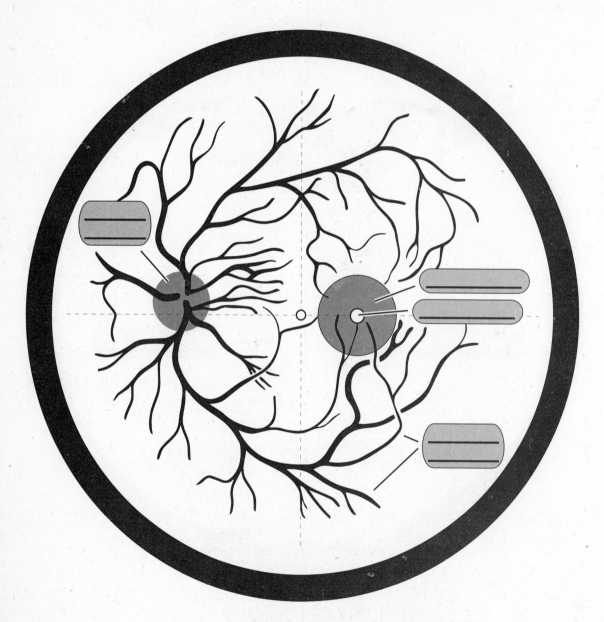

Optic Axis
(at center of crossed dashed lines)

RETINA AND OPTIC NERVE

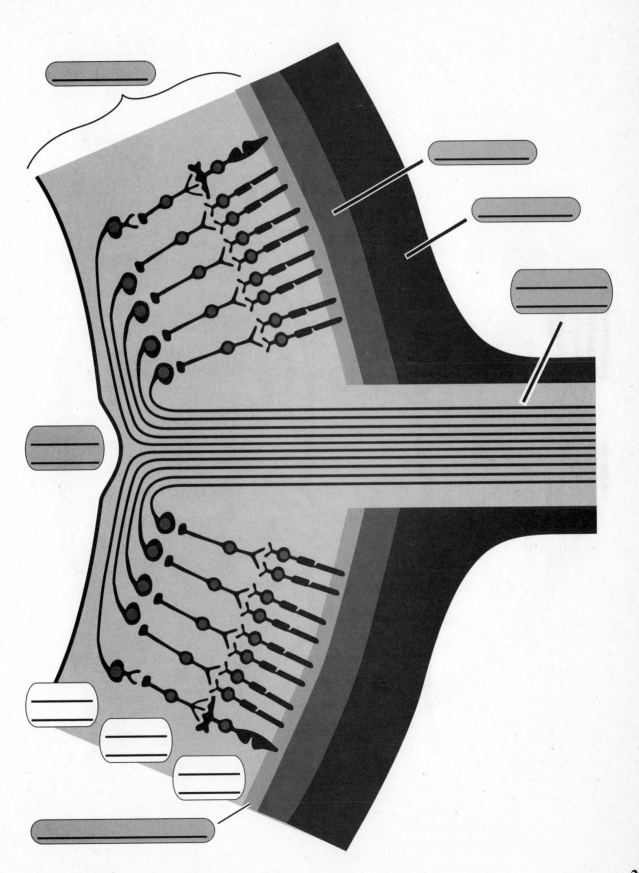

RETINA ULTRASTRUCTURE

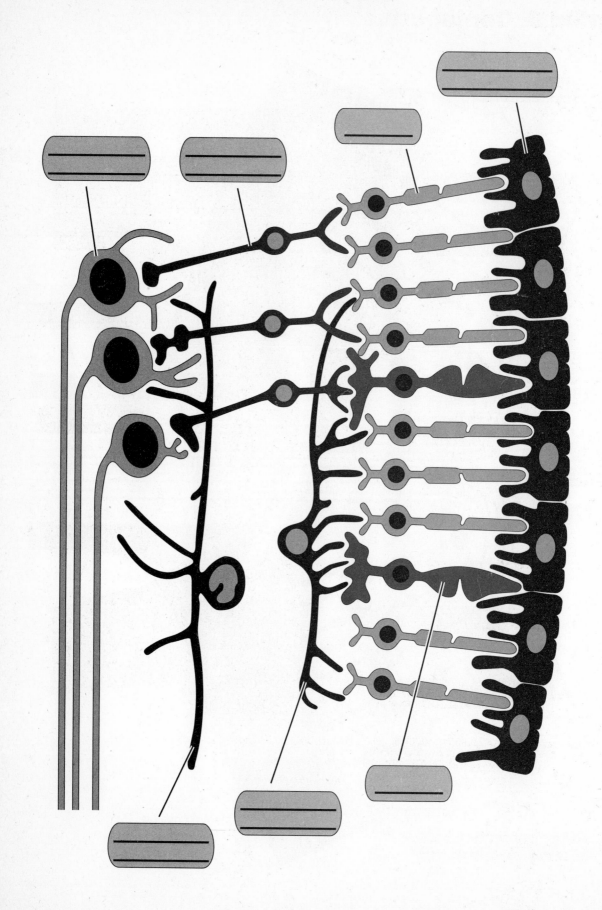

EYE : Accessory Structures
Eyelid & Conjunctiva

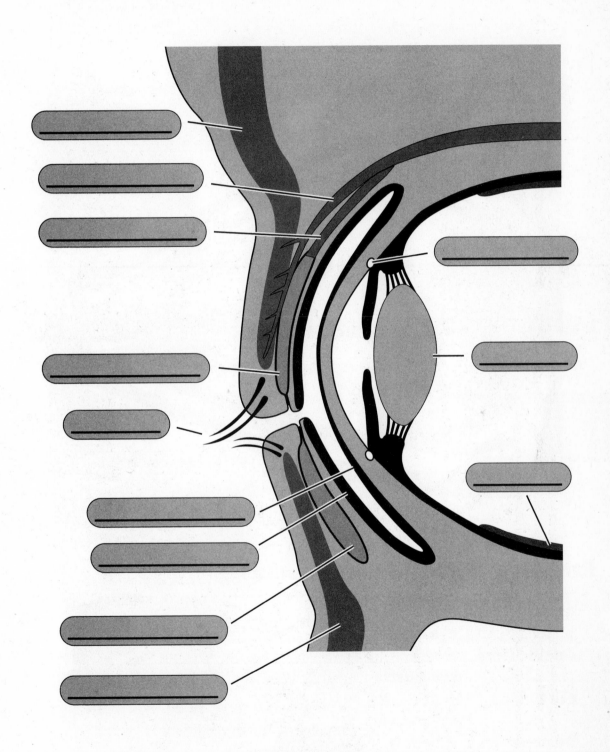

EYE MUSCLES
6 muscles that move the eyeball
(and the levator palpebrae superioris, which raises the upper eyelid)

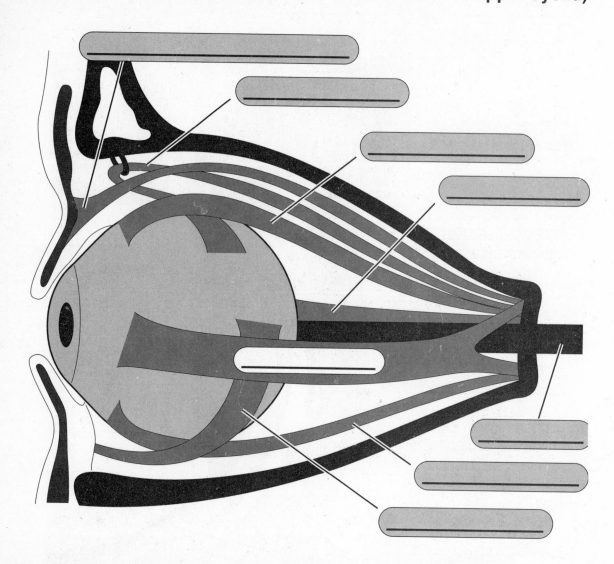

Primary Actions of Eye Muscles

Abduction   action: _____

              eye muscle : _____

Adduction   action: _____

              eye muscle : _____

Elevation   action: _____

              eye muscles : _____

Depression   action: _____

              eye muscles : _____

LACRIMAL APPARATUS

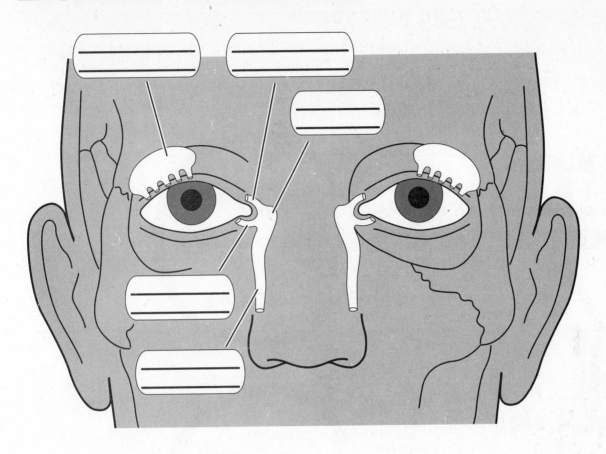

Cranial Nerves to the Eye Muscles

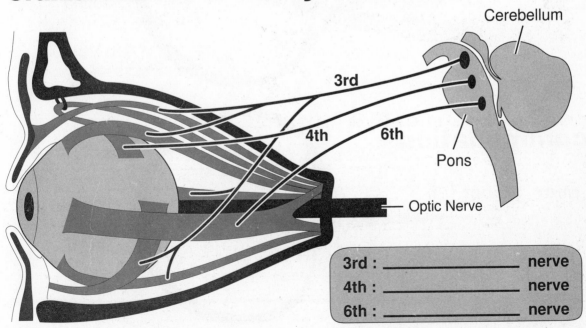

Cerebellum

3rd

4th   6th

Pons

Optic Nerve

3rd : _____ nerve
4th : _____ nerve
6th : _____ nerve

LENS ACCOMMODATION

When the eye focuses on near objects, _____ muscles contract, relaxing the tension on the _____ of the lens. This allows the elastic lens to contract and bulge, becoming more _____ .

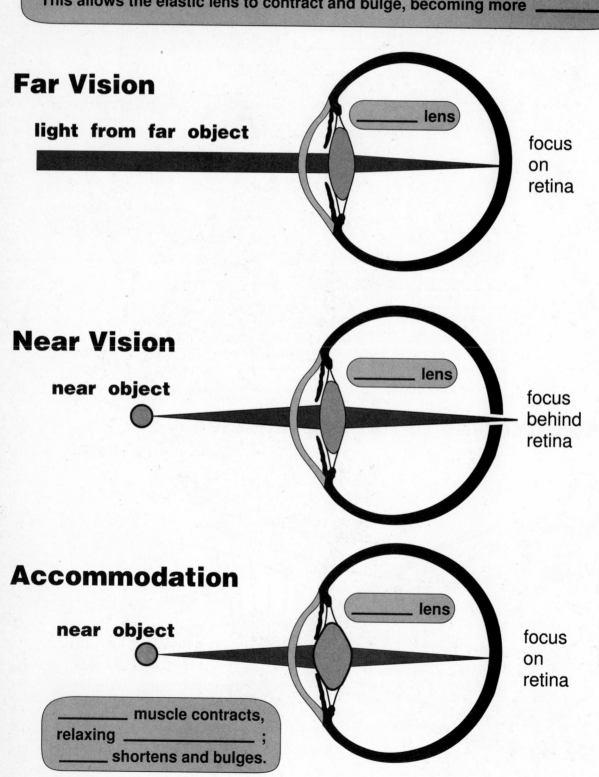

Far Vision

light from far object

_____ lens

focus on retina

Near Vision

near object

_____ lens

focus behind retina

Accommodation

near object

_____ lens

focus on retina

_____ muscle contracts, relaxing _____ ; _____ shortens and bulges.

CILIARY MUSCLES

For near vision, the ciliary muscles contract.
This decreases the tension on the suspensory ligaments;
the elastic lens bulges, becoming more rounded.

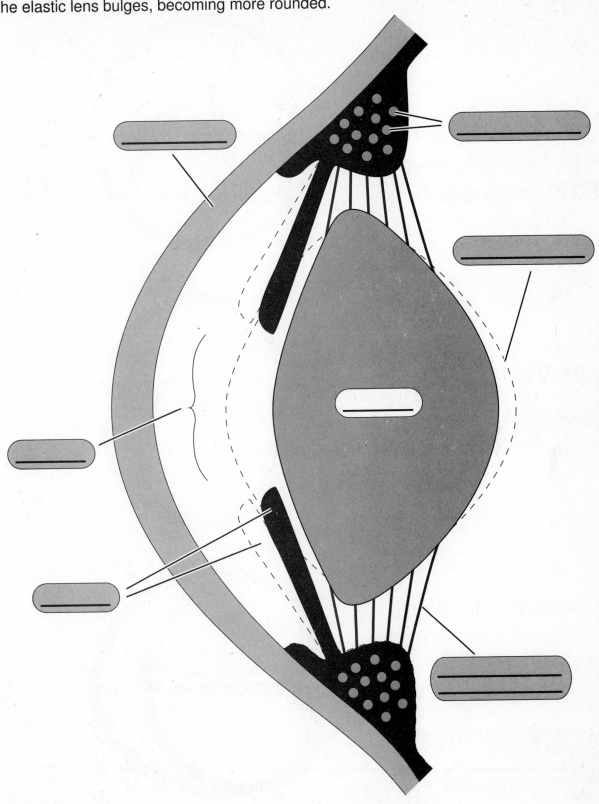

EYEBALL SHAPES

The focus of light rays on the retina is affected by the length of the optic axis.

Normal Eye

(Emmetropic Eye)

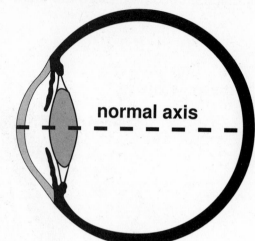

normal axis

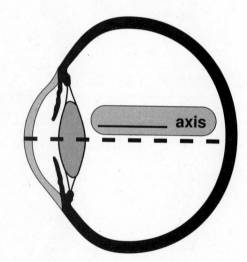

_____ sighted Eye

(_____ Eye)

_____ axis

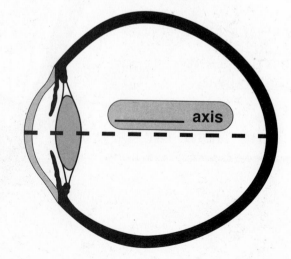

_____ sighted Eye

(_____ Eye)

_____ axis

NEARSIGHTED EYE (Myopic Eye)
far objects unclear

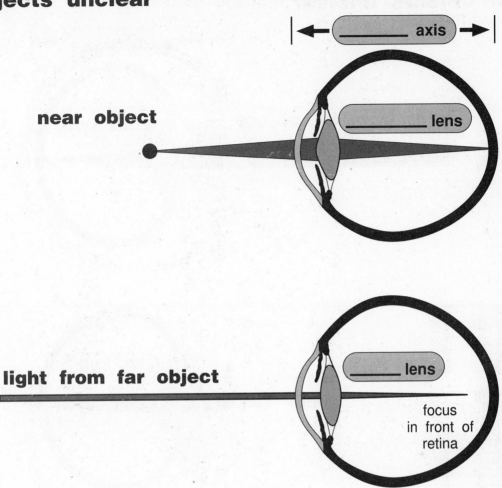

near object

axis

_____ lens

light from far object

_____ lens

focus
in front of
retina

Corrected Vision :

concave glass lens
corrects focus

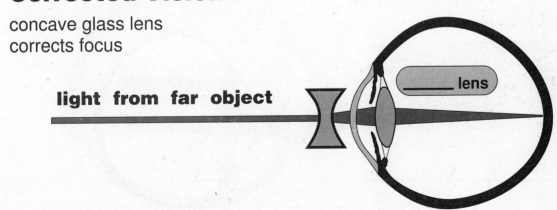

light from far object

_____ lens

FARSIGHTED EYE (Hypermetropic Eye)
near objects unclear

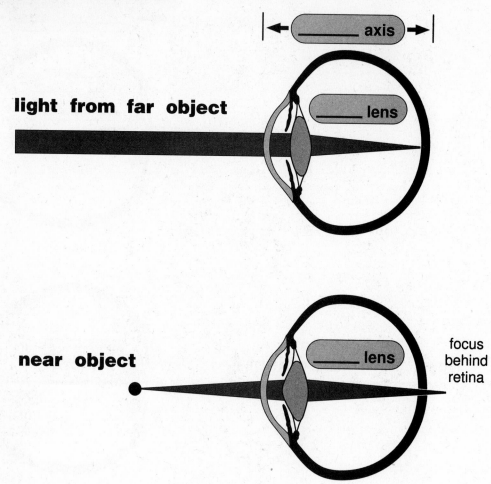

axis

light from far object

lens

near object

lens

focus
behind
retina

Corrected Vision :

convex glass lens
corrects focus

near object

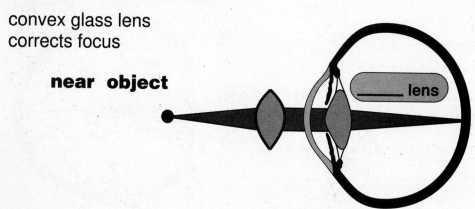

lens

RODS : Rhodopsin Cycle

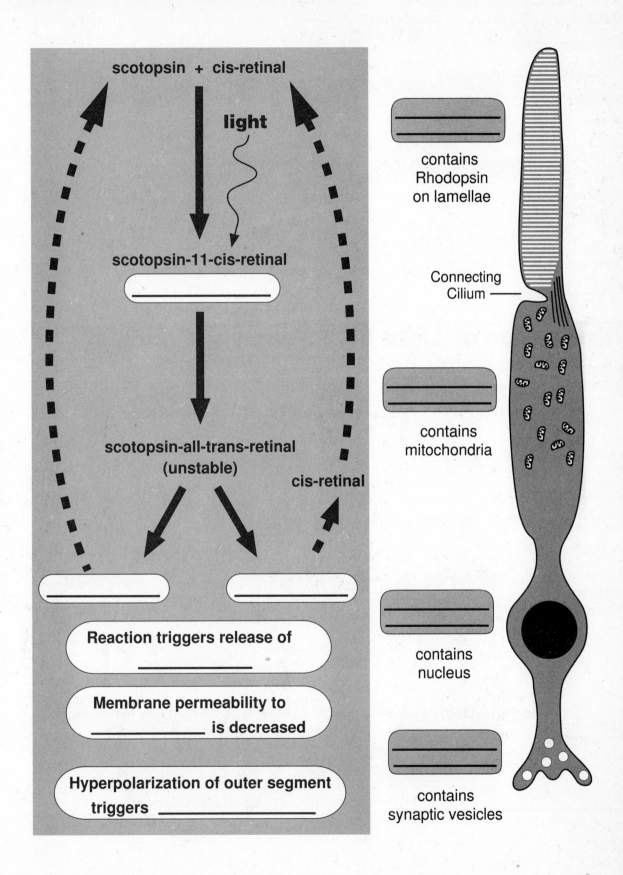

scotopsin + cis-retinal

light

scotopsin-11-cis-retinal

scotopsin-all-trans-retinal
(unstable)

cis-retinal

Reaction triggers release of
_____

Membrane permeability to
_____ **is decreased**

Hyperpolarization of outer segment
triggers _____

contains
Rhodopsin
on lamellae

Connecting
Cilium

contains
mitochondria

contains
nucleus

contains
synaptic vesicles

CONES : Color Perception

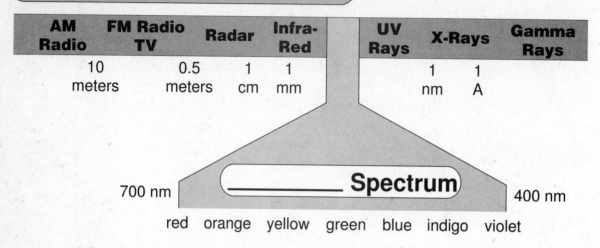

_____ **Spectrum**

AM Radio	FM Radio TV	Radar	Infra-Red		UV Rays	X-Rays	Gamma Rays
10 meters	0.5 meters	1 cm	1 mm		1 nm	1 A	

_____ Spectrum

700 nm   400 nm

red   orange   yellow   green   blue   indigo   violet

Absorption of Light by 3 Types of Cones

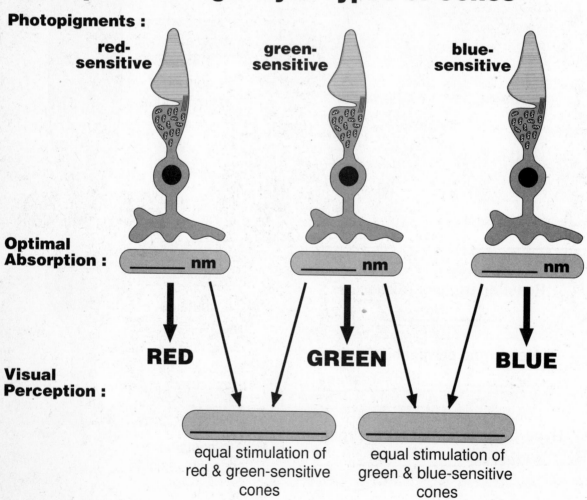

Photopigments :

red-sensitive   green-sensitive   blue-sensitive

Optimal Absorption :

_____ nm   _____ nm   _____ nm

RED   **GREEN**   **BLUE**

Visual Perception :

_____   _____

equal stimulation of red & green-sensitive cones   equal stimulation of green & blue-sensitive cones

VISUAL PATHWAY

Visual information received by the right side of each retina travels to the _____ lobe of the brain.

Visual information received by the left side of each retina travels to the _____ lobe of the brain.

Retina
(right eye)

(left eye)

crossing over
of optic nerves

(part of thalamus)

(in the midbrain)

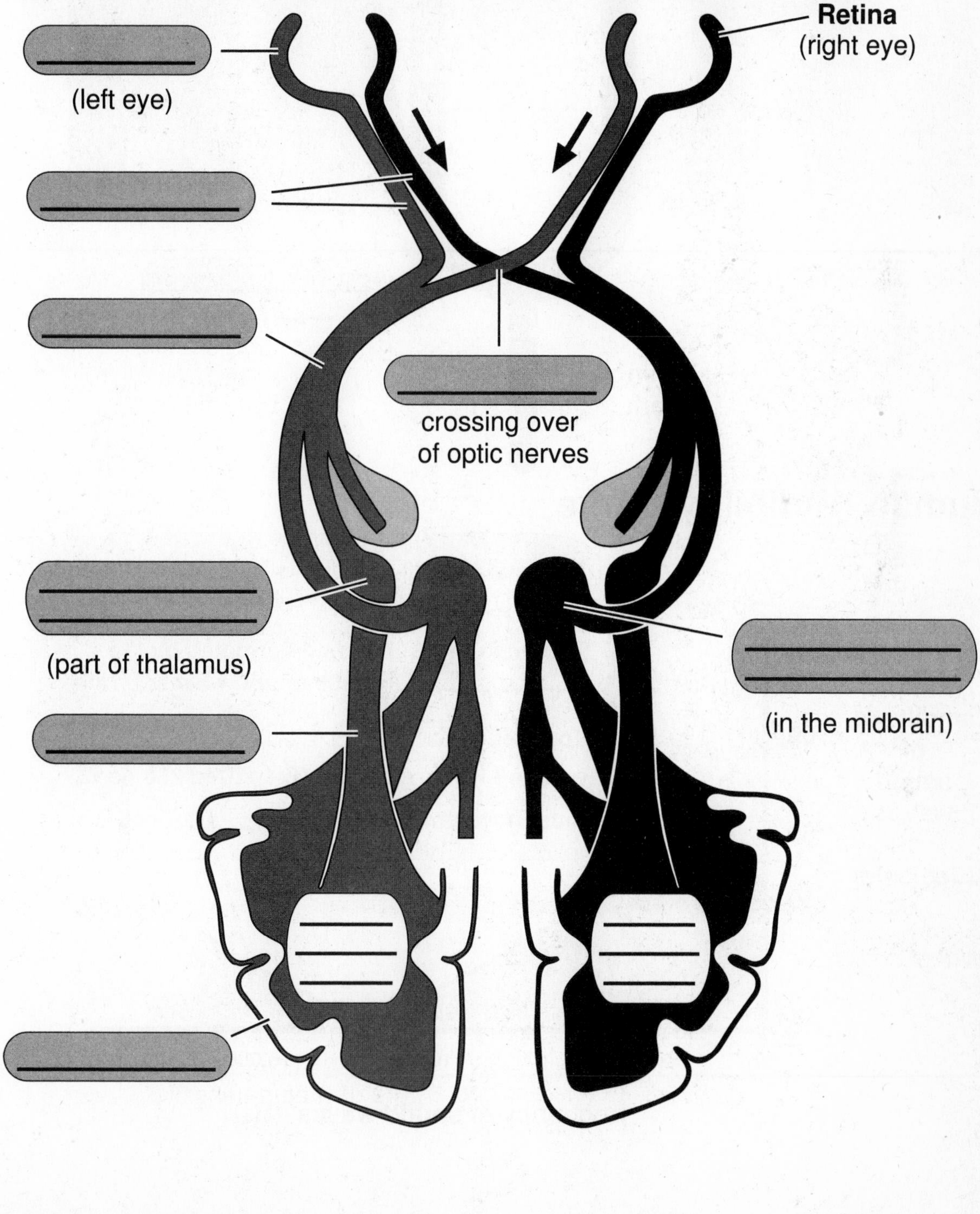

THE NATURE OF SOUND

Vibrations

vibrations produce areas of
rarefaction & compression

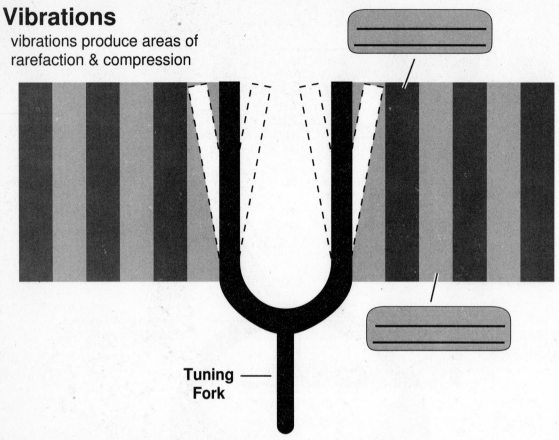

Tuning —
Fork

Human Audibility Curve

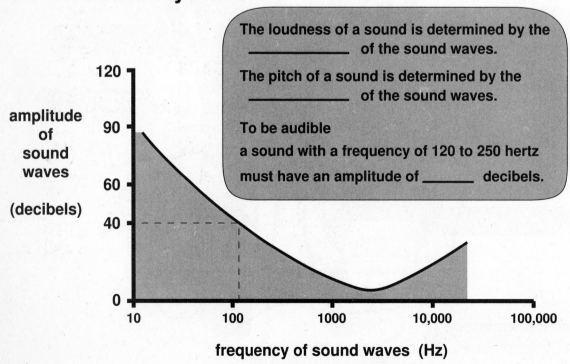

The loudness of a sound is determined by the
_____ of the sound waves.

The pitch of a sound is determined by the
_____ of the sound waves.

To be audible
a sound with a frequency of 120 to 250 hertz
must have an amplitude of _____ decibels.

amplitude
of
sound
waves

(decibels)

120

90

60

40

0

10   100   1000   10,000   100,000

frequency of sound waves (Hz)

EAR ANATOMY

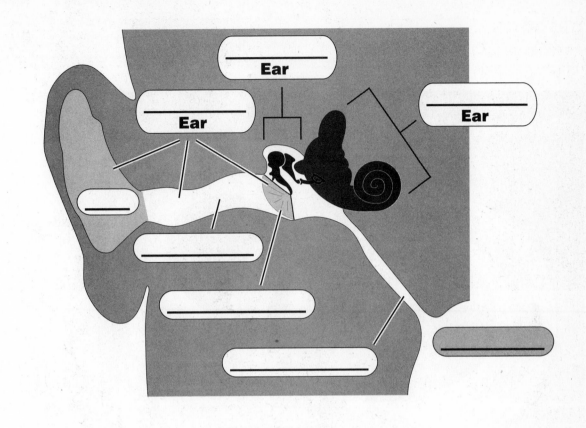

_____ Ear

_____ Ear

_____ Ear

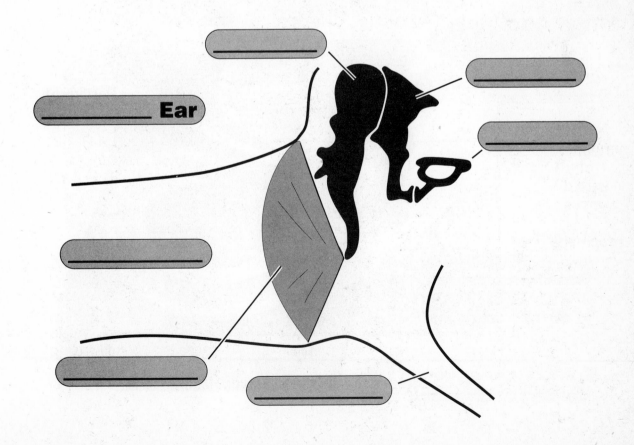

_____ Ear

INTERNAL (INNER) EAR

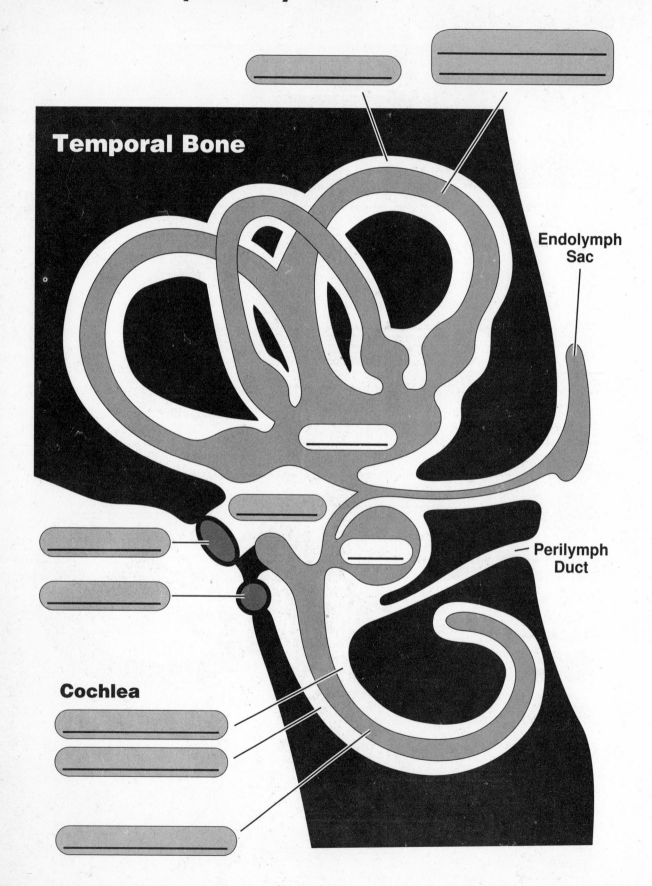

Temporal Bone

Endolymph Sac

Perilymph Duct

Cochlea

COCHLEA
cross section

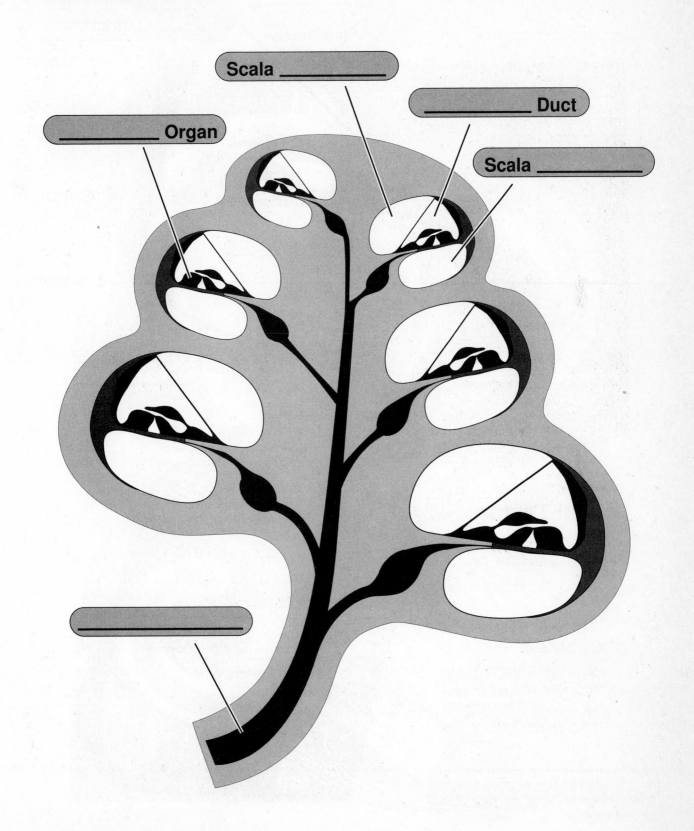

Scala _____

_____ Duct

_____ Organ

Scala _____

_____

SPIRAL ORGAN (organ of Corti)

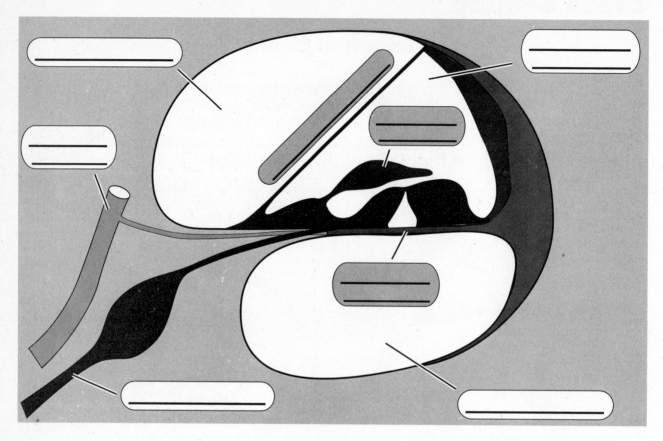

Spiral Organ

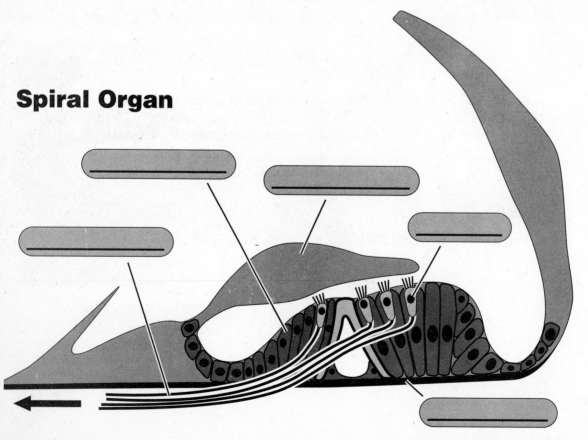

SOUND TRANSMISSION (in Cochlea)

uncoiled Cochlea (schematic)

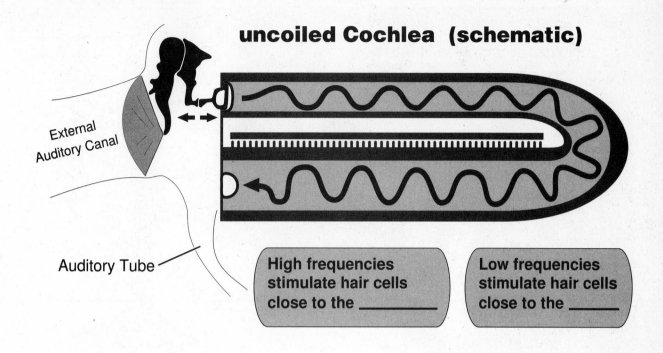

External
Auditory Canal

Auditory Tube

| High frequencies stimulate hair cells close to the _____ | Low frequencies stimulate hair cells close to the _____ |

cross section of cochlea

longitudinal section through the dashed line

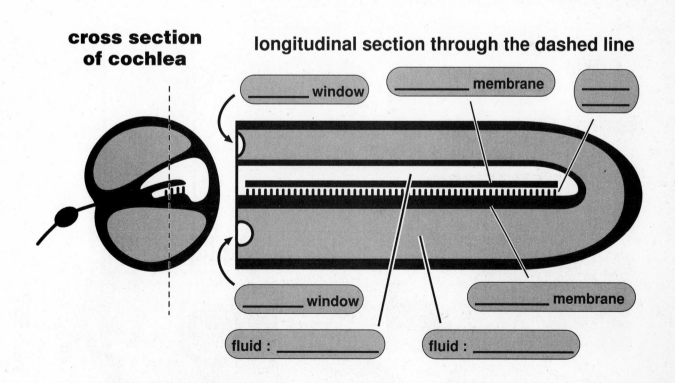

_____ window

_____ membrane

_____

_____ window

_____ membrane

fluid : _____

fluid : _____

CRISTA   (ampulla organ)

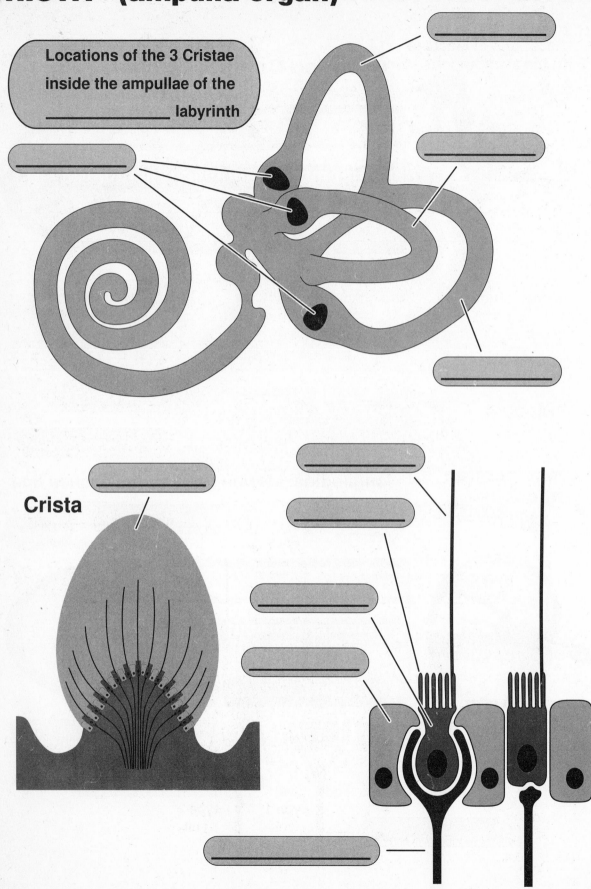

Locations of the 3 Cristae inside the ampullae of the _____ labyrinth

Crista

MACULA (utricle organ)

**Locations of Maculae
in the Membranous Labyrinth**

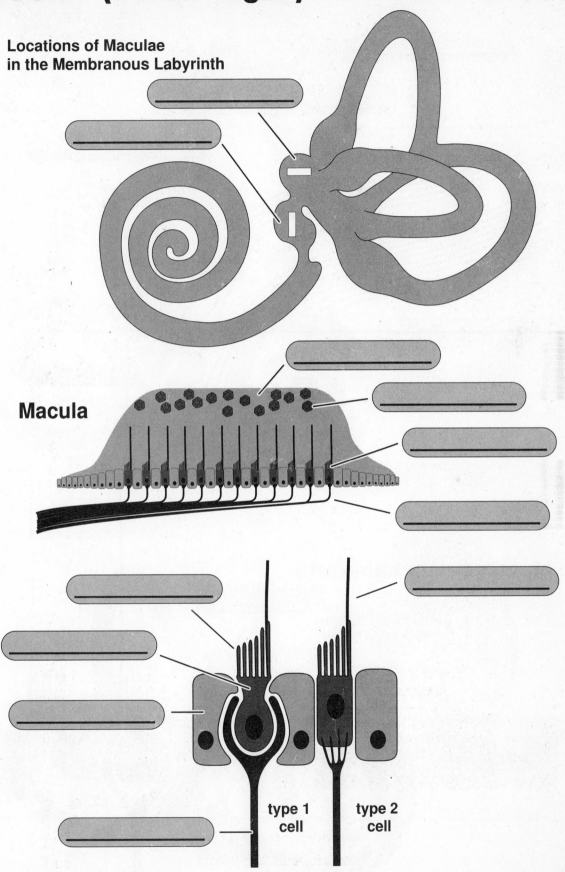

Macula

type 1
cell

type 2
cell

VESTIBULO-COCHLEAR NERVE

_____ Nerve

_____ Nerve

_____

_____ Nerve

Membranous Labyrinth

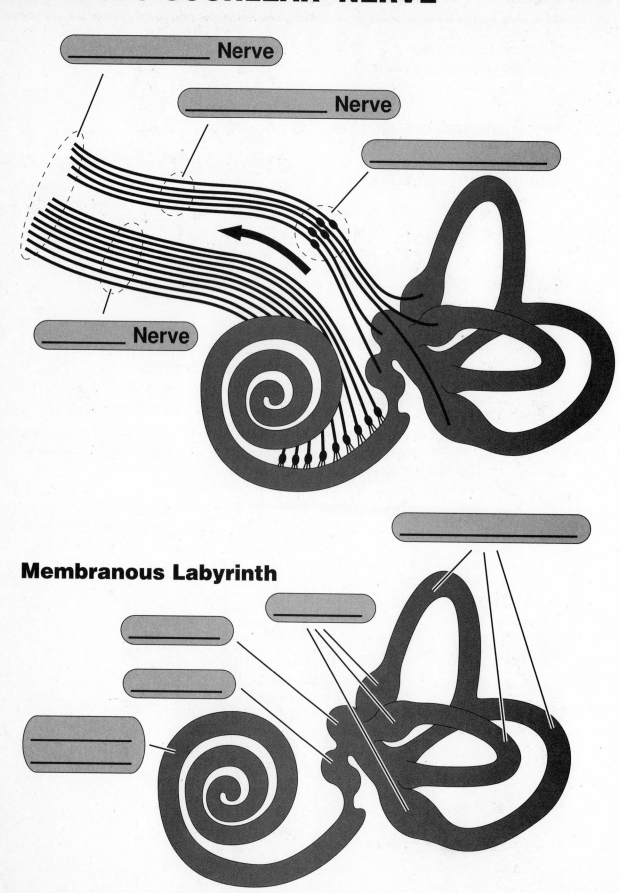

312

Part III : Terminology

Pronunciation Guide

acetylcholine as′ - ē - til - KŌ - lēn

acetylcholinesterase as′ - ē - til - kō′ - lin - ES - ter - ās

adenylate cyclase a - DEN - i - lāt SĪ - klās

adrenal a - DRĒ - nal

adrenaline a - DREN - a - lin

adrenergic ad′ - ren - ER - jik

afferent AF - er - ent

alpha AL - fa

ampulla am - POOL - la

analgesia an - al - JĒ - zē - a

anion AN - ī - on

antebrachial an′ - tē - BRĀ - kē - al

aortic ā - OR - tik

apneustic ap - NOO - stik

aqueous AK - wē - us

arachnoid a - RAK - noyd

astrocyte AS - trō - sīt

auditory AW - di - tō - rē

Auerbach OW - er - bak

auricular aw - RIK - yoo - lar

autonomic aw′ - tō - NOM - ik

axillary AK - si - lar - ē

axon AK - son

basilar BĀS - i - lar

beta BĀ - ta

brachial BRĀ - kē - al

Broca BRŌ - ka

carotid ka - ROT - id

cauda equina KAW - da ē - KWĪ - na

caudate KAW - dāt′

celiac SĒ - lē - ak

cerebellar ser - e - BEL - ar

cerebellum ser - e - BEL - um

cerebral SER - e - bral (se - RĒ - bral)

cerebrospinal se - rē′ - brō - SPĪ - nal

cerebrum SER - e - brum (se - RĒ - brum)

cerumen se - ROO - min

ceruminous se - ROO - mi - nus

cervical SER - vi - kul

chemoreceptor kē′ - mō - rē - SEP - tor

cholinergic kō′ - lin - ER - jik

choroid KŌ - royd

ciliary SIL - ē - ar′ - ē

circumflex SER - kum - fleks

circumvallate ser - kum - VAL - āt

coccygeal kok - SIJ - ē - al

coccyx KOK - six

cochlea KOK - lē - a

colliculi ko - LIK - yoo - lī

colliculus ko - LIK - yoo - lus

commissure KOM - mi - shur

communicans kō - MYOO - ni - kanz

communicantes kō - myoo - ni - KAN - tēz

conjunctiva kon′ - junk - TĪ - va

contralateral kon′ - tra - LAT - er - al

conus medullaris KŌ - nus med - yoo - LAR - is

cornea KOR - nē - a

corpora KOR - po - ra

corpus callosum KOR - pus kal - LŌ - sum

corpus striatum KOR - pus strī - Ā - tum

Corti KOR - tē

craniosacral krā - nē - ō - SĀ - kral

crista KRIS - ta

cuneatus kyoo - nē - Ā - tus

cutaneous kyoo′ - TĀ - nē - us

decussation dē′ - ku - SĀ - shun

dendrite DEN-drīt
denticulate den-TIK-yoo-lāt
dermatome DER-ma-tōm
diencephalon dī'-en-SEF-a-lon
dura mater DYOO-ra MĀ-ter
efferent EF-er-ent
emmetropic em'-e-TROP-ik
endoneurium en'-dō-NYOO-rē-um
endorphins en-DOR-fins
enkephalins en-KEF-a-lins
ependymal e-PEN-de-mal
epinephrine ep-ē-NEF-rin
epineurium ep'-i-NYOO-rē-um
Eustachian yoo-STĀ-kē-an
exteroceptor eks'-ter-ō-SEP-tor
falx cerebelli FALKS ser'-e-BEL-ē
falx cerebri FALKS SER-e-brē
fascicle FAS-i-kul
fasciculi fa-SIK-yoo-lī
fasciculus fa-SIK-yoo-lus
fenestra cochlea fe-NES-tra KOK-lē-a
fenestra vestibuli fe-NES-tra ves-TIB-yoo-lē
filiform FIL-i-form
filum terminale FĪ-lum ter-mi-NAL-ē
fissure FISH-ur
fornix FOR-niks
fovea FŌ-vē-a
fungiform FUN-ji-form
gamma aminobutyric GAM-ma am-i-nō-byoo-TIR-ik
ganglia GANG-glē-a
ganglion GANG-glē-on
geniculate je-NIK-yoo-lāt
genitofemoral jen'-i-tō-FEM-or-al
glia GLĒ-a
glial GLĒ-al
gluteal GLOO-tē-al
gnostic NOS-tik
Golgi GOL-jē
gracilis gra-SIL-is
gustatory GUS-ta-tō-rē
gyri JĪ-rī
gyrus JĪ-rus
hypermetropia hī'-per-me-TRŌ-pē-a
hyperpolarization hī'-per-POL-a-ri-zā'-shun
hypothalamus hī'-pō-THAL-a-mus
iliohypogastric il'-ē-ō-hī-pō-GAS-trik
ilioinguinal il'-ē-ō-IN-gwi-nal
insula IN-su-la
intercostal in'-ter-KOS-tal
intrafusal in'-tra-FYOO-zal
ion Ī-on
ipsilateral ip'-si-LAT-er-al
kinesthesia kin-is-THĒ-szē-a
labyrinth LAB-i-rinth

lacrimal LAK-ri-mal
lemniscus lem-NIS-kus
lumbar LUM-bar
lumbo–sacral LUM-bō-SĀ-kral
macula lutea MAK-yoo-la LOO-tē-a
mechanoreceptor mek'-a-nō-rē-SEP-tor
medulla oblongata me-DUL-la ob'-long-GA-ta
Meibomian mī-BŌ-mē-an
Meissner MĪS-ner
membranous MEM-bra-nus
meninges me-NIN-jēz
meninx MEN-inks
Merkel MER-kel
mesencephalon mes'-en-SEF-a-lon
metencephalon met'-en-SEF-a-lon
microglia mī-KROG-lē-a
modality mō-DAL-i-tē
monoamine oxidase mon-ō-AM-ēn OK-si-dās
muscarinic mus'-ka-RIN-ik
musculocutaneous mus'-kyoo-lō-kyoo-TĀN-ē-us
myelencephalon mī-el-en-SEF-a-lon
myelin MĪ-e-lin
myoneural mī-ō-NOO-ral
myopia mī-Ō-pē-a
neurofibral noo-rō-FĪ-bral
neurofibril noo-rō-FĪ-bril
neuroglia noo-ROG-lē-a
neurohypophysis noo-rō-hī-POF-i-sis
neurolemma noo-rō-LEM-ma
neurolemmocyte noo-rō-LE-mō-sīt
neuromuscular noo-rō-MUS-kyoo-lar
neuron NOO-ron
neuropeptide noo-rō-PEP-tīd
neurosecretory noo-rō-SĒK-re-tō-rē
nicotinic nik'-ō-TIN-ik
Nissl NIS-l
nociceptor nō-sē-SEP-tor
noradrenaline nor-a-DREN-a-lin
norepinephrine nor'-ep-ē-NEF-rin
nuclei NOO-klē-ī
nucleus NOO-klē-us
obturator OB-too-rā'-tor
occipital ok'-SIP-i-tal
olfactory ol-FAK-tō-rē
oligodendrocyte OL-i-gō-den'-drō-sīt
ophthalmology of'-thal-MOL-ō-jē
optic chiasma OP-tik kī-AZ-ma
ossicle OS-si-kul
otolith Ō-tō-lith
oxytocin ok'-sē-TŌ-sin
Pacinian pa-SIN-ē-an
palpebrae PAL-pe-brē
papilla pa-PIL-a
papillae pa-PIL-ē

parasympathetic par′-a-sim-pa-THET-ik
patellar pa-TELL-ar
pectoral PEK-tō-ral
peduncle pe-DUNG-kul
perforating PER-fō-rā-ting
perikaryon per′-i-KAR-ē-on
perilymph PER-i-lymf
perineurium per′-i-NYOO-rē-um
peripheral pe-RIF-er-al
peroneal per′-ō-NĒ-al
phrenic FREN-ik
pia mater PĪ-a MĀ-ter
piriformis pir-i-FORM-is
pituitary pi-TOO-i-tar′-ē
plantar PLAN-ter
plexus PLEK-sus
pneumotaxic noo-mō-TAK-sik
pons PONZ
postganglionic pōst′-gang-lē-ON-ik
postsynaptic pōst′-sin-AP-tik
preganglionic prē-gang-lē-ON-ik
presbyopia prez-bē-Ō-pē-a
presynaptic prē-sin-AP-tik
prevertebral prē-VERT-e-bral
proprioception prō-prē-ō-SEP-shun
prosencephalon prōs′-en-SEF-a-lon
pterygopalatine ter′-i-gō-PAL-a-tin
pudendal pyoo-DEN-dal
Purkinje pur-KIN-jē
putamen pu-TĀ-men
pyramid PIR-a-mid
pyramidal pi-RAM-i-dal
quadratus femoris kwad-RĀ-tus FEM-or-is
quadrigemina kwad-ri-JEM-in-a
rami RĀ-mī
ramus RĀ-mus
Ranvier RON-vē-ā
reciprocal innervation re-SIP-rō-kal in-ner-VĀ-shun
recruitment rē-KROOT-ment
refraction rē-FRAK-shun
refractory re-FRAK-to-rē
reticular re-TIK-yoo-lar
retina RET-i-na
retinal RE-ti-nal
rhodopsin rō-DOP-sin
rhombencephalon rom′-ben-SEF-a-lon
Ruffini roo-FĒ-nē
saccule SAK-yool
sacral SĀ-kral
saltatory sal-ta-TŌ-rē
satiety sa-TĪ-e-tē
scala tympani SKĀ-la TIM-pan-ē
scala vestibuli SKĀ-la ves-TIB-yoo-lē
scapular SKAP-yoo-lar

Schlemm SHLEM
Schwann SCHVON
sciatic sī-AT-ik
sclera SKLE-ra
scleral SKLE-ral
sebaceous se-BĀ-shus
segmental seg-MEN-tal
sinus SĪ-nus
somatic sō-MAT-ik
splanchnic SPLANK-nik
stereognosis ste′-rē-og-NŌ-sis
subarachnoid sub′-a-RAK-noyd
subclavius sub-KLĀ-vē-us
subdural sub-DOO-ral
submucosal sub-myoo-KŌ-sal
subscapular sub-SKAP-yoo-lar
substantia nigra sub-STAN-shē-a NĪ-gra
sulci SUL-sī
sulcus SUL-kus
supraclavicular soo′-pra-kla-VIK-yoo-lar
suprascapular soo′-pra-SKAP-yoo-lar
sympathomimetic sim′-pa-thō-mi-MET-ik
synapse SIN-aps
synaptic sin-AP-tik
tactile TAK-tīl
tectorial tek-TŌ-rē-al
telencephalon tel-en-SEF-a-lon
tentorium ten-TŌ-rē-um
thalami THAL-a-mī
thalamus THAL-a-mus
thoracic thō-RAS-ik
thoracolumbar thō′-ra-kō-LUM-bar
tibial TIB-ē-al
tympanic tim-PAN-ik
ulnar UL-nar
utricle YOO-tri-kul
uvea YOO-vē-a
ventral VEN-tral
ventricle VEN-tri-kul
vermis VER-mis
vesicle VES-i-kul
vestibular ves-TIB-yoo-lar
viscera VIS-er-a
visceral VIS-er-al
visceroceptor vis-er-ō-SEP-tor
viscus VIS-kus
vitreous VIT-rē-us
Wernicke VER-ni-kē
Zeis ZĪS

Glossary of Terms

Absolute refractory period   A refractory period is the time during which a neuron membrane is unresponsive to stimuli. The *absolute* refractory period is the portion of a refractory period during which a second action potential cannot be generated, even with a very strong (suprathreshold) stimulus.

Acetylcholine (ACh)   A neurotransmitter released by many PNS neurons and some CNS neurons. It is excitatory at neuromuscular junctions, where it acts directly to open chemically gated cation channels.

Acetylcholinesterase (AChE)   An enzyme that inactivates acetylcholine.

Accommodation   A change in the curvature of the eye lens to adjust for vision at various distances; focusing.

Action potential   A change in the neuron membrane potential from -70 mV to +30 mV and then back to -70 mV. Each action potential has a duration of 1 msec and a magnitude of 100 mV. An action potential self-propagating along the surface of a neuron axon is called a *nerve impulse*.

Adaptation   The adjustment of the pupil of the eye to light variations. A change in the sensitivity of a sensory receptor to a long-lasting stimulus; usually a decrease in sensitivity.

Adenylate cyclase   An enzyme in the postsynaptic membrane of an effector cell; it is activated when neurotransmitters bind to their receptors. This enzyme converts ATP to cyclic AMP, which triggers a series of reactions that lead to some change in effector cell activity. (Effector cells are muscle or gland cells.)

Adrenal medulla   The inner portion of an adrenal gland. It consists of modified postganglionic sympathetic neurons that secrete the hormones epinephrine & norepinephrine.

Adrenergic fiber   A nerve fiber that releases norepinephrine (also called noradrenaline) from its synaptic end bulbs.

Adrenergic receptors   Receptors in postsynaptic membranes that bind the neurotransmitter norepinephrine (also called noradrenaline).

Afferent neuron   A neuron that carries impulses from sensory receptors into the CNS. Also called a *sensory neuron*.

A fibers   The largest nerve fibers (5 to 20 micrometers in diameter). All are myelinated and conduct impulses very quickly (from 12 to 130 meters per second). They include: sensory fibers that relay information about touch, pressure, temperature, & joint position; somatic motor fibers that carry impulses to skeletal muscles.

Agonist   A chemical that enhances synaptic transmission or mimics a natural neurotransmitter. For example, amphetamine is a dopamine agonist; it causes an increase in the amount of dopamine released at synapses (especially in the limbic system) and produces symptoms of schizophrenia.

All-or-none principle   All action potentials have the same magnitude and duration (unless fatigue or toxic chemicals alter membrane properties). An action potential either occurs or it does not occur; there is no partial action potential. This distinguishes action potentials from graded potentials.

Alpha-adrenergic receptor   A receptor found on the cells of internal (visceral) organs. Stimulation by sympathetic postganglionic neurons usually leads to excitation.

Ampulla   A saclike dilation of a semicircular canal in the internal ear.

Antagonist   A chemical that blocks or inhibits synaptic transmission. For example, botulinus toxin, which is produced by the bacterium Clostridium botulinum, blocks the release of acetylcholine.

Anterior   Nearer to the front; opposite of posterior. Also called *ventral*.

Anterior Cavity   The region inside the eyeball between the lens and the cornea that is filled with a watery fluid called the aqueous humor. It is divided into the anterior chamber (between the cornea and the iris) and the posterior chamber (between the iris and the suspensory ligaments).

Anterior nucleus   A nucleus of the thalamus that is concerned with emotions and memory.

Anterior root   A spinal nerve has two points of attachment to the spinal cord: an anterior root and a posterior root. The anterior root contains motor (efferent) fibers. Also called the *ventral root*.

Aortic body   A receptor on the aortic arch that responds to changes in blood levels of oxygen, carbon dioxide, and hydrogen ions.

Aqueous humor   The watery fluid that fills the anterior cavity of the eye. It is secreted by the ciliary processes.

Arachnoid   The middle membranous covering of the brain and spinal cord. It is between the dura mater & pia mater.

Ascending (sensory) pathways   Two general pathways that lead from sensory receptors to the cerebral cortex : the posterior column-medial lemniscal pathway and the anterolateral (spinothalamic) pathways.

Association areas   Areas of the cerebral cortex that are concerned with memory, reasoning, will, judgment, personality, motor patterns, and concepts of word-hearing and word-seeing. The main association areas include the somatosensory, visual, auditory, gnostic, premotor, and frontal eye field.

Association fibers   Myelinated axons that transmit impulses between gyri in the same cerebral hemisphere.

Association neurons   Neurons lying completely within the brain or spinal cord. They integrate incoming sensory information and send out instructions via motor neurons.

Astrocyte   A neuroglial cell having a star shape that supports neurons in the brain and spinal cord and attaches the neurons to blood vessels.

Auditory association area   Inferior to the primary auditory area in the cortex of the temporal lobe. It determines whether sound is speech, music, or noise. It also determines the meaning of speech by translating words into thoughts. Also called *Wernicke's area*.

Auditory ossicles   The 3 small bones of the middle ear. They include the malleus, incus, and stapes.

Auditory tube   The tube that connects the middle ear with the nasal cavity and throat. Also called the *Eustachian tube*.

Auricle   The elastic, cartilagenous flap of the ear that is designed to funnel sound waves into the external auditory canal. One of the 3 structures of the external ear; the others are the external auditory canal and the eardrum. Also called the *pinna*.

Autonomic ganglia   Clusters of autonomic neuron cell bodies located outside the brain and spinal cord. There are 3 general types of autonomic ganglia: sympathetic trunk ganglia, prevertebral ganglia (sympathetic), and terminal ganglia (parasympathetic).

Autonomic motor pathways   These pathways consist of 2 motor (efferent) neurons in series (one following the other). The first is called a preganglionic neuron, the second is called a postganglionic neuron.

Autonomic nervous system (ANS)   One of the 2 major subdivisions of the peripheral nervous system. Its sensory (afferent) neurons conduct impulses to the CNS from visceral organs (internal organs: heart, lungs, bladder, etc.). Its motor (efferent) neurons conduct impulses from the CNS to smooth muscle, cardiac muscle, and glands. The ANS is divided into the sympathetic and parasympathetic divisions.

Axon   A long process extending out from a neuron cell body. It conducts impulses away from the cell body to other cells (muscle cells, gland cells, or other neurons).

Axon terminals   The fine processes at the ends of axons and their collaterals. The expanded ends of axon terminals are called synaptic end bulbs.

Axonal transport   There are 2 types of transport systems that carry materials between the cell body and the axon terminals. *Slow axonal transport* conveys the cytoplasm (axoplasm) from the cell body toward the axon terminals. *Fast axonal transport* conveys materials in both directions along the surfaces of microtubules.

Baroreceptors   Stretch receptors in the walls of the heart and blood vessels that respond to changes in blood pressure. They are also called *pressoreceptors*.

Basal ganglia   Several groups of nuclei in each cerebral hemisphere. Also called the *cerebral nuclei*.

Basilar membrane   A membrane in the cochlea of the internal ear. The spiral organ (organ of Corti) rests on the basilar membrane. It separates the cochlear duct from the scala tympani.

Beta-adrenergic receptor   A receptor found on the cells of visceral organs. Stimulation by sympathetic postganglionic neurons usually leads to inhibition.

B fibers   Intermediate sized nerve fibers (less than 3 micrometers in diameter). All are myelinated and conduct impulses up to 15 meters per second. They include: sensory fibers that relay information from viscera to the CNS; motor fibers that carry impulses from the CNS to autonomic ganglia.

Blind spot   *See* Optic disc.

Blood-brain barrier (BBB)   An anatomical and physiological barrier that prevents the passage of harmful substances and pathogens from the blood into most parts of the brain.

Bony labyrinth   A series of cavities within the temporal bone. It forms the vestibule, cochlea, and semicircular canals of the internal ear.

Bowman's glands   *See* Olfactory glands.

Brachial plexus   The network of nerves that supplies the upper extremity. These nerves branch from the ventral rami of spinal nerves C5 - C8 & T1. *Brachial* = arm.

Brain   A mass of nervous tissue located in the cranial cavity. Its main parts are the cerebrum, diencephalon, brain stem, and cerebellum.

Brain stem   This part of the brain consists of the midbrain, pons, and medulla oblongata. The medulla oblongata is continuous with the spinal cord.

Broca's area   *See* Motor speech area.

Brain vesicles   Brain vesicles are bulges in the neural tube that occur during embryonic development. The primary brain vesicles include the prosencephalon (forebrain), mesencephalon (midbrain), and rhombencephalon (hindbrain).

Canal of Schlemm   *See* Scleral venous sinus.

Cardiovascular center   A region within the medulla oblongata that regulates the force and rate of heart contractions and the diameter of blood vessels.

Carotid body   A receptor on or near the carotid sinus that responds to changes in levels of oxygen in the blood.

Carotid sinus   A dilated region of the carotid artery that contains receptors that monitor blood pressure.

Cauda equina   The roots of lumbar and sacral spinal nerves that fill the dural sac on either side of the filum terminale. Its shape is like a horse's tail. *Cauda* = tail; *Equina* = horse.

Cell body   The part of a neuron that includes the nucleus and the cytoplasm immediately surrounding it. It contains the usual cell organelles: mitochondria, endoplasmic reticulum, etc. Also called the *soma* or *perikaryon*.

Central canal   A small tube that runs the length of the spinal cord in the gray commissure; it is filled cerebrospinal fluid.

Central fovea   A cuplike depression in the center of the macula lutea of the retina. Since it contains only cones, it is the best retinal area for color vision and acute (sharp) vision.

Central nervous system (CNS)   One of the 2 major divisions of the nervous system. It includes the brain and spinal cord.

Central sulcus   A groove in the cerebral hemispheres that separates the frontal lobe from the parietal lobes.

Cerebellar peduncles   Three paired bundles of nerve fibers that connect the right and left sides of the cerebellum with the brain stem.

Cerebellum   The second largest part of the brain. It is located posterior to the medulla and pons and inferior to the occipital lobes of the cerebrum. The cerebellum compares intended movements with what is actually happening; it helps to smooth and coordinate complex sequences of skeletal muscle contractions and maintains normal posture and balance.

Cerebral cortex   The thin layer of gray matter (about 3 mm thick) that covers the cerebral hemispheres. It is divided into three main functional areas: sensory, motor, and association areas.

Cerebral peduncle   A pair of fiber bundles in the midbrain; they contain motor and sensory fibers that carry impulses between upper parts of the brain and lower parts of the brain and spinal cord.

Cerebrospinal fluid (CSF)   A fluid produced by the choroid plexuses, which are located in the four ventricles of the brain. It circulates in the ventricles of the brain and in the subarachnoid space surrounding the brain and spinal cord.

Cerebrum   The largest part of the brain. It consists of two cerebral hemispheres and each hemisphere is divided into 4 lobes.

Ceruminous glands   Modified sweat glands in the external auditory canal whose secretions and those of sebaceous (oil) glands combine to form cerumen (ear wax).

Cervical ganglia   The 3 pairs of cervical ganglia are part of the sympathetic trunk ganglia. They are located on both sides of the vertebral column in the neck. They consist of clusters of postganglionic sympathetic neuron cell bodies.

Cervical plexus A network of nerves on each side of the neck that supplies the skin and muscles of the head, neck, and upper part of the shoulders. The phrenic nerves arise from the cervical plexuses and supply motor fibers to the diaphragm. The cervical plexus is formed by the ventral rami of the first five cervical nerves (C1–C5). *Cervical* = neck.

C fibers The smallest nerve fibers (0.5 to 1.5 micrometers in diameter). All are unmyelinated and conduct impulses from 0.5 to 2 meters per second. They include: sensory fibers that relay information about pain, touch, pressure, & temperature from the skin to the CNS; motor fibers that carry impulses from autonomic ganglia to their effectors (cardiac muscle, smooth muscle, or glands).

Chemically gated ion channels Ion channels in plasma membranes that respond to specific chemical stimuli. For example, in some postsynaptic membranes the interaction of the neurotransmitter acetylcholine with receptors opens cation channels.

Chemoreceptor A receptor on or near the carotid and aortic bodies that responds to chemical changes in the blood.

Cholinergic fibers Nerve fibers that release acetylcholine from their synaptic end bulbs. They include all autonomic preganglionic fibers, all parasympathetic postganglionic fibers, and a few sympathetic postganglionic fibers (those that lead to sweat glands and some that lead to blood vessels in skeletal muscles). Also called *cholinergic neurons*.

Cholinergic receptors Receptors in postsynaptic cells that bind acetylcholine. There are 2 types: nicotinic (found on postganglionic neurons) and muscarinic (found on all effectors innervated by parasympathetic postganglionic fibers or cholinergic sympathetic fibers).

Cholinesterase An enzyme that breaks down acetylcholine.

Choroid One of the 3 portions of the middle, vascular layer of the eyeball. It lines the internal surface of the sclera.

Choroid plexuses Specialized networks of capillaries located in the 4 brain ventricles; they produce cerebrospinal fluid.

Chromatophilic substance Rough endoplasmic reticulum in the cell bodies of neurons. Also called *Nissl bodies*.

Ciliary body One of the 3 portions of the middle, vascular layer of the eyeball. It is located between the choroid and the iris. It consists of ciliary processes that secrete aqueous humor and ciliary muscle that controls the shape of the lens.

Circumvallate papilla A papilla is an elevation on the tongue that contains taste buds. Circumvallate papillae are the largest of the 3 types of papillae and are located on the posterior portion of the tongue.

Cochlea The cochlea is located in the internal ear. It is one of the 3 parts of the bony labyrinth. The other two parts are the vestibule and the semicircular canals.

Cochlear duct The membranous cochlea, consisting of a spirally arranged tube enclosed in the bony cochlea and lying along its outer wall. Contains a fluid called endolymph. Also called the *scala media*.

Colliculi (superior & inferior) Two pairs of swellings on the roof of the midbrain: the superior colliculi are reflex centers for movements of the head and eyeballs in response to visual stimuli; the inferior colliculi are reflex centers for movements of the head and trunk in response to auditory stimuli. Also called the *corpora quadrigemina*.

Columns (of spinal cord) The anterior and posterior gray horns divide the white matter on each side of the spinal cord into three broad areas called columns. Also called *funiculi*.

Commissural fibers Myelinated axons that transmit impulses from the gyri in one cerebral hemisphere to the corresponding gyri in the opposite hemisphere. The 3 main groups of commissural fibers are the corpus callosum, the anterior commissure, and the posterior commissure.

Cones The light-sensitive receptors in the retina concerned with color vision and visual acuity in bright light.

Conjunctiva A thin, protective mucous membrane that lines the inner aspect of the eyelids and the anterior surface of the eyeball.

Continuous conduction How nerve impulses are transmitted on unmyelinated fibers. It is the step-by-step depolarization of each adjacent segment of the plasma membrane. (Saltatory conduction occurs on myelinated fibers.)

Contralateral reflex arc A type of spinal reflex arc in which impulses enter one side of the spinal cord and leave on the opposite side.

Conus medullaris The tapered inferior end of the spinal cord. Located near the 1st lumbar vertebra.

Converging circuit One of the 5 basic types of neuronal circuits found in the CNS. Several presynaptic neurons synapse with a single postsynaptic neuron.

Cornea The anterior transparent portion of the fibrous coat of the eyeball. (The posterior portion of the fibrous coat is the sclera.)

Corpora quadrigemina Four small elevations on the dorsal region of the midbrain; they are concerned with visual and auditory reflexes. Also called the *superior and inferior colliculi*.

Corpus callosum A large region above the 3rd ventricle of the brain consisting of myelinated axons that carry impulses between the two cerebral hemispheres. It is one of the 3 main groups of commissural fibers in the brain.

Corpuscle of touch A sensory receptor for the sensation of touch; found in the dermal papillae, especially in palms and soles. Also called a *Meissner's corpuscle*.

Corpus striatum A region of striated gray matter in each cerebral hemisphere. It consists of the caudate and lenticular nuclei and the white matter of the internal capsule.

Cranial cavity The subdivision of the dorsal body cavity formed by the cranial bones; it contains the brain.

Cranial nerves The 12 pairs of nerves that emerge from the brain. They are divided into 3 main groups based upon the types of fibers they contain : purely sensory, primarily motor, and mixed (contain both sensory and motor fibers).

Craniosacral outflow The autonomic nerve fibers that emerge from the brain via cranial nerves 3, 7, 9, & 10 and from the spinal cord via spinal sacral nerves 2, 3, & 4. All of these fibers are the axons of preganglionic parasympathetic neurons. Their cell bodies are located in nuclei in the brain stem or in the lateral gray horns of the spinal cord.

Crista The sensory organ for dynamic equilibrium. It is a small elevation in the membranous ampulla of each semicircular duct. It is composed of receptor cells (hair cells), supporting cells, and a mass of gelatinous material called the cupula.

Crossed extensor reflex A balance-maintaining spinal reflex. This reflex results in the synchronized extension of one limb and the flexion of the opposite limb.

Current Electrical current is the flow of electrons. The electrochemical current involved in nerve physiology is the flow of ions.

Cutaneous sensations Sensations that arise in the skin. They include tactile, thermal, and pain sensations.

Decussation Crossing over; refers to the crossing over of most of the fibers in the large descending tracts. It occurs in the medulla oblongata.

Dendrites Highly branched cytoplasmic processes extending out from the neuron cell body. Specialized for detecting changes in the environment or for responding to input from other neurons.

Depolarization The process by which a membrane becomes more positive on the inside. During the first part of an action potential the plasma membrane responds to a stimulus by opening its voltage-gated sodium ion channels. This allows sodium ions to flow into the cell (driven by their concentration and electric gradients). The movement of positively charged sodium ions into the cell reverses the polarity of the cell membrane (-70 mV to +30 mV).

Dermatome An area of the skin that receives most of its innervation from one spinal nerve.

Descending (motor) pathways Descending (motor) pathways may be divided into two categories: the direct or pyramidal pathways and the indirect or extrapyramidal pathways. The direct pathways transmit impulses down the spinal cord via the corticospinal and corticobulbar tracts. The indirect pathways transmit impulses down the spinal cord via 5 major tracts: rubrospinal, tectospinal, vestibulospinal, lateral reticulospinal, and anterior reticulospinal.

Descending (motor) tract A descending tract is the portion of a descending pathway that extends from the brain to lower motor neuron cell bodies in the brain stem or spinal cord. (The remainder of the pathway consists of the axon of the lower motor neuron, which carries the impulse to a skeletal muscle in a spinal or cranial nerve.)

Diencephalon The part of the brain between the cerebrum (forebrain) and the midbrain. It is derived from the gray matter surrounding the 3rd ventricle, and its main structures are the thalamus and hypothalamus.

Direct (pyramidal) pathways Transmit impulses from the motor cortex to skeletal muscles. While in the CNS these pathways transmit their impulses via 3 major tracts: lateral corticospinal, anterior corticospinal, and corticobulbar. They control precise, voluntary movements.

Diverging circuit One of the 5 basic types of neuronal circuits found in the CNS. One presynaptic neuron synapses with several postsynaptic neurons.

Dorsal Nearer to the back; opposite of ventral. Also called *posterior*.

Dual innervation Most visceral organs receive input from both sympathetic and parasympathetic fibers. In general, the input from one type of fiber stimulates a particular organ and input from the other type of fiber inhibits it.

Dura mater The outer membrane covering the brain and spinal cord. One of the 3 meninges (membranes) that surround the structures of the CNS. The other two meninges are the pia mater and arachnoid.

Dynamic equilibrium The maintenance of body position, mainly the head, in response to sudden movements such as rotation, acceleration, and deceleration. The sensory organ for dynamic equilibrium is located in the internal ear and is called the crista.

Efferent neuron A neuron that carries impulses away from the brain or spinal cord toward an effector (muscle or gland). Also called a *motor neuron*.

Endoneurium The connective tissue that surrounds individual nerve fibers in a nerve.

End organ of Ruffini *See* Type II cutaneous mechanoreceptor.

Ependyma Neuroglial cells that line the ventricles of the brain and assist in the circulation of the cerebrospinal fluid by ciliary action.

Epidural space The region outside the dura mater of the spinal cord, between the dura mater and the bony walls of the vertebrae; it is filled with fat tissue that cushions the cord.

Epinephrine A hormone secreted by the adrenal medulla. It is produced by modified sympathetic postganglionic neurons and has effects that are similar to those that result from sympathetic stimulation. Also called *adrenaline*.

Epineurium The connective tissue surounding the entire nerve; it includes the external fibrous coat and the tissue surrounding fascicles (bundles of nerve fibers).

Eustachian tube *See* Auditory tube.

Excitability The ability of nerve and muscle cells to respond to certain stimuli by producing impulses (propagated action potentials). It is made possible by the presence of voltage-gated ion channels in the plasma membranes.

Excitatory postsynaptic potential (EPSP) A slight depolarization of the postsynaptic membrane that occurs at excitatory synapses. EPSPs generate local currents that flow toward the initial segment of the axon. If the local currents are strong enough to generate a threshold potential at the initial segment, an action potential will result.

External auditory canal A canal in the temporal bone that transmits sound waves from the auricle to the tympanic membrane. Also called the the *external auditory meatus*.

External ear It consists of 3 parts: the auricle (pinna), external auditory canal (external auditory meatus), and tympanic membrane (eardrum). Also called the *outer ear*.

Exteroceptor A sensory receptor adapted for the reception of stimuli from outside the body (the external environment).

Falx cerebelli A fold of dura mater projecting inward between the two cerebellar hemispheres.

Falx cerebri A fold of dura mater extending down into the longitudinal fissure between the two cerebral hemispheres.

Fascicle A small bundle of nerve fibers wrapped in a connective tissue called the perineurium. Nerve fibers in both the spinal and cranial nerves are bundled in fascicles. Also called a *fasciculus* (plural: fasciculi).

Fibrous tunic The outer coat of the eyeball; the posterior portion is the sclera and the anterior portion is the cornea.

Fight-or-flight response Stimulation of the sympathetic division of the autonomic nervous system leads to a vast array of responses that prepare the body for stress-related behavior, such as fighting or running.

First-order neurons Sensory neurons that carry impulses into the CNS. Their cell bodies are in the posterior (dorsal) root ganglia of spinal nerves. Sensory pathways are composed of 3-neuron sets. The 2nd and 3rd-order neurons are inside the CNS.

Fissure A groove or deep depression in a cerebral hemisphere. Fissures serve as landmarks for regions of the cerebral cortex. The *longitudinal fissure* separates the right and left cerebral hemispheres; the *central sulcus* separates the frontal lobe from the parietal lobes; the *lateral sulcus* separates the temporal lobe from the frontal and parietal lobes; and the *parieto-occipital fissure* marks the border between the occipital and parietal lobes. Also called a *sulcus* (plural: *sulci*).

Flexor reflex   A protective spinal reflex. It results in the synchronized contraction of flexor muscles to avoid pain and the relaxation of extensor muscles (antagonists). It is also called the *withdrawal reflex.*

Free nerve endings   Sensory neuron endings (dendrites) that have no anatomical specializations. They respond to pain, temperature changes, tickle, and itch. They are also called *naked nerve endings.*

Fornix   A tract of association fibers in the brain. It connects the hippocampus with the mammillary bodies. It is visible below the corpus callosum in a midsagittal section of the brain.

Ganglion (plural: ganglia)   A cluster of neuron cell bodies that lies outside the CNS. There are 4 main types of ganglia. Posterior (dorsal) root ganglia contain the cell bodies of sensory neurons. The cell bodies of autonomic postganglionic neurons are found in sympathetic trunk ganglia, prevertebral ganglia, and terminal ganglia.

Gated ion channels   Ion channels in plasma membranes that open and close in response to specific stimuli. The categories of stimuli include voltage, chemical, mechanical pressure, and light.

General sensations   The sensations of touch, pressure, vibration, temperature, pain, tickle, itch, and proprioception. Also called *somatic senses.*

General somatic motor (efferent)neurons   Carry impulses from the CNS to skeletal muscles.

General somatic sensory (afferent)neurons   Carry impulses for limb position from muscles and joints into the CNS; they also carry impulses for pain, temperature, touch, vibration, and pressure from the skin into the CNS.

General visceral motor (efferent) neurons   The output component of the autonomic nervous system. Carry impulses to smooth muscle, cardiac muscle, and glands.

General visceral sensory (afferent) neurons   The input component of the autonomic nervous system. They are associated with chemoreceptors that monitor changes in the chemical composition of the body fluids or with mechanoreceptors that monitor the degree of stretch in blood vessels and visceral organs.

Generator potential   The electrical response of a sensory receptor to a stimulus. It is a graded potential, which means that its magnitude varies with the strength and duration of the stimulus. If the generator potential is strong enough to reach threshold it will trigger (generate) an action potential in a sensory (afferent) neuron. Also called a *receptor potential.*

Gland of Zeis   *See* Sebaceous ciliary gland.

Glia   *See* Neuroglia.

Gnostic area   An association area of the cerebral cortex. It is located among the somatosensory, visual, and auditory association areas. It integrates sensory information from many different sources so that a common thought can be formed. It then transmits signals to other parts of the brain to cause the appropriate response.

Golgi tendon organ   *See* Tendon organ.

Graded potentials   Electrical responses in plasma membranes that vary in size. The size (or magnitude) of a graded potential depends upon how many gated ion channels have opened and how long each one is open. EPSPs, IPSPs, and generator potentials are examples of graded potentials.

Gray matter   Aggregations of neuron cell bodies or bundles of unmyelinated axons and neuroglia in the CNS. The outer shell of the brain (the cortex) is gray matter, while the inner region of the spinal cord is gray matter.

Gray ramus communicans   One of the two structures that connect a sympathetic trunk ganglion to a spinal nerve. It contains sympathetic postganglionic fibers that carry impulses via spinal nerves to the skin (arrector pili muscles and sweat glands) and to blood vessels. It is gray because the postganglionic fibers are unmyelinated.

Gustatory pathway   The sensations of taste are transmitted to the medulla oblongata of the brain via 3 cranial nerves: the facial nerve (VII) transmits impulses from the anterior 2/3 of the tongue; the glossopharyngeal nerve (IX) transmits impulses from the posterior 1/3 of the tongue; the vagus (X) transmits impulses from the throat and epiglottis.

Gustatory sensations   There are 4 primary taste sensations: sour, salty, bitter, and sweet. All other tastes are combinations of these four, modified by accompanying olfactory sensations.

Gyrus (plural: gyri)   A ridge or elevated region in a cerebral hemisphere. Gyri serve as landmarks for regions of the cerebral cortex. The postcentral gyrus is the location of the primary somatosensory area; the precentral gyrus is the location of the primary motor area. Also called a *convolution.*

Hair cells   Sensory receptors for taste, equilibrium, and hearing.

Hypermetropia   Farsightedness. A condition in which visual images of near objects are focused behind the retina, resulting in blurred vision. A common cause is a short anterior-posterior eyeball axis.

Hyperpolarization   The process by which a membrane potential becomes more negative than the resting potential. It results from an increased outflow of potassium ions.

Hypothalamus   A portion of the diencephalon. It is located beneath the thalamus (*hypo* = below) and forms the floor and part of the walls of the 3rd ventricle. It consists of about 12 nuclei divided among 4 major regions: mammillary, tuberal, supraoptic, & preoptic regions. It is the most important region of the brain for regulating the internal environment.

Impulse frequency   The number of impulses conducted along a nerve fiber per unit time. Since all action potentials are the same (all-or-none principal), the message transmitted is determined by impulse frequency. Impulse frequencies range between 10 and 1000 impulses per second.

Indirect (extrapyramidal) pathways   Transmit impulses from the brain stem to skeletal muscles. While in the CNS these pathways transmit their impulses via 5 major spinal cord tracts: rubrospinal, tectospinal, vestibulospinal, lateral reticulospinal, and anterior reticulospinal.

Inhibitory postsynaptic potential (IPSP)   An IPSP increases the negativity of the membrane potential, making it more difficult for the postsynaptic membrane to reach threshold and fire. At inhibitory synapses the neurotransmitter generates an IPSP in the postsynaptic membrane by opening the chemically gated Cl⁻ or K⁺ channels; both actions increase the negativity inside the postsynaptic cell.

Innervation   The nerve supply of a given structure.

Insula   A triangular area of the cerebral cortex that lies deep within the lateral sulcus (fissure) and cannot be seen in an external view of the brain.

Intercostal nerves   The ventral rami (branches) of thoracic spinal nerves that pass between the ribs. Unlike the other spinal nerves, they do not form plexuses. They are also called *thoracic nerves*.

Intermediate mass   A bridge of nervous tissue that passes through the 3rd ventricle and joins the right and left portions of the thalamus.

Internal capsule   A thick sheet of white matter made up of myelinated fibers connecting various parts of the cerebral cortex. It is located between the thalamus and the lenticular nuclei.

Internal ear   The internal ear consists of two labyrinths, one inside the other. The bony labyrinth is a complex group of communicating passages in the temporal bone. The membranous labyrinth is a series of sacs and tubes that lie within the bony labyrinth and have approximately the same shape. The internal ear contains the sense organs for hearing, dynamic equilibrium, and static equilibrium. It is also called the *inner ear*.

Intrafusal fibers   Three to ten specialized skeletal muscle fibers called intrafusal fibers are partially enclosed in a spindle-shaped connective tissue capsule; the entire structure is called a muscle spindle. Muscle spindles are stretch receptors, monitoring the length of the muscle.

Ion channels   Channels in plasma membranes that control the movement of ions in and out of a cell. There are 2 basic types: leakage channels (nongated) and gated channels. Leakage channels are always open. Gated channels open and close depending upon the influence of 4 types of stimuli: electrical, chemical, mechanical pressure, and light.

Ipsilateral reflex arc   A type of reflex arc in which impulses enter and leave the spinal cord on the same side.

Joint kinesthetic receptors   Proprioceptive receptors located within and around articular capsules of synovial joints. They are sensitive to joint movement.

Kinesthesia   The awareness of the directions of movement.

Lacrimal apparatus   A group of structures in the region of the eyes that produces and drains tears.

Lamellated corpuscle   An oval pressure receptor located in the subcutaneous layer of the skin. Also called a *Pacinian corpuscle*.

Lateral cerebral sulcus   A groove that separates the frontal lobe from the temporal lobe in each hemisphere.

Lateral geniculate nucleus   A nucleus in each half of the thalamus that relays visual information to the auditory cortex of the occipital lobes.

Lateralization   Structural and functional differences between the left and right cerebral hemispheres.

Leakage (nongated) ion channels   Ion channels in plasma membranes that are always open. Plasma membranes of neurons have many more K⁺ leakage channels than Na⁺ leakage channels; that is why the membrane permeability to

K⁺ is much higher.

Lens   An elastic, transparent, biconvex structure located posterior to the iris and anterior to the vitreous body of the eye. It is suspended from the ciliary body by suspensory ligaments. The lens fine-tunes focusing of light rays for clear vision.

Lenticular nucleus   A nucleus located in each cerebral hemisphere; it is subdivided into a lateral portion called the putamen and a medial portion called the globus pallidus. It is part of a group of nuclei referred to as the basal ganglia. Also called the *lentiform nucleus*.

Light-gated ion channels   Ion channels that close in response to light. Na⁺ channels located in the plasma membranes of rods close when light strikes the retina.

Limbic system   A ring of interconnected structures in the cerebrum and diencephalon that function in emotional aspects of behavior related to survival. The structures include the limbic lobe, dentate gyrus, amygdaloid body, septal nuclei, mammillary bodies, anterior nucleus of the thalamus, olfactory lobes, and bundles of interconnecting myelinated axons.

Lobes (of the cerebrum)   Each cerebral hemisphere is divided into 4 lobes: frontal, parietal, temporal, and occipital.

Lower motor neurons   Lower motor neurons have their cell bodies in cranial nerve motor nuclei or in spinal cord anterior gray horns; their axons extend to skeletal muscle fibers. (The simplest descending pathways of the CNS consist of two sets of neurons. Upper motor neuron cell bodies are in the cerebral cortex or in brain stem nuclei. Their axons extend down the spinal cord to lower motor neurons.)

Lumbar plexus   A network of nerves formed by the ventral rami of spinal nerves L1—L4.

Macula lutea   A yellow spot in the center of the retina. The fovea centralis, which contains only cones, is in the center of the macula lutea.

Mechanically gated ion channels   Ion channels that open or close in response to mechanical pressure or vibration. Examples: responses to touch or sound waves.

Mechanoreceptor   A receptor that detects mechanical deformation of the receptor itself or of adjacent cells. The stimuli of mechanoreceptors include touch, pressure, vibration, proprioception, hearing, equilibrium, and blood pressure.

Medial geniculate nucleus   A nucleus in each half of the thalamus that relays auditory information to the auditory cortex of the temporal lobes.

Medial lemniscus   A flat band of myelinated nerve fibers extending through the medulla, pons, and midbrain and terminating in the thalamus on the same side. Sensory neurons in this tract transmit impulses for proprioception, fine touch, pressure, and vibration sensations.

Medulla oblongata   The most inferior of the three parts of the brain stem. (The other parts are the midbrain and the pons.) Nuclei in the medulla control vital respiratory and cardiovascular functions. The nuclei of several cranial nerves are located in the medulla.

Meibomian gland   *See* Tarsal gland.

Meissner's corpuscle   *See* Corpuscle of touch.

Membrane potential   The voltage present at any instant across a plasma membrane. The resting membrane potential for a neuron is usually -70 mV. During an action potential the membrane potential changes from -70 mV to +30 mV and back to -70 mV in 1 msec.

Membranous labyrinth   The portion of the internal ear that is located inside the bony labyrinth. It consists of the membranous semicircular canals, the saccule and utricle, and the cochlear duct.

Meninges   Three membranes covering the brain and spinal cord. Moving from the innermost membrane outward, they include the pia mater, arachnoid, and dura mater.

Merkel's disc   *See* Tactile disc or Type I cutaneous mechanoreceptor.

Mesencephalon   *See* Midbrain.

Microglia   Neuroglial cells of the CNS that carry on phagocytosis. Also called *brain macrophages*.

Midbrain   The part of the brain between the pons and the diencephalon. The corpora quadrigemina is located on the dorsal region. Also called the *mesencephalon*.

Middle ear   A small epithelial-lined cavity in the temporal bone. It is separated from the external ear by the eardrum and from the internal ear by a thin bony partition containing the oval and round windows. The 3 auditory ossicles extend across the middle ear connecting the eardrum to the oval window. Also called the *tympanic cavity*.

Mixed nerves   Cranial nerves that contain both sensory (afferent) and motor (efferent) fibers. They include the trigeminal (V), facial (VII), glossopharyngeal (IX), and vagus (X) nerves.

Modality   A specific kind of sensory information; a type of sensation (vision, hearing, taste, etc.). Sensory receptors respond vigorously to one particular kind of stimulus and weakly or not at all to others.

Motor areas   The regions of the cerebral cortex that govern the movement of skeletal muscles. The primary motor area, located on the precentral gyrus of the frontal lobe, is the major region for the initiation of voluntary movements.

Motor end plate   The portion of the plasma membrane (sarcolemma) of a muscle fiber that is adjacent to the synaptic end bulb of a motor neuron. It is part of a neuromuscular junction.

Motor neuron   A neuron that conducts impulses from the CNS to an effector (muscle or gland). Also called an *efferent neuron*.

Motor (descending) pathway   The route followed by a nerve impulse as it travels from the brain to a muscle or gland.

Motor speech area   The motor speech area is concerned with the translation of thoughts into speech. Also called *Broca's area*.

Muscarinic receptors   One of the 2 types of receptors that bind acetylcholine. They are found on all autonomic effectors innervated by parasympathetic postganglionic fibers and some effectors innervated by sympathetic postganglionic fibers.

Muscle spindle   An encapsulated receptor located between normal muscle fibers. It consists of three to ten specialized skeletal muscle fibers called intrafusal fibers partially enclosed in a spindle-shaped connective tissue capsule. It is a stretch receptor, monitoring the length of a muscle.

Myelin sheath   Up to 100 layers of neurolemmocyte (Schwann cell) plasma membrane wrapped tightly around an axon. The myelin sheath electrically insulates the axon and increases the speed of nerve impulse transmission.

Myenteric plexus   A network of autonomic nerve fibers located in the muscular layer of the small intestine. Also called *plexus of Auerbach*.

Myopia   Nearsightedness. A condition in which visual images of far objects are focused in front of the retina, resulting in blurred vision. A common cause is a long anterior-posterior eyeball axis.

Near point vision   The minimum distance from the eye that an object can be clearly focused with maximum effort. For a normal eye it is about 4 inches (10 cm).

Negative feedback   The principle governing most control systems. It is a response mechanism in which the stimulus initiates actions that reverse or reduce the stimulus. This is the primary mechanism for maintaining homeostasis. For example, as blood pressure increases, nerve impulses travel to centers in the brain, which send out instructions to decrease the force and rate of heart contractions.

Nerve   A cordlike bundle of nerve fibers and their associated connective tissue coursing together outside the CNS.

Nerve impulse   Self-propagating action potentials that move along the surface of nerve fibers. Nerve impulses on myelinated fibers travel by saltatory conduction, the action potentials "jumping" from node to node. Nerve impulses on unmyelinated fibers travel by continuous conduction, each action potential triggering an action potential in the adjacent plasma membrane.

Neural tube   A tube of nervous tissue that forms along the dorsal surface of the embryo at about 3 weeks. All the structures of the CNS are derived from the neural tube.

Neuroendocrine cells   Nerve cells in the hypothalamus that secrete hormones.

Neurofibral node   A space along a myelinated nerve fiber between the individual neurolemmocytes (Schwann cells) that form the myelin sheath. In saltatory conduction action potentials "jump" from node to node. Also called *node of Ranvier*.

Neurofibril   One of the delicate threads that forms a complicated network in the cytoplasm of the cell body and processes of a neuron.

Neuroglia   Cells of the nervous system that are specialized to perform the functions of connective tissue. The neuroglia of the CNS include astrocytes, oligodendrocytes, microglia, and ependyma. The neuroglia of the PNS include neurolemmocytes (Schwann cells) and the ganglion satellite cells. Also called *glial cells* and *glia*.

Neurohypophysis   *See* Posterior pituitary gland.

Neurolemma   The outermost, nucleated cytoplasmic layer of a neurolemmocyte (Schwann cell). It surrounds the myelin sheath. When a nerve fiber is injured, the neurolemma aids regeneration. Also called *sheath of Schwann*.

Neurolemmocyte   A neuroglial cell of the PNS that forms the myelin sheath and neurolemma of a nerve fiber by wrapping around a nerve fiber in a jelly-roll fashion. Also called a *Schwann cell*.

Neuromodulators   Chemicals secreted by neurons that influence the signaling of neighboring or distant neurons, magnifying or dampening their response to other neurotransmitters.

Neuromuscular junction   The area of contact between the synaptic end bulb of a motor neuron and a portion of the muscle cell plasma membrane called the motor end plate.

Neuron   A nerve cell. It has 3 main parts: cell body, dendrites, and axon.

Neuronal circuits   Neuronal pools in the CNS are arranged in patterns called neuronal circuits. The 5 basic types of neuronal circuits include: simple series, diverging, converging, reverberating, and parallel after-discharge.

Neuronal pools   The billions of neurons in the CNS are arranged into complicated patterns called neuronal pools.

Neuropeptides   One of the 4 basic chemical classifications for neurotransmitters. Neuropeptides are chains of 2 to about 40 amino acids that occur naturally in the brain.

Neurosecretory cell   A neuron in the hypothalamus that produces antidiuretic hormone (ADH) or oxytocin. These hormones are stored in the axon terminals, which are located in the posterior pituitary gland.

Neurotransmitters   Molecules that transmit impulses across synapses from a presynaptic neuron to a postsynaptic neuron or effector cell. The 4 chemical types of neurotransmitters include: acetylcholine, amino acids, biogenic amines, and neuropeptides.

Nicotinic receptor   One of the 2 types of receptors that bind acetylcholine. Found on all autonomic postganglionic neurons and on the motor end plates of neuromuscular junctions.

Nissl bodies   *See* Chromatophilic substance.

Nociceptor   A receptor that detects pain.

Node of Ranvier   *See* Neurofibral node.

Norepinephrine   A chemical that functions as a neurotransmitter and a hormone. Most sympathetic postganglionic neurons release norepinephrine. The exceptions are the sympathetic postganglionic fibers that lead to sweat glands and those that lead to some blood vessels in skeletal muscle. The hormone norepinephrine is released by modified sympathetic postganglionic neurons in the adrenal medulla. Also called *noradrenaline*.

Nucleus (in the CNS)   A cluster of neuron cell bodies in the brain or spinal cord that have a common function.

Nucleus cuneatus   A cluster of neurons in the medulla oblongata. Fibers of the fasciculus cuneatus terminate here.

Nucleus gracilis   A cluster of neurons in the medulla oblongata. Fibers of the fasciculus gracilis terminate here.

Olfactory   Pertaining to smell.

Olfactory bulb   The mass of gray matter at the end of each olfactory nerve. Olfactory bulbs are located beneath the frontal lobe of the cerebrum on either side of the crista galli of the ethmoid bone.

Olfactory glands   Glands located among the epithelial cells of the mucous membrane lining the nose. They secrete mucus that moistens the surface of the olfactory epithelium and dissolves odorant gases. Also called *Bowman's glands*.

Olfactory receptors   Bipolar neurons located in the mucous membrane lining the upper portion of each nasal cavity. They are chemoreceptors.

Olfactory nerves   The unmyelinated axons of olfactory receptors unite to form the olfactory nerves, which pass through multiple foramina (holes) in the cribriform plate of the ethmoid bone and terminate in the olfactory bulbs.

Olfactory tract   A bundle of axons that extends from each olfactory bulb posteriorly to the olfactory portions of the cerebral cortex. The olfactory tract divides into two pathways: one leads to the thalamus and then to the cortex of the frontal lobes; another leads to primitive regions of the cortex on the inferior surface of the brain.

Oligodendrocyte   A neuroglial cell that supports neurons and produces a phospholipid myelin sheath around axons of neurons of the CNS.

One-way propagation   A nerve impulse moves in only one direction along a nerve fiber. This is because the membrane is refractory behind the leading edge of an action potential.

One-way synaptic transmission   Nerve impulses can be transmitted across synapses in only one direction. This is because the neurotransmitter is located in the synaptic end bulbs of presynaptic neurons and only the postsynaptic membranes have the correct receptor proteins to recognize and bind the neurotransmitter.

Optic   Pertaining to the eye, vision, or the properties of light.

Optic chiasma   Where fibers from the nasal (medial) portion of both retinas cross over. Visual information from the nasal portion of the left retina is transmitted to the right occipital lobe and vice versa. It is located just anterior to the pituitary gland.

Optic disc   A small area of the retina just medial to the posterior end of the optic axis. It is the location where optic nerve fibers and blood vessels exit and enter the eyeball, and there are no photoreceptor cells present. Also called the *blind spot*.

Optic tracts   After passing through the optic chiasma, the fibers of the optic nerves become part of the two optic tracts. The optic tracts enter the brain and terminate in the lateral geniculate nuclei of the thalamus.

Orbit   The bony, pyramid-shaped cavity of the skull that holds the eyeball.

Organ of Corti   *See* Spiral organ.

Otoliths   Particles of calcium carbonate embedded in the otolithic membrane of the internal ear. They are involved in the maintenance of static equilibrium.

Otolithic membrane   A thick, gelatinous, glycoprotein layer located directly over the hair cells of the maculae. Maculae are the sense organs for static equilibrium and are located in the utricle and saccule of the internal ear.

Oval window   A membrane-covered opening in the thin, bony partition between the middle and internal ear. The base or footplate of the stapes is attached to this membrane. Also called the *fenestra vestibuli*.

Oxytocin   A hormone secreted by neurosecretory cells in the paraventricular nucleus of the hypothalamus.

Pacinian corpuscle   *See* Lamellated corpuscle.

Pain   Pain is classified as acute or chronic. Acute pain is sharp, fast, pricking pain. Chronic pain is burning, aching, throbbing, slow pain. Pain sensations result from tissue damage, excessive stimulation of any type, excessive distention of a structure, prolonged muscular contraction, muscle spasms, inadequate blood flow to a structure, or certain chemicals released during inflammation (prostaglandins & kinins).

Palpebrae   Eyelids.

Papillae   Elevations on the upper surface of the tongue. There are 3 types: circumvallate, fungiform, & filiform. Circumvallate and fungiform papillae contain taste buds.

Parasympathetic division   One of the 2 subdivisions of the autonomic nervous system. Pathways consist of two sets of neurons: preganglionic neurons and postganglionic neurons. Preganglionic axons exit from the CNS via cranial nerves 3, 7, 9, & 10; and via spinal nerves S2—S4. It is primarily concerned with activities that restore and conserve body energy.

Parasympathetic responses   Responses that restore and conserve body energy during times of rest or recovery.

They are summarized by the acronym "SLUD": Salivation, Lacrimation, Urination, & Defecation. Concerned primarily with the digestive and urinary systems.

Patellar reflex Extension of the lower leg by contraction of the quadriceps femoris muscle in response to tapping the patellar ligament. An example of a stretch reflex. Also called the *knee jerk reflex*.

Perception A conscious sensation. We are consciously aware of sensations associated with the external environment. For the most part, we are unaware of sensations involving the internal environment, such as changes in blood pressure or the chemical composition of the blood.

Perikaryon *See* Cell body.

Perilymph The fluid contained in the bony labyrinth of the internal ear. It surrounds the membranous labyrinth.

Perineurium The connective tissue forming a sheath around each fascicle (bundle of nerve fibers) in a nerve.

Peripheral nervous system One of the 2 major divisions of the nervous system; the part that lies outside the CNS. It consists of nerves and ganglia.

Photopigment A substance that can absorb light and undergo structural changes that can lead to the development of a receptor potential in photoreceptor cells (rods and cones). Photopigments are integral proteins in the plasma membrane of the outer segment of rods and cones. They are made of retinal (derived from vitamin A) and an opsin (the variable portion of the molecule). *Rhodopsin* is the photopigment found in rods.

Photoreceptor A receptor cell that detects light on the retina of the eye. Rods and cones.

Plexus A network of nerves, veins, or lymphatics.

Plexus of Auerbach *See* Myenteric plexus.

Plexus of Meissner *See* Submucosal plexus.

Polarized Opposite effects or states existing at the same time. A polarized plasma membrane has the outer surface positively charged and the inner surface negatively charged.

Pons The portion of the brain stem that forms a "bridge" between the medulla and the midbrain. It is anterior to the cerebellum.

Positive feedback When a response enhances the original effects of a stimulus. For example, during an action potential if a stimulus causes a neuron membrane to depolarize enough to reach threshold, the change in voltage causes a further depolarization. Depolarization stimulates more depolarization.

Postcentral gyrus A gyrus immediately posterior to the central sulcus. It contains the primary somatosensory area of the cerebral cortex.

Posterior Nearer to the back; opposite of anterior. Also called *dorsal*.

Posterior cavity The space between the lens and the retina of the eye, which is filled with a jellylike substance called the vitreous body. Also called the *vitreous chamber*.

Posterior pituitary gland The posterior part of the pituitary gland. Neuron cell bodies of the supraoptic and paraventricular nuclei of the hypothalamus produce the hormones vasopressin and oxytocin, which are transported down axons to the posterior pituitary. These hormones are released when appropriate stimuli from the blood or brain reach the hypothalamus. Also called *neurohypophysis*.

Posterior root A spinal nerve has two points of attachment to the spinal cord: a posterior root and an anterior root. The posterior root contains sensory (afferent) fibers. Also called the *dorsal root*.

Posterior root ganglion A ganglion located in the posterior root that contains the cell bodies of sensory neurons. Also called the *dorsal root ganglion*.

Postganglionic neuron The second visceral motor neuron in an autonomic pathway. Its cell body is located in an autonomic ganglion and its axon terminates on an autonomic effector (smooth muscle, cardiac muscle, or gland).

Postsynaptic membrane The portion of the plasma membrane of a postsynaptic neuron that is adjacent to the synaptic end bulb of the presynaptic neuron. It contains the receptor proteins that recognize and bind neurotransmitter. Also called the *subsynaptic membrane*.

Postsynaptic neuron The neuron that is activated by the release of a neurotransmitter from a presynaptic neuron. It carries an impulse away from the synapse.

Postsynaptic potentials One of the two types of graded potentials (the other type of graded potential is a generator potential). It occurs on a postsynaptic membrane in response to the action of neurotransmitters.

Precentral gyrus A gyrus immediately anterior to the central sulcus. It contains the primary motor area of the cerebral cortex.

Preganglionic fibers The axons of the first visceral motor neurons that emerge from the CNS. Sympathetic preganglionic fibers are called the thoracolumbar outflow. Parasympathetic preganglionic fibers are called the craniosacral outflow.

Preganglionic neuron The first visceral motor neuron in an autonomic pathway. Its cell body is in the brain or spinal cord, and its myelinated axon terminates at an autonomic ganglion, where it synapses with a postganglionic neuron.

Presbyopia A loss of elasticity of the lens of the eye due to advancing age. It results in the inability to focus clearly on near objects.

Presynaptic facilitation When the amount of neurotransmitter released from the end bulb of a presynaptic neuron is increased. The increased release of neurotransmitter is the result of an excitatory input from a third neuron that synapses near the end bulb of the presynaptic neuron.

Presynaptic inhibition When the amount of neurotransmitter released from the end bulb of a presynaptic neuron is decreased. The decreased release of neurotransmitter is the result of an inhibitory input from a third neuron that synapses near the end bulb of the presynaptic neuron.

Presynaptic neuron A neuron that carries impulses toward a synapse.

Prevertebral ganglia Clusters of cell bodies of postganglionic sympathetic neurons located anterior to the vertebral column and close to the abdominal arteries. Also called the *collateral ganglia*.

Primary motor area A region of the cerebral cortex in the precentral gyrus of the frontal lobe of the cerebrum. It controls the actions of specific muscles or groups of muscles.

Primary somatosensory area A region of the cerebral cortex in the postcentral gyrus of the parietal lobe of the cerebrum. It localizes exactly the points of the body where sensations originate. Also called the *general sensory area*.

Primary vesicles The 3 bulges that appear in the neural tube during the fourth week of embryonic development: forebrain (prosencephalon), midbrain (mesencephalon), and hindbrain (rhombencephalon).

Projection The process by which the brain refers a sensation to its point of stimulation.

Projection fibers Myelinated axons that transmit impulses from the cerebrum and other parts of the brain to the spinal cord or from the spinal cord to the brain.

Proprioception The awareness of the precise position of body parts.

Proprioceptors Sensory receptors located in muscles (muscle spindles), tendons (tendon organs), or joints (joint kinesthetic receptors) that provide information about body position and movements.

Pupil The hole in the center of the iris. After passing through the pupil, light rays pass through the lens and the vitreous body of the posterior cavity before striking the retina.

Pyramids Two bulges on the ventral surface of the medulla oblongata. The largest descending (motor) tracts run from the cerebral cortex, through the pyramids, and down the spinal cord. Most of the fibers in the left pyramid cross over to the right side, descend in the lateral white columns of the spinal cord, and end in the anterior gray horns; most of the fibers in the right pyramid cross over to the left side.

Pyramidal pathways Collections of motor nerve fibers arising in the brain and passing down the spinal cord to motor neurons in the anterior gray horns.

Ramus (plural: rami) A branch.

Receptors There are 2 basic types of receptors: A sensory receptor is the peripheral end of a sensory neuron or a specialized cell modified to respond to a specific sensory modality, such as touch, pressure, cold, light, or sound. A protein receptor is a protein molecule designed to combine with a substance that has a complementary shape. For example, receptors in the postsynaptic membranes of neuromuscular junctions are designed to bind with acetylcholine.

Receptor potential *See* Generator potential.

Reciprocal innervation When nerve impulses stimulate the contraction of one muscle and simultaneously inhibit the contraction of antagonistic muscles.

Recruitment The process of increasing the number of active motor units.

Red nucleus A cluster of neuron cell bodies in the midbrain. Fibers originating in the red nucleus form the rubroreticular and rubrospinal tracts.

Referred pain Pain that is felt at a site remote from the place of origin.

Reflex An automatic, fast response to a change in the internal or external environment.

Reflex arc The basic structural and functional unit of the nervous system. It consists of 5 basic components: receptor, sensory (afferent) pathway, integrating center, motor (efferent) pathway, and effector.

Refraction The bending of light as it passes from one medium to another of a different density, as from air into glass.

Refractory period The period of time immediately following an action potential, when an excitable cell is unresponsive to stimuli. During the absolute refractory period a neuron membrane is unresponsive to all stimuli; it lasts about 1 msec. During the relative refractory period, which lasts for 10 to 15 msec after the absolute refractory period, the membrane will respond if the stimulus is suprathreshold.

Repolarization Restoration of the resting membrane potential. During the second half of an action potential the plasma membrane becomes highly permeable to K^+ and relatively impermeable to Na^+. The increased rate of diffusion of K^+ out of the cell restores the resting membrane potential.

Respiratory center A region of gray matter in the medulla oblongata that controls the basic rhythm of breathing.

Resting membrane potential The voltage that exists between the inside and outside of a neuron cell membrane when the neuron is not responding to a stimulus. It is about -70 mV, with the inside negative relative to the outside.

Reticular activating system (RAS) A part of the reticular formation. When the RAS is activated, a generalized alert or arousal behavior results.

Reticular formation A large portion of the brain stem, consisting of small areas of gray matter interspersed among the white matter. It also extends into the spinal cord and diencephalon. It receives input from higher brain regions that control skeletal muscles and contributes to regulating muscle tone.

Retina The inner coat of the eyeball, which lines most of the posterior cavity. It is a thin layer of neural tissue that contains the photoreceptors (rods & cones). Also called the *nervous tunic*.

Retinal The pigment portion of the photopigment rhodopsin. (The protein portion of rhodopsin is scotopsin.)

Rhodopsin A photopigment located in the rods of the retina. It consists of 2 parts: a protein called scotopsin and a pigment called retinal. It is sensitive to low levels of illumination.

Rod A visual receptor in the retina of the eye. It is specialized for vision in dim light.

Round window A small opening in the bony partition that separates the middle and internal ears. It is just below the oval window and is covered by a membrane. Also called the *fenestra cochlea*.

Saccule One of the two chambers in the membranous labyrinth of the internal ear. It contains the sensory organ for static equilibrium (the macula).

Sacral parasympathetic outflow The parasympathetic preganglionic fibers that emerge from the CNS in spinal nerves S2—S4. Collectively they form the pelvic splanchnic nerves, which innervate smooth muscle and glands in the colon, ureters, urinary bladder, & reproductive organs.

Sacral plexus A network formed by the ventral rami of spinal nerves L4 through S4.

Saltatory conduction The propagation of an action potential along the exposed portions of a myelinated nerve fiber. The nerve impulse seems to jump (*saltare* = to jump) from one neurofibral node to the next.

Satellite cell A type of neuroglial cell found in ganglia of the peripheral nervous system.

Scala tympani The lower spiral-shaped channel of the bony cochlea in the internal ear. It extends from the tip of the spiral cavity to the round window (the secondary tympanic membrane), and is filled with a fluid called perilymph.

Scala vestibuli The upper spiral-shaped channel of the bony cochlea in the internal ear. It extends from the region of the vestibule adjacent to the oval window to the tip of the spiral cavity, and is filled with a fluid called perilymph.

Schwann cell *See* Neurolemmocyte.

Sclera The posterior portion of the fibrous tunic of the eyeball. It is the tough, white, outer coat, which helps protect the eyeball and maintain its shape; it is visible as the "white" of the eye. (The anterior portion of the fibrous tunic is the cornea, which is transparent.)

Scleral venous sinus A sinus or canal through which aqueous humor drains from the anterior chamber of the eyeball into the blood. Its opening is located at the junction of the sclera and the cornea. Also called *canal of Schlemm.*

Scotopsin The protein portion of the visual pigment rhodopsin. Found in rods of the retina.

Sebaceous ciliary glands Sebaceous glands at the base of the hair follicles of eyelashes; they secrete lubricating fluid into the follicles. Also called *glands of Zeis.*

Semicircular canals The portion of the bony labyrinth in the internal ear that contains the three semicircular ducts. It consists of three channels in the petrous portion of the temporal bone. The channels are semicircular, oriented in three perpendicular planes, and filled with a fluid called perilymph.

Semicircular ducts The membranous, fluid-filled ducts (or tubes) located inside the semicircular canals. They contain the organs for dynamic equilibrium, which are located in a dilated portion of each duct called the ampulla. (The organs for dynamic equilibrium are called cristae.)

Sensation The conscious or unconscious awareness of external or internal stimuli.

Sensory areas Regions of the cerebral cortex concerned with the interpretation of sensory impulses. The five primary sensory areas include: somatosensory (general sensory), visual, auditory, gustatory, and olfactory.

Sensory neuron A neuron that conducts impulses from a sensory receptor into the CNS. Also called an *afferent neuron.*

Sensory (ascending) pathway The route followed by a nerve impulse as it travels from a sensory receptor to the brain.

Sensory receptor A sensory neuron or specialized epithelial cell that is sensitive to a certain type of stimulus.

Sheath of Schwann *See* Neurolemma.

Smooth muscle An organ specialized for contraction, composed of smooth muscle fibers (cells). Found in the walls of hollow internal organs, and innervated by visceral motor neurons.

Sodium-potassium pump An active transport system located in plasma membranes that transports sodium ions out of the cell and potassium ions into the cell. This mechanism maintains a relatively constant sodium ion concentration across the membrane, which is necessary for normal impulse transmission.

Somatic nervous system (SNS) One of the two major subdivisions of the peripheral nervous system. In the SNS sensory (afferent) neurons carry information from the receptors for general senses (touch, pressure, vibration, temperature, pain, & proprioception) and the special senses (smell, taste, vision, hearing, & equilibrium). All motor (efferent) neurons of the SNS innervate skeletal muscles. In the SNS sensations are consciously perceived and actions are voluntary.

Somatic spinal reflexes Spinal reflexes that result in the contraction of skeletal muscles. Some examples are the stretch reflex, tendon reflex, flexor reflex, and crossed extensor reflex.

Somatosensory cortex Located in the postcentral gyrus of the cerebral cortex. Its function is to localize exactly the points of the body where sensations originate.

Somesthetic Pertaining to sensations and sensory structures of the body.

Special senses The special senses include: smell, taste, vision, hearing, and equilibrium.

Special somatic sensory (afferent) neurons Sensory neurons that carry impulses for vision, hearing, & equilibrium to the CNS via cranial nerves.

Special visceral motor (efferent)neurons Carry impulses from the CNS to skeletal muscles via cranial nerves; control facial expression and position of the jaw, neck, larynx, and pharynx.

Special visceral sensory (afferent)neurons Carry impulses for taste and smell to the CNS via cranial nerves.

Spinal cord A mass of nerve tissue extending from the base of the cranium to the first lumbar vertebra in the lower back. It is a continuation of the medulla of the brain stem and serves as a pathway for nerve impulses traveling to and from the brain; it also serves as an integrating center for spinal reflexes.

Spinal meninges Three layers of membranes that envelop the spinal cord; a continuation of the meninges that surround the brain. They include the dura mater, arachnoid, and pia mater.

Spinal nerves The 31 pairs of nerves that emerge from the spinal cord. They include: 8 cervical, 12 thoracic, 5 lumbar, 5 sacral, and 1 coccygeal. All are mixed nerves, containing both sensory (afferent) and motor (efferent) fibers. Each spinal nerve is attached to the spinal cord by two roots, an anterior (ventral) root and a posterior (dorsal) root.

Spinal reflexes Reflexes are fast, predictable, automatic responses to changes in the environment that help maintain homeostasis. Reflexes in which the spinal cord functions as the integrating center are called spinal reflexes.

Spinal reflex arcs Reflex arcs describe the pathway of the nerve impulses during a spinal reflex. There are five basic types of spinal reflex arcs: monosynaptic, polysynaptic, ipsilateral, contralateral, and intersegmental.

Spinal segment The region of the spinal cord from which a given pair of spinal nerves emerge. For example, the first pair of thoracic nerves emerge from spinal segment T1.

Spinocerebellar tracts The anterior and posterior spinocerebellar tracts convey nerve impulses for subconscious muscle and joint sense to the cerebellum.

Spiral organ The organ of hearing. It is located in the cochlear duct of the membranous labyrinth in the internal ear. It consists of hair cells (sensory receptors), supporting cells, a tectorial membrane, and a basilar membrane. Also called the *organ of Corti.*

Static equilibrium The maintenance of posture in response to changes in the orientation of the body, mainly the head, relative to the ground.

Stereognosis The ability to recognize the size, shape, and texture of an object by touch.

Stimulus Any change in the internal or external environments capable of altering the membrane potential on a receptor cell. The stimulus changes the membrane permeability to ions, opening or closing specific gated ion channels.

Stretch receptors Sensory receptors that respond when stretched. They are located in muscles (muscle spindles) and in the walls of respiratory tubes and blood vessels.

Stretch reflex A monosynaptic reflex triggered by a sudden stretch of a muscle, and ending with a contraction of that same muscle. An important clinical example is the patellar or knee jerk reflex. Also called a *tendon jerk.*

Subarachnoid space   A space between the arachnoid and the pia mater. Provides a space for the circulation of cerebrospinal fluid around the brain and spinal cord.

Subdural space   A space between the arachnoid and the dura mater. Contains a small amount of fluid.

Submucosal plexus   A network of autonomic nerve fibers located in the outer portion of the submucous layer of the small intestine. Also called the *plexus of Meissner.*

Subthreshold stimulus   A stimulus of such weak intensity that it cannot initiate an action potential. Also called a *subliminal stimulus.*

Sulcus (plural: sulci)   A groove in the surface of the cerebrum or cerebellum. Also called a *fissure.*

Summation   The algebraic addition of the excitatory and inhibitory effects of many stimuli applied to a neuron cell body.

Sympathetic division   One of the 2 subdivisions of the autonomic nervous system. Pathways consist of two sets of neurons: preganglionic neurons and postganglionic neurons. Preganglionic axons exit from the spinal cord via spinal nerves T1 — L2. It is primarily concerned with processes involving the expenditure of energy (fight-or-flight responses). Also called the *thoracolumbar division.*

Sympathetic innervation   Refers to an organ that receives autonomic input from sympathetic fibers only. Examples of organs that receive only sympathetic innervation include: most blood vessel walls, sweat glands, arrector pili muscles, adipose cells, and kidneys. (In dual innervation an organ receives input from both sympathetic and parasympathetic fibers.)

Sympathetic responses   Responses that expend body energy during times of stress. Often referred to as fight-or-flight responses or "E" situations: Emergency, Exercise, and Embarrassment.

Sympathetic trunk ganglia   Clusters of postganglionic sympathetic neuron cell bodies. They form a chain of ganglia on each side of the vertebral column from the neck to the coccyx. Also called *paravertebral* or *vertebral chain ganglia.*

Sympathomimetic drugs   Chemicals that mimic the effects brought about by nerves of the sympathetic division.

Synapse   The contact point between a neuron and another cell (another neuron or a muscle or gland cell). The place where one neuron releases neurotransmitter that diffuses across a space called the synaptic cleft and affects the activity of an adjacent cell. It has 3 main parts: synaptic end bulb, synaptic cleft, and postsynaptic membrane.

Synaptic cleft   The narrow gap that separates the synaptic end bulb of one neuron from the cell membrane of another neuron, muscle cell, or gland cell. Neurotransmitter diffuses across the synaptic cleft.

Synaptic delay   Time required for synaptic transmission at a chemical synapse. Usually about 0.5 msec.

Synaptic end bulb   The expanded end of an axon terminal. It contains synaptic vesicles filled with neurotransmitter. It is one of the 3 parts of a synapse, the other two parts are the synaptic cleft and the postsynaptic membrane. Also called *synaptic knob* or *end foot.*

Synaptic gutters   Invaginated portions of the motor end plate. (The motor end plate is the portion of a muscle cell membrane directly adjacent to the synaptic end bulb.) Also called *synaptic troughs.*

Synaptic transmission   The series of events that occur between the arrival of a nerve impulse at an axon terminal and the activation of the postsynaptic membrane.

Synaptic vesicle   A membrane-enclosed sac that stores neurotransmitters. When an action potential reaches the synaptic end bulb, a synaptic vesicle fuses with the cell membrane and releases neurotransmitters by exocytosis.

Tactile   Pertaining to the sense of touch.

Tactile disc   A modified epidermal cell located in hairless skin that serves as a receptor for discriminative touch. Also called *type I cutaneous mechanoreceptor* or *Merkel's disc.*

Tactile sensations   All sensations detected by mechanoreceptors: touch, pressure, vibration, itch, and tickle.

Tarsal gland   Sebaceous (oil) gland that opens on the edge of each eyelid. Also called a *Meibomian gland.*

Tarsal plate   A thin, elongated sheet of connective tissue, one in each eyelid, giving the eyelid form and support. The aponeurosis (sheet of tendon) of the levator palpebrae superioris is attached to the tarsal plate of the superior eyelid.

Taste buds   Structures located on the tongue, soft palate, larynx, and pharynx that contain the sensory receptors for taste. They consist of three kinds of epithelial cells: gustatory receptor cells, supporting cells, and basal cells.

Tectorial membrane   A gelatinous membrane projecting over and in contact with the hair cells of the spiral organ in the cochlear duct. The bending of hairs against the tectorial membrane triggers action potentials in hair cells.

Tendon organ   A sensory organ responsive to changes in muscle tension and force of contraction. Found near the junction between a tendon and muscle. Also called *Golgi tendon organ.*

Tendon reflex   A polysynaptic, ipsilateral reflex triggered by increased tension in a tendon. The response causes the relaxation of the attached muscle. It is designed to protect tendons and their associated muscles. The receptors involved are called tendon organs.

Tentorium cerebelli   A transverse shelf of dura mater that forms a partition between the occipital lobes of the cerebral hemispheres and the cerebellum.

Terminal ganglia   Clusters of cell bodies of postganglionic parasympathetic neurons. They are located within or close to the walls of the visceral organs that the postganglionic fibers innervate. Also called *intramural ganglia.*

Thalamus (plural: thalami)   Paired oval masses of mostly gray matter organized into nuclei. Located above the midbrain, and forming the lateral walls of the 3rd ventricle. The thalamus is the principal relay station for sensory impulses that reach the cerebral cortex from the spinal cord.

Thermoreceptors   Receptors located in the skin that detect changes in temperature. There are 2 types: hot and cold.

Third ventricle   A slitlike cavity between the right and left halves of the thalamus and between the lateral ventricles.

Thoracolumbar outflow   The fibers of the sympathetic preganglionic neurons. They have their cell bodies in the lateral gray horns of the thoracic segments and the first two lumbar segments of the spinal cord.

Threshold potential   The membrane voltage that must be reached in order to trigger an action potential. For neurons it is about − 55 mV (15 mV more positive than the resting membrane potential).

Threshold stimulus   Any stimulus strong enough to initiate an action potential. Also called a *liminal stimulus.*

Tract A bundle of nerve fibers in the brain or spinal cord.

Transduction Conversion of a stimulus into a generator potential in a receptor cell.

Translation Conversion of sensory nerve impulses into conscious sensations in the cerebral cortex.

Transverse fissure The deep cleft that separates the cerebrum from the cerebellum.

Trigger zone The junction of an axon hillock and the initial segment of an axon. It is the region where local currents generated by excitatory and inhibitory synaptic events are added together; if the summation reaches threshold the first action potential occurs at the trigger zone. Voltage-gated channels are clustered most densely in this region.

Tympanic membrane A thin, semitransparent partition of fibrous connective tissue that separates the external auditory canal from the middle ear. Its function is to convert sound waves into vibrations and transfer the vibrations to the auditory ossicles of the middle ear. Also called the *eardrum*.

Type I cutaneous mechanoreceptor *See* Tactile disc.

Type II cutaneous mechanoreceptor Receptor that detects heavy and continuous touch sensations. Located in the dermis (the skin layer between the epidermis and the subcutaneous layer). Also called *end organ of Ruffini*.

Upper motor neurons The simplest descending pathways of the CNS consist of two sets of neurons. Upper motor neuron cell bodies are in the cerebral cortex or in brain stem nuclei. Their axons extend down the spinal cord to lower motor neurons. (Lower motor neurons have their cell bodies in cranial nerve motor nuclei or in the spinal cord anterior gray horns and their axons extend to skeletal muscle fibers.)

Utricle One of the two chambers in the membranous labyrinth of the internal ear. It contains the sensory organ for static equilibrium (the macula).

Uvea *See* Vascular tunic.

Vascular tunic The middle layer of the eyeball; composed of the choroid, ciliary body, and iris. Also called the *uvea*.

Ventral Nearer to the front; opposite of dorsal. Also called *anterior*.

Ventral anterior nuclei Nuclei in the thalamus that are centers for synapses in the somatic motor system. They are involved in voluntary motor actions and arousal.

Ventral lateral nuclei Nuclei in the thalamus that are centers for synapses in the somatic motor system. They are involved in voluntary motor actions and arousal.

Ventral posterior nuclei Nuclei in the thalamus that relay sensory input concerning taste and somatic sensations.

Ventral ramus The anterior branch of a spinal nerve, containing sensory and motor fibers to the muscles and skin of the anterior surface of the head, neck, trunk, and the extremities.

Ventricles Four cavities in the brain where cerebrospinal fluid is produced by specialized capillary beds called choroid plexuses. (Also, the two inferior chambers of the heart.)

Vermis The central constricted area of the cerebellum that separates the two cerebellar hemispheres. It is divided into lobules.

Vertebral canal A cavity within the vertebral column that contains the spinal cord. Formed by the vertebral foramina of all the vertebrae. Also called the *spinal canal*.

Vertebral column The 33 vertebrae. The 5 sacral vertebrae are fused and the 4 coccygeal vertebrae are fused, so the total number of separate vertebral bones is 26. It encloses and protects the spinal cord. The vertebrae serve as points of attachment for the ribs and back muscles. Also called the *backbone, spinal column,* and *spine*.

Vestibular membrane The membrane in the internal ear that separates the upper spiral-shaped channel called the scala vestibuli from the cochlear duct.

Vestibule One of the three main parts of the bony labyrinth of the internal ear. The other two parts are the cochlea and the semicircular canals. *Vestibule* = entrance hall.

Viscera (singular: viscus) The organs inside the ventral body cavity.

Visceral Pertaining to the organs or to the covering of an organ.

Visceral autonomic reflexes Reflexes that result in the contraction or relaxation of smooth or cardiac muscle or a change in the rate of secretion by a gland. They help regulate heart action, blood pressure, respiration, digestion, defecation, and urinary bladder functions.

Visceral effectors Cardiac muscle, smooth muscle, and glandular epithelium.

Visceral sensations Sensations that originate in the viscera (internal organs). Often the impulses do not reach the cerebral cortex, so there is no conscious perception.

Visceroreceptor Receptor that provides information about the body's internal environment.

Visual field The visual field of each eye is divided into two regions: the nasal (medial) half and the temporal (lateral) half. Light rays from an object in the nasal half of the visual field fall on the temporal half of the retina, and vice versa.

Visual pathway The pathway followed by nerve impulses as they travel from the retina of the eye to the visual cortex of the occipital lobes.

Vitreous body A soft, jellylike substance that fills the posterior cavity of the eyeball. It helps to maintain the shape of the retinal surface.

Voltage The measure of the electrical potential energy. The greater the voltage, the greater the potential energy. Voltage measures the difference in charge on either side of an insulated barrier. The insulated barrier in the case of a neuron is the high fat content of the plasma membrane.

Voltage-gated ion channels Ion channels in a plasma membrane that open or close in response to changes in the membrane potential. Their presence in muscle and nerve cell plasma membranes makes them "excitable" cells.

Voltage-gated Na⁺ channels These ion channels have two separate gates: inactivation gates and activation gates. Inactivation gates are open when the neuron is inactive (resting). Many of the activation gates open at threshold, triggered by membrane depolarization (the threshold potential).

Wernicke's area *See* Auditory association area.

White matter Aggregations or bundles of myelinated axons located in the brain or spinal cord.

White ramus communicans One of the two structures that connect a sympathetic trunk ganglion to a spinal nerve. It contains sympathetic preganglionic fibers that carry impulses from the anterior ramus of a spinal nerve to the nearest sympathetic trunk ganglion. It is white in appearance because its fibers are myelinated.

Bibliography

Bustamante, Jairo B.   *Neuroanatomia Funcional.*
Bogota : Fondo Educativo Interamericano, 1978.

Dorland, William Alexander.   *Dorland's Illustrated Medical Dictionary,* 27th ed.
Philadelphia : W. B. Saunders, 1988.

Ganong, William F.   *Review of Medical Physiology*, 15th ed.
Norwalk, Connecticut : Appleton & Lange, 1991.

Junqueira, L. Carlos, Jose Carneiro, and Robert O. Kelley.   *Basic Histology*, 6th ed.
Norwalk, Connecticut : Appleton & Lange, 1989.

Kapit, Wynn and Lawrence M. Elson.   *The Anatomy Coloring Book.*
New York : Harper & Row, 1977.

Melloni, B. J., Ida Dox, and Gilbert Eisner.   *Melloni's Illustrated Medical Dictionary,* 2nd ed.
Baltimore : Williams & Wilkins, 1985.

Moore, Keith.   *Clinically Oriented Anatomy*, 3rd ed.
Baltimore : Williams & Wilkins, 1992.

Netter, Frank H.   *Atlas of Human Anatomy.*
Summit, N.J. : Ciba-Geigy, 1989.

Tortora, Gerard J. and Sandra Reynolds Grabowski.   *Principles of Anatomy and Physiology,* 7th ed.
New York : HarperCollins, 1993.

Vander, Arthur J., James H. Sherman, and Dorothy S. Luciano.   *Human Physiology,* 5th ed.
New York : McGraw-Hill, 1990.